2011
YEAR BOOK OF
HAND AND UPPER
LIMB SURGERY®

The 2011 Year Book Series

Year Book of Anesthesiology and Pain Management™: Drs Chestnut, Abram, Black, Gravlee, Lien, Mathru, and Roizen

Year Book of Cardiology®: Drs Gersh, Cheitlin, Elliott, Gold, Graham, and Thourani

Year Book of Critical Care Medicine®: Drs Dellinger, Parrillo, Balk, Dorman, Dries, and Zanotti-Cavazzoni

Year Book of Dermatology and Dermatologic Surgery™: Dr Del Rosso

Year Book of Diagnostic Radiology®: Drs Osborn, Abbara, Elster, Manaster, Oestreich, Offiah, Rosado de Christenson, Stephens, and Walker

Year Book of Emergency Medicine®: Drs Hamilton, Bruno, Handly, Mullin, Quintana, and Ramoska

Year Book of Endocrinology®: Drs Schott, Apovian, Clarke, Eugster, Ludlam, Meikle, Schinner, Schteingart, and Toth

Year Book of Gastroenterology™: Drs Talley, DeVault, Harnois, Murray, Pearson, Philcox, Picco, and Smith

Year Book of Hand and Upper Limb Surgery®: Drs Yao and Steinmann

Year Book of Medicine®: Drs Barker, Garrick, Gersh, Khardori, LeRoith, Seo, Talley, and Thigpen

Year Book of Neonatal and Perinatal Medicine®: Drs Fanaroff, Benitz, Donn, Neu, Papile, Polin, and van Marter

Year Book of Neurology and Neurosurgery®: Drs Klimo and Rabinstein

Year Book of Obstetrics, Gynecology, and Women's Health®: Drs Dungan and Shulman

Year Book of Oncology®: Drs Arceci, Bauer, Chiorean, Gordon, Lawton, Murphy, Thigpen, and Tsao

Year Book of Ophthalmology®: Drs Rapuano, Cohen, Flanders, Hammersmith, Milman, Myers, Nelson, Penne, Pyfer, Sergott, Shields, and Vander

Year Book of Orthopedics®: Drs Morrey, Beauchamp, Huddleston, Swiontkowski, and Trigg

Year Book of Otolaryngology-Head and Neck Surgery®: Drs Sindwani, Balough, Franco, Gapany, and Mitchell

Year Book of Pathology and Laboratory Medicine®: Drs Raab, Parwani, Bejarano, and Bissell

Year Book of Pediatrics®: Dr Stockman

Year Book of Plastic and Aesthetic Surgery™: Drs Miller, Gosain, Gurtner, Gutowski, Ruberg, Salisbury, and Smith

Year Book of Psychiatry and Applied Mental Health®: Drs Talbott, Ballenger, Buckley, Frances, Krupnick, and Mack

Year Book of Pulmonary Disease®: Drs Barker, Jones, Maurer, Raza, Tanoue, and Willsie

Year Book of Sports Medicine®: Drs Shephard, Cantu, Feldman, Jankowski, Khan, Lebrun, Nieman, Pierrynowski, and Rowland

Year Book of Surgery®: Drs Copeland, Behrns, Daly, Eberlein, Fahey, Huber, Klodell, Mozingo, and Pruett

Year Book of Urology®: Drs Andriole and Coplen

Year Book of Vascular Surgery®: Drs Moneta, Gillespie, Starnes, and Watkins

2011

The Year Book of HAND AND UPPER LIMB SURGERY®

Editors

Jeffrey Yao, MD
Assistant Professor of Orthopaedic Surgery, Robert A. Chase Hand and Upper Limb Center, Stanford, California

Scott P. Steinmann, MD
Professor, Department of Orthopedic Surgery, Mayo Clinic College of Medicine, Rochester, Minnesota

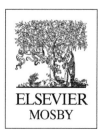

ELSEVIER
MOSBY

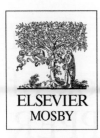

ELSEVIER
MOSBY

Vice President, Continuity: Kimberly Murphy
Developmental Editor: Teia Stone
Production Supervisor, Electronic Year Books: Donna M. Skelton
Electronic Article Manager: Mike Sheets
Illustrations and Permissions Coordinator: Dawn Vohsen

Composition by TNQ Books and Journals Pvt Ltd, India

Editorial Office:
Elsevier
Suite 1800
1600 John F. Kennedy Blvd.
Philadelphia, PA 19103-2899

International Standard Serial Number: 1551-7977
International Standard Book Number: 978-0-323-08415-4

Printed and bound by CPI Group (UK) Ltd, Croydon, CR0 4YY

Transferred to Digital Print 2011

Editors Emeritus

Peter C. Amadio, MD
Lloyd A. and Barbara A. Amundson Professor of Orthopedics; Consultant, Department of Orthopedic Surgery, Mayo Clinic, Rochester, Minnesota

Richard A. Berger, MD, PhD
Professor of Orthopedic Surgery and Anatomy; Dean, Mayo School of Continuous Professional Development; Chair, Division of Hand Surgery, Mayo Clinic, Rochester, Minnesota

James Chang, MD
Professor of Surgery and Orthopedic Surgery, Chief of Plastic Surgery, Stanford University Medical Center, Stanford, California

Robert A. Chase, MD
Emile Holman Professor of Surgery (Emeritus), Stanford University School of Medicine, Stanford, California

James H. Dobyns, MD
Emeritus Professor (Academic) of Orthopedic Surgery, United States Air Force, Emeritus Professor (Academic) of Orthopedic Surgery, Mayo Foundation, Rochester, Minnesota; Emeritus Professor (Clinical) of Orthopedic Surgery, University of Texas Health Science Center, San Antonio, Texas

Vincent R. Hentz, MD
Emeritus Professor of Surgery, Stanford University School of Medicine, Robert A. Chase Hand and Upper Limb Center, Division of Plastic Surgery, Stanford University Medical Center, Stanford, California

Amy L. Ladd, MD
Professor of Orthopaedic Surgery and Plastic Surgery, Robert A. Chase Hand and Upper Limb Center; Chief, Pediatric Hand Clinic, Lucile Packard Children's Hospital, Stanford, California

Contributing Editors

Julie E. Adams, MD
Assistant Professor of Orthopaedic Surgery, University of Minnesota, Minneapolis, Minnesota

Samuel A. Antuña, MD, PhD, FEBOT
Shoulder and Elbow Unit, Hospital Universitario La Paz, Madrid, Spain

Philip Blazar, MD
Assistant Professor of Orthopaedic Surgery, Harvard Medical School, Brigham and Women's Hospital, Boston, Massachusetts

Jonathan T. Bravman, MD
Sports Medicine Fellow, Department of Orthopaedic Surgery, Massachusetts General Hospital, Boston, Massachusetts

Charles Carroll IV, MD
Northwestern Orthopedic Institute, Illinois Hand Center; Associate Professor of Clinical Orthopedic Surgery, Feinberg School of Medicine, Chicago, Illinois

Emilie Cheung, MD
Assistant Professor, Shoulder and Elbow Surgery, Department of Orthopedic Surgery, Stanford University Medical Center, Stanford, California

Patrick Y. K. Chin, MD, MBA, Dip Sport Med, FRCS(C)
Division of Arthroscopic Reconstruction and Joint Preservation Surgery, Clinical Instructor, Department of Orthopaedic Surgery, University of British Columbia, Vancouver, British Columbia, Canada

Matthew Seung Suk Choi, MD
Associate Professor, Chief, Department of Plastic and Reconstructive Surgery, Hanyang University Guri Hospital, Guri, Gyunggi-do, Korea

Alphonsus Chong, MD
Consultant Hand Surgeon, Department of Hand and Reconstructive Microsurgery, National University Hospital, Singapore; Assistant Professor, Department of Orthopedic Surgery, Yong Loo Lin School of Medicine, National University of Singapore, Singapore

Kevin Chung, MD
Professor of Surgery, Section of Plastic Surgery, Department of Surgery, Assistant Dean for Faculty Affairs University of Michigan Medical School, Ann Arbor, Michigan

Akin Cil, MD
Assistant Professor of Orthopedics, Truman Medical Centers, University of Missouri-Kansas City, Kansas City, Missouri

Catherine Curtin, MD
Assistant Professor, Robert A. Chase Hand and Upper Limb Center, Division of Plastic Surgery, Stanford University Medical Center, Stanford, California

David G. Dennison, MD
Assistant Professor of Orthopedic Surgery, Mayo Clinic, Rochester, Minnesota

Scott F. M. Duncan, MD, MPH, MBA

Department of Orthopedic Surgery, Mayo Clinic Health System, Mayo Clinic College of Medicine, Rochester, Minnesota

Thomas R. Duquin, MD

Clinical Assistant Professor, University at Buffalo Department of Orthopaedic Surgery, Buffalo, New York

Scott G. Edwards, MD

Associate Professor, Department of Orthopaedic Surgery, Chief, Division of Hand and Elbow Surgery, Medical Director, the Center for Hand and Elbow Specialists, Georgetown University, Washington, District of Columbia

John C. Elfar, MD

Assistant Professor of Orthopaedic Surgery, Division of Hand and Upper Extremity Surgery, University of Rochester Medical Center, Strong Memorial Hospital, Rochester, New York

Bassem Elhassan, MD

Assistant Professor of Orthopedic Surgery, Mayo Clinic, Rochester, Minnesota

Antonio M. Foruria, MD, PhD

Shoulder and Elbow Reconstructive Surgery Unit, Department of Orthopaedic Surgery, Fundación Jiménez Díaz-Capio, Madrid, Spain

Tyler J. Fox, MD

Shoulder and Elbow Fellow, Department of Orthopaedic Surgery, Massachusetts General Hospital, Boston, Massachusetts

Ruby Grewal, MD, MSc, FRCSC

Assistant Professor, Division of Orthopedic Surgery, University of Western Ontario, Hand and Upper Limb Center, St Joseph's Health Care, London, Ontario, Canada

Thomas B. Hughes, MD

Assistant Professor of Orthopaedic Surgery, Drexel University College of Medicine, Allegheny Orthopaedic Associates, Allegheny General Hospital, Pittsburgh, Pennsylvania

Justin Jacobson, MD

Shoulder and Elbow Reconstruction Fellow, Mayo Clinic, Rochester, Minnesota

Ryosuke Kakinoki, MD, PhD

Associate Professor, Chief, Hand Surgery and Microsurgery, Department of Orthopedic Surgery and Rehabilitation Medicine, Graduate School of Medicine, Kyoto University, Kyoto, Japan

Steve K. Lee, MD

Associate Attending Orthopaedic Surgeon, Hand Surgery Service, Hospital for Special Surgery, New York, New York

Mark I. Loebenberg, MD

Chief of the Shoulder and Elbow Service, Rabin Medical Center, Aviv University School of Medicine, Petach Tikvah, Israel

John C. Macy, MD

Clinical Instructor, University of Vermont; Attending Surgeon, Fletcher Allen Health Care, Burlington, Vermont, Associates in Orthopedic Surgery, PC, South Burlington, Vermont

Pierre Mansat, MD, PhD
Professor, Service d'Orthopédie-Traumatologie, CHU-Purpan, Toulouse, France

Daniel J. Mastella, MD
The Hand Center, Assistant Director, University of Connecticut/Connecticut Combined Hand Surgery Fellowship, Assistant Clinical Professor, University of Connecticut Department of Orthopaedics, Hartford, Connecticut

Timothy R. McAdams, MD
Assistant Professor, Robert A. Chase Hand and Upper Limb Center, Department of Orthopaedic Surgery, Stanford, California

Kai Megerle, MD
Postdoctoral Fellow, Division of Plastic Surgery, Stanford University Medical Center, Stanford, California

Peter M. Murray, MD
Director for Education, Mayo Clinic Florida; Professor of Orthopaedic Surgery, College of Medicine, Consultant in Orthopaedic Surgery, Hand and Microvascular Surgery, Mayo Clinic, Jacksonville, Florida

Luke S. Oh, MD
Attending Orthopaedic Surgeon, Department of Orthopaedic Surgery, Massachusetts General Hospital, Boston, Massachusetts

Marianne Outzen, MS, OTR/L, CHT
Certified Hand Therapist, California Pacific Medical Center, Davies Campus, Hand Therapy Center, San Francisco, California

Kevin J. Renfree, MD
Assistant Professor, Department of Orthopaedic Surgery, Mayo Clinic Hospital, Phoenix, Arizona

Tamara D. Rozental, MD
Assistant Professor, Harvard Medical School, Beth Israel Deaconess Medical Center, Department of Orthopaedic Surgery, Boston, Massachusetts

Eon K. Shin, MD
Assistant Professor in Orthopaedic Surgery, Thomas Jefferson University Hospital, The Philadelphia Hand Center, PC, Philadelphia, Pennsylvania

Steven S. Shin, MD, MMS
Director, Hand Surgery, Chief Financial Officer, Kerlan-Jobe Orthopaedic Clinic, Los Angeles, California

Adam M. Smith, MD
Private Practice, West Tennessee Bone and Joint Clinic, Jackson, Tennessee

Jin Bo Tang, MD
Professor and Chair, Department of Hand Surgery, Affiliated Hospital of Nantong University; Chair, Hand Surgery Research Center, Nantong University, Jiangsu, China

Roger van Riet, MD, PhD
Elbow Surgery, Monica Hospital, MoRe Foundation, Deurne, Belgium; Professor of Orthopedic Surgery, Université Libre Bruxelles, Brussels, Belgium

J. Michael Wiater, MD
Associate Professor of Orthopaedic Surgery, Oakland University William Beaumont School of Medicine, Rochester, Michigan; Chief, Shoulder and Elbow Surgery, Department of Orthopaedic Surgery, Beaumont Health System, Royal Oak, Michigan

Thomas W. Wright, MD
Professor of Orthopaedic Surgery, University of Florida, Gainesville, Florida

David S. Zelouf, MD
Clinical Instructor, Department of Orthopaedic Surgery, Thomas Jefferson University Hospital, The Philadelphia Hand Center, Philadelphia, Pennsylvania

Dan Zlotolow, MD
Hand and Upper Extremity Surgeon, Shriners Hospital for Children, Philadelphia, Pennsylvania

Journals Represented

Journals represented in this YEAR BOOK are listed below.
American Journal of Emergency Medicine
American Journal of Sports Medicine
Annals of Plastic Surgery
Annals of Thoracic Surgery
Arthroscopy
Clinical Biomechanics
Clinical Orthopaedics and Related Research
Injury
Journal of Bone and Joint Surgery
Journal of Bone and Joint Surgery (American Volume)
Journal of Bone and Joint Surgery (British Volume)
Journal of Bone and Mineral Research
Journal of Hand Surgery
Journal of Hand Surgery (American Volume)
Journal of Hand Therapy
Journal of Orthopaedic Research
Journal of Orthopaedic Trauma
Journal of Pediatric Orthopaedics
Journal of Plastic, Reconstructive & Aesthetic Surgery
Journal of Trauma
Microsurgery
Neurosurgery
Orthopedics
Pharmacotherapy
Plastic and Reconstructive Surgery
Skeletal Radiology
Transplantation Proceedings

STANDARD ABBREVIATIONS

The following terms are abbreviated in this edition: acquired immunodeficiency syndrome (AIDS), cardiopulmonary resuscitation (CPR), central nervous system (CNS), cerebrospinal fluid (CSF), computed tomography (CT), deoxyribonucleic acid (DNA), electrocardiography (ECG), health maintenance organization (HMO), human immunodeficiency virus (HIV), intensive care unit (ICU), intramuscular (IM), intravenous (IV), magnetic resonance (MR) imaging (MRI), ribonucleic acid (RNA), and ultrasound (US).

NOTE

To facilitate the use of the YEAR BOOK OF HAND AND UPPER LIMB SURGERY® as a reference tool, all illustrations and tables included in this publication are now identified as they appear in the original article. This change is meant to help the reader recognize that any illustration or table appearing in the YEAR BOOK OF HAND AND UPPER LIMB SURGERY® may be only one of many in the original article. For this reason, figure and table numbers will often appear to be out of sequence within the YEAR BOOK OF HAND AND UPPER LIMB SURGERY®.

Introduction

Over the past several years, there has been a continued interest in disorders of the entire upper extremity. Many surgeons have an interest in learning and treating disorders of the entire upper extremity from the shoulder to the hand. The 2011 YEAR BOOK OF HAND AND UPPER LIMB SURGERY continues to follow this trend.

The articles surveyed by the YEAR BOOK cover a wide variety of subjects, including brachial plexus and wrist and forearm reconstruction. Many interesting articles have addressed complex forearm trauma and reconstructive options in addition to standard areas of interest, including distal radius fracture treatment.

This year there was a significant effort by the contributing editors to the YEAR BOOK. The YEAR BOOK would be unable to perform its mission if the contributing editors, who are known for their national and international expertise, were unable to comment on the various manuscripts. We are certainly indebted to them for their commentary every year. The YEAR BOOK will continue to evolve its electronic format, which will hopefully progress toward a real-time format. In years to come, we strive to make the YEAR BOOK more accessible for the interested upper limb surgeon. We thank Debora Dellapena for her significant contributions in guiding the YEAR BOOK process, and we are grateful for the efforts and exciting stewardship provided by Teia Stone.

Scott P. Steinmann, MD
Jeffrey Yao, MD

1 Hand Trauma

An Evidence-Based Approach to Metacarpal Fractures
Friedrich JB, Vedder NB (Univ of Washington, Seattle)
Plast Reconstr Surg 126:2205-2209, 2010

The Maintenance of Certification module series is designed to help the clinician structure his or her study in specific areas appropriate to his or her clinical practice. This article is prepared to accompany practice-based assessment of preoperative assessment, anesthesia, surgical treatment plan, perioperative management, and outcomes. In this format, the clinician is invited to compare his or her methods of patient assessment and treatment, outcomes, and complications, with authoritative, information-based references.

This information base is then used for self-assessment and benchmarking in parts II and IV of the Maintenance of Certification process of the American Board of Plastic Surgery. This article is not intended to be an exhaustive treatise on the subject. Rather, it is designed to serve as a reference point for further in-depth study by review of the reference articles presented.

▶ This systematic review provides an evidence-based update of a very common hand injury.

Summarizing the latest research on this condition, the authors note a lack of prospective studies comparing operative with nonoperative treatment for this fracture. In addition, there are few studies comparing the different fixation modalities. Based on available evidence, the authors suggest that metacarpal fractures may be treated nonoperatively with some form of immobilization if good reduction is obtained. If the fracture reduction remains stable, there are data to suggest that mobilization may be begun as early as 2 weeks. This article provides a useful update on this condition. As the authors point out, the article is not exhaustive. Readers unfamiliar with the condition would find it helpful to read a textbook before this update. For those who see and treat this problem in their practice, it does provide some helpful treatment guides based on the latest evidence.

A. Chong, MD

Pull-Out Wire Fixation for Acute Mallet Finger Fractures With K-Wire Stabilization of the Distal Interphalangeal Joint

Zhang X, Meng H, Shao X, et al (Second Hosp of Qinhuangdao, Changli, Hebei, People's Republic of China; Third Hosp of Hebei Med Univ, Shijiazhuang, People's Republic of China)

J Hand Surg 35A:1864-1869, 2010

Purpose.—The aim of this study was to describe and assess a surgical technique for the treatment of mallet finger fractures using a pull-out wire with K-wire stabilization of the distal interphalangeal (DIP) joint in extension.

Methods.—From May 2003 to January 2008, we performed pull-out wire fixation of the fracture fragment with stabilization of the DIP joint using a K-wire in 65 closed mallet finger fractures in 65 patients with a mean age of 32 years (range, 18—48). The mean time between the injury and surgery was 8 days (range, 0—19 d). In this cohort, the mean joint surface involvement was 39% (range, 30% to 49%) and all injuries were associated with DIP joint subluxation. Fifteen days after surgery, the digits were assessed for skin necrosis, skin breakdown, and wound and wire track infection. Patient follow-up lasted 24 to 27 months, with a mean period of 25.5 months. The fingers were assessed for loss of extension and flexion of the DIP joints. We graded the results using Crawford's criteria.

Results.—Fracture reduction was maintained and all fractures united. We found no skin necrosis, skin breakdown, infection, or nail deformities. At the final follow-up, the mean extensor loss of the DIP joints was 7° (range, 0° to 37°). The mean flexion loss of the DIP joints was 1° (range, 0° to 15°). We noted extensor loss of the joint less than 10° in 57 digits and 10° to 15° (mean, 13°) in 8 digits. Based on Crawford's criteria, 52 digits were excellent, 8 were good, 4 were fair, and one was poor.

Conclusions.—Pull-out wire fixation of the reduced fracture fragment and K-wire stabilization of the DIP joint is a useful technique for the treatment of mallet finger fractures.

Type of Study/Level of Evidence.—Therapeutic IV.

▶ This article presents a retrospective review of a pull-out wire and K-wire technique for fixation of the potentially difficult fractures. The article documents reasonable results and should be considered when treating a mallet fracture surgically. The study size was significant, and the results are clearly documented. Fragment size averaged 39% of the articular surface. Further study is warranted to compare this technique with others. The diagrams are helpful and can be used to plan the procedure. The study warrants consideration by the surgeon considering operative care of these common fractures.

C. Carroll IV, MD

Decreasing Incidence and Changing Pattern of Childhood Fractures: A Population-Based Study
Mäyränpää MK, Mäkitie O, Kallio PE (Univ of Helsinki, Finland)
J Bone Miner Res 25:2476-2483, 2010

Fractures are common in children, and some studies suggest an increasing incidence. Data on population-based long-term trends are scarce. In order to establish fracture incidence and epidemiologic patterns, we carried out a population-based study in Helsinki, Finland. All fractures in children aged 0 to 15 years were recorded from public health care institutions during a 12-month period in 2005. Details regarding patient demographics, fracture site, and trauma mechanism were collected. All fractures were confirmed from radiographs. Similar data from 1967, 1978, and 1983 were used for comparison. In 2005, altogether 1396 fractures were recorded, 63% in boys. The overall fracture incidence was 163 per 10,000. Causative injuries consisted of mainly falls when running or walking or from heights less than 1.5 m. Fracture incidence peaked at 10 years in girls and 14 years in boys. An increase in fracture incidence was seen from 1967 to 1983 (24%, $p < .0001$), but a significant decrease (18%, $p < .0001$) was seen from 1983 to 2005. This reduction was largest in children between the ages of 10 and 13 years. Despite the overall decrease and marked decrease in hand (-39%, $p < .0001$) and foot (-48%, $p < .0001$) fractures, the incidence of forearm and upper arm fractures increased significantly by 31% ($p < .0001$) and 39% ($p = .021$), respectively. Based on these findings, the overall incidence of childhood fractures has decreased significantly during the last two decades. Concurrently, the incidence of forearm and upper arm fractures has increased by one-third. The reasons for these epidemiologic changes remain to be elucidated in future studies.

▶ In this well-designed prospective population-based study, the investigators collected data on the incidence of all pediatric fractures (aged younger than 16 years) in Helsinki in 2005. The peak fracture incidence occurred around the age of 10 years for girls and 14 years for boys. Boys sustained nearly two-thirds of all fractures. Almost 20% of children had had a previous fracture, with 3 or more fractures in 2% of patients. Refractures made up only 0.4% of all fractures. Nearly 75% of all pediatric fractures were of the upper extremity, with distal radius, hand, and finger fractures making up over 50% of all fractures. The incidence was 122 upper extremity fractures per 10 000 children per year. Overall, the incidence of upper extremity fractures declined modestly (7%), while lower extremity fractures decreased dramatically (34%) between 1983 and 2005. While it is difficult to universalize the results of a regionally discreet incidence assessment, their overall trends do match those of previously published studies from around the world. Given that the average medical student and primary care physician in the United States have no formal exposure to hand surgery, and that there are fewer than 15 surgeons in the United States who specialize solely in pediatric hand surgery, this population seems grossly underserved. Fortunately, most pediatric upper extremity fractures do relatively well with benign neglect. However, for the many children with complex upper extremity injuries, appropriate care by an orthopedist familiar with the pediatric upper extremity is critical.

D. A. Zlotolow, MD

Distal Radial Fractures in the Elderly: Operative Compared with Nonoperative Treatment
Egol KA, Walsh M, Romo-Cardoso S, et al (New York Univ Hosp for Joint Diseases)
J Bone Joint Surg Am 92:1851-1857, 2010

Background.—There is much debate regarding the optimal treatment of displaced, unstable distal radial fractures in the elderly. The purpose of this retrospective review was to compare outcomes for elderly patients with a displaced distal radial fracture who were treated with or without surgical intervention.

Methods.—This case-control study examined ninety patients over the age of sixty-five who were treated with or without surgery for a displaced distal radial fracture. All fractures were initially treated with closed reduction and splinting. Patients who failed an acceptable closed reduction were offered surgical intervention. Patients who did not undergo surgery were treated until healing with cast immobilization. Patients who underwent surgery were treated with either plate-and-screw fixation or external fixation. Baseline radiographs and functional scores were obtained prior to treatment. Follow-up was conducted at two, six, twelve, twenty-four, and fifty-two weeks. Clinical and radiographic follow-up was completed at each visit, while functional scores were obtained at the twelve, twenty-four, and fifty-two-week follow-up evaluations. Outcomes at fixed time points were compared between groups with standard statistical methods.

Results.—Forty-six patients with a mean age of seventy-six years were treated nonoperatively, and forty-four patients with a mean age of seventy-three years were treated operatively. Other than age, there was no difference with respect to baseline demographics between the cohorts. At twenty-four weeks, patients who underwent surgery had better wrist extension (p = 0.04) than those who had not had surgery. At one year, this difference was not seen. No difference in functional status based on the Disabilities of the Arm, Shoulder and Hand scores and pain scores at any of the follow-up points was seen between the groups. Grip strength at one year was significantly better in the operative group. Radiographic outcome was superior for the patients in the operative group at each follow-up interval. There was no difference between the groups with regard to complications.

Conclusions.—Our findings suggest that minor limitations in the range of wrist motion and diminished grip strength, as seen with nonoperative care, do not seem to limit functional recovery at one year.

Level of Evidence.—Therapeutic <u>Level III</u>. See Instructions to Authors for a complete description of levels of evidence.

▶ There is a paradigm shift in the treatment of elderly patients with distal radius fractures. The traditional approach in treating patients with unstable distal radius fractures demonstrates adequate functional recovery despite radiographic evidence of fracture collapse. In other words, although surgical treatments give more precise anatomic reduction, better anatomic reduction of the fractures in the elderly population does not often equate with better outcomes. This is a nicely done study in which the authors evaluated 46 patients treated nonoperatively and 44 patients treated operatively. Patients were older than 65 years and were followed up at set intervals with radiographic and functional measurements. Surprisingly, despite better radiographic reduction with surgical treatments, the 2 groups fare equally well in outcomes assessment at 1 year, despite the nonoperative group having slightly less wrist motion and grip strength at the 3-month mark.

This study demonstrated that perhaps because the elderly patients have less functional demand, the less-than-optimal radiographic reduction does not necessarily mean that these patients will have poor functional outcomes at 1 year. The real question is whether the earlier recovery of function with surgical treatment may be associated with better patient satisfaction and less impairment time, because many of these patients live alone and require earlier recovery of function. This article is yet another well-performed study to critically evaluate the treatment of distal radius fractures in the elderly. An ambitious 21-center clinical trial on the treatment of distal radius fractures in the elderly will soon be conducted to answer some of the vexing questions surrounding the most optimal treatment for elderly patients presenting with distal radius fractures.

K. Chung, MD

Manipulation of Objects with and without the Use of the Index Finger: Implications for Digital Amputations
Hammond ERA, Szturm T, Shay BL (Univ of Manitoba, Winnipeg, Canada)
J Hand Ther 23:352-360, 2010

Study Design.—Clinical Measurement.

Purpose.—To evaluate changes in temporal and amplitude movement accuracy with tasks requiring fine motor manipulation with and without the use of the index finger (WIF).

Participants.—Twenty right-handed participants (10 males, 10 females, aged 24—47 years) were recruited.

Methods.—Three objects, ranging in weight and size, that required the use of 2 or 3 fingers were selected for this study. Motor performance was quantified during manipulation of a pen, cork, and wine glass using a computerized visual guided tracking task. The miniBird (Ascension Technology, Burlington, VT, USA) miniature motion tracking sensor was attached to each object to measure and record the 3D linear and angular motion.

Results.—Task performance and temporal accuracy of the pen task in the normal condition was more accurate ($P = .033$). During the WIF condition there was significantly more motion performing the wine task ($P < .001$).

Conclusions.—The protocol directly measures the ability of the hand to coordinate movement in response to a visual tracking target. Both temporal accuracy and amplitude consistency can be objectively evaluated. The current study evaluates the ability of the hand to manipulate 3 objects used in fine motor manipulation, using motion analysis and visual tracking.

Level of Evidence.—3b.

▶ This is a study that shows that in the normal hand, manipulating objects without the index finger is slower and less accurate, most importantly, manipulating a wine glass. Clinically, patients with index finger amputation actually recover quite well, primarily because the middle finger is so adept at taking over the responsibilities of the index finger. In my practice, patients with index finger—only amputation generally do not need a lot of retraining to regain the use of the affected hand for daily activities. Fine motor coordination timed tasks, such as the Purdue Peg Task, are a great treatment modality for this patient population because it is a race against the clock and allows for improvement in dexterity with each trial. For the patient with a dominant hand index finger amputation, handwriting retraining is important; beginning with a large-diameter pen or pencil offers a smoother transition to handwriting independently. Drinking wine, my most favorite activity of daily living, should be assessed first and foremost after an index finger amputation. It is unfortunate that as a hand therapist I have failed to keep wine glasses, corks, and wine bottle openers in the clinic. Improving accuracy in manipulating a wine glass from hand to mouth is an excellent treatment plan, 0-spill frequency is the measurable outcome, and clinking wine glasses with 100% accuracy with the therapist and surgeon is the ultimate goal.

M. Outzen, MS, OTR/L, CHT

2 Hand: Arthritis and Arthroplasty

Suture Button Compared With K-Wire Fixation for Maintenance of Posttrapeziectomy Space Height in a Cadaver Model of Lateral Pinch
Yao J, Zlotolow DA, Murdock R, et al (Stanford Univ Med Ctr, Redwood City, CA; Univ of Maryland School of Medicine, Baltimore)
J Hand Surg 35A:2061-2065, 2010

Purpose.—Hematoma distraction arthroplasty has regained popularity as a treatment for thumb carpometacarpal arthritis with reports of satisfactory results. Our goal was to investigate the use of a suture button device to maintain the posttrapeziectomy space height of the thumb metacarpal. Our hypothesis is that a suture button that suspends the thumb metacarpal from the second metacarpal, when applied to the hematoma distraction arthroplasty technique, would provide subsidence resistance comparable to traditional K-wire fixation.

Methods.—Ten fresh frozen matched pairs of human cadaveric arms were used. After open trapeziectomy, suspension of the thumb metacarpal was performed with either a 1.4-mm (0.045-inch) K-wire advanced through the base of the thumb metacarpal into the second metacarpal shaft or a suture button device that suspended the thumb metacarpal from the second metacarpal shaft. Cyclic pinch was simulated by using a lateral pinch model previously described and validated. Lateral pinch is simulated by loading the extensor pollicis longus, adductor pollicis, abductor pollicis brevis, and flexor pollicis longus in a 1:5:6:10 ratio. Dynamic pinch is achieved with cyclic unloading of the abductor pollicis brevis, adductor pollicis, and flexor pollicis longus tendons. Measurements were made of the height of excised trapeziums, the distance from the metacarpal base to the scaphoid after trapeziectomy (trapeziectomy space height) at time zero, both loaded and unloaded, and at sequential loading cycles of 1,000, 2,000, 3,000, 4,000, 5,000, and 10,000 cycles.

Results.—Student *t*-test evaluation showed no significant differences between the groups in initial trapeziectomy space height (p = .10), postfixation trapeziectomy space height (p = .10), or loss of trapeziectomy space height between precycling and after 10,000 cycles (p = .80).

Conclusions.—Suture button fixation maintains similar posttrapeziectomy space height and prevents subsidence of the thumb metacarpal when compared with K-wire fixation in this model. This technique may allow for earlier range of motion after the hematoma distraction arthroplasty.

▶ Hand surgeons continue to search for the optimal technique in surgical treatment of the arthritic basilar joint of the thumb. Suture button fixation was shown in a cadaveric model to maintain similar posttrapeziectomy joint space when compared with Kirschner wire fixation following cyclical loading and stress. The authors present that this technique may allow for earlier motion in the postoperative care of these operative procedures. The technique requires clinical validation but adds to the existing knowledge base for caring for this common arthritic problem in the hand.

C. Carroll IV, MD

A Systematic Review of Conservative Interventions for Osteoarthritis of the Hand

Valdes K, Marik T (Hand Works Therapy, Sarasota, FL; Apple Physical Therapy, Tacoma, WA)

J Hand Ther 23:334-351, 2010

Study Design.—Systematic Review.

Introduction.—Hand therapy interventions for patients with hand osteoarthritis (OA) can include splinting, joint protection technique instruction, paraffin, exercises, and provision of a home exercise program.

Purpose.—Examine the quality of the evidence regarding the hand therapy interventions for hand OA.

Methods.—Twenty-one studies dated between 1986 and 2009 were included in the systematic review for analysis.

Results.—The current evidence provides varied support for the interventions of orthotics, hand exercises, joint protection techniques, the utilization of adaptive devices, and paraffin. Findings for the use of joint protection techniques are supported for improvements in function and pain reduction. Minimal evidence exists for paraffin used for the treatment of hand OA.

Conclusions.—The current literature supports the use of orthotics, hand exercises, application of heat, and joint protection education combined with provision of adaptive equipment to improve grip strength and function.

Level of Evidence.—2A.

▶ The authors present a comprehensive review of the literature for treatment of carpometacarpal (CMC) osteoarthritis (OA). In clinical practice, hand therapy for CMC OA is most effective in early stages. Splinting appropriately, often inclusive of the wrist for night wear (based on an article from last year[1]); joint protection technique training, training in adaptive devices (such as built up keys or large diameter pens), and training in self-application of moist heat modalities (such as paraffin wax) seems to provide the most immediate pain relief and return to function. Modalities, such as ultrasound or laser light, unfortunately, have shown little benefit beyond being snake oil or billing tools. Once one of these modalities is initiated, it becomes difficult to not repeat it on subsequent visits. Patients often become easily entranced by the magical effects of the miracle modality and may want to extend reasonable numbers of treatment visits solely for the application of the modality. Otherwise, early CMC OA conservative treatment can be completed in 1 to 4 visits. Strengthening with therapy is warranted if the patient's pinch is pain free and stable. Analyze the base of the metacarpal subluxation on the CMC joint; if it is most commonly dorsal, avoid repetitive pinch and consider strengthening CMC extension/ abduction (without interphalangeal involvement). For additional information, Judy Colditz's[2] Thumb Mechanics self-study course offers a thorough understanding of the biomechanics and treatment of the painful CMC joint.

M. Outzen, MS, OTR/L, CHT

References

1. Rannou F, Dimet J, Boutron I, et al. Splint for base-of-thumb osteoarthritis: a randomized trial. *Ann Intern Med.* 2009;150:661-669.
2. Colditz JC. Thumb Mechanics: Linking Anatomy & Treatment of CMC Osteoarthritis. http://www.handlab.com/product-detail.asp?productid=40. Accessed April 22, 2011.

3 Hand: Bone and Ligament

Scapholunate Stabilization With Dynamic Extensor Carpi Radialis Longus Tendon Transfer

Peterson SL, Freeland AE (Portland Veterans Administration Med Ctr, OR; Univ of Mississippi Med Ctr, Jackson)
J Hand Surg 35A:2093-2100, 2010

Dynamic extensor carpi radialis longus tendon transfer to the distal pole of the scaphoid acts synchronously and synergistically with wrist motion to restore the slider crank mechanism of the scaphoid after scapholunate interosseous ligament (SLIL) injury. The procedure is designed to simulate a hypothetical dorsal radioscaphoid ligament that more closely approximates the normal viscoelastic forces acting on the scaphoid throughout all phases of wrist motion than does the static checkrein effect and motion limitations of capsulodesis or tenodesis. Extensor carpi radialis longus transfer may be independently sufficient to support normal or near-normal scapholunate and midcarpal kinematics and prevent further injury propagation in patients with partial SLIL tears and dynamic scapholunate instability. Extensor carpi radialis longus transfer alone may improve carpal congruity in patients with static scapholunate instability, but SLIL and dorsal lunate ligament repair or reconstruction is essential for favorable durable outcomes. Extensor carpi radialis longus transfer offers a simple and reasonable alternative to capsulodesis or tenodesis to support these ligament repairs or reconstructions, does not require intercarpal fixation, and allows rehabilitation to proceed expeditiously at approximately 1 month after surgery.

▶ I commend the authors for the innovative thinking to try to reconstruct scapholunate joint instability using a new technique. The idea of transferring the extensor carpi radialis longus (ECRL) to the distal dorsal aspect of the scaphoid is very interesting. The procedure is simple, does not require pinning of the intercarpal joints, and allows earlier restoration of range of motion. The dart motion of the wrist consists of wrist extension—radial deviation and ulnar deviation with wrist flexion. The ECRL can act both as a static and dynamic stabilizer of the scaphoid throughout this motion. However, despite the fact that the authors reported a case example of their procedure, we still do not have a long-term outcome on a large enough number of patients to justify us to recommend this procedure for the treatment of scapholunate joint instability.

B. Elhassan, MD

Management of Peripheral Triangular Fibrocartilage Complex Tears in the Ulnar Positive Patient: Arthroscopic Repair Versus Ulnar Shortening Osteotomy

Papapetropoulos PA, Wartinbee DA, Richard MJ, et al (Duke Univ Med Ctr, Durham, NC)
J Hand Surg 35A:1607-1613, 2010

Purpose.—One pattern of injury to the triangular fibrocartilage complex (TFCC) is a traumatic peripheral tear located at the ulnar end of the TFCC. Since 1989, this specific injury has been classified as a Palmer type 1B lesion. Various treatment options have been described for 1B injuries, yet when there is coexistent ulnar positive variance, it can make the choice of treatment difficult. The purpose of this article is to help the surgeon decide how to treat type 1B lesions in ulnar positive patients by directly comparing arthroscopic repair (repair) to ulnar shortening osteotomy (USO). The null hypothesis was that repair and USO would provide equivalent postoperative improvement with regard to motion; Disability of the Arm, Shoulder, and Hand (DASH) score; visual analog scale (VAS) score; and grip strength.

Methods.—We tested our hypothesis by retrospectively reviewing prospectively collected data from 51 patients treated surgically between 2000 and 2006 with type 1B tears in the setting of ulnar positive variance. Of these 51 patients, 27 were treated with arthroscopic repair and 24 with USO. All patients were evaluated before surgery as well as at final follow-up for active range of motion measurements, grip strength, DASH score, and VAS score. Radiographs were taken of all patients before surgery to confirm the presence of ulnar positive variance, and after surgery in the USO group to evaluate for bony union.

Results.—At the final follow-up, we found no statistically significant difference between the repair and USO groups with regard to flexion, extension, pronation, supination, radial deviation, or ulnar deviation. Likewise, there was no significant difference in grip strength, DASH scores, or VAS scores. When analyzing each cohort individually, both groups improved significantly after surgery with regard to DASH score, VAS score, and wrist extension. There was also a trend toward improved motion in all other directions except for an insignificant decrease in post-operative pronation in the repair group. Two patients in the USO group required additional surgery, with one revision performed for nonunion and one for painful hardware, which caused extensor carpi ulnaris tendonitis.

Conclusions.—The results of our study suggest that type 1B TFCC tears in the ulnar positive patient can be managed equivalently well with repair or USO.

Type of Study/Level of Evidence.—Therapeutic III.

▶ The authors present their results after reviewing the treatment of peripheral triangular fibrocartilage complex (TFCC) tears in ulnar positive patients. Their conclusion was that there was no clear superiority of either arthroscopic peripheral TFCC repair or ulnar shortening osteotomy. Their results were concluded after reviewing 1-year follow-up of motion; disabilities of the arm, shoulder, and hand; and grip strengths scores, and all their patients had to have a stable distal radioulnar joint for inclusion within the study.

There were some limitations of the study that should be considered, given the conclusions. This study was nonrandomized, and the patients with type 1B injury did not have instability. All patients also had to have an MR arthrogram demonstrating a TFCC injury and no sign of degenerative changes in the lunate or triquetrum suggestive of ulnar impaction syndrome. On physical examination, they were required to have pain with ulnar deviation against resistance. It was not clarified if this was done with axial load, pronation, and ulnar deviation, suggesting that the pain could be considered to be present with ulnar impaction.

This study did involve women to men in the ratio 2:1. The arthroscopic repair group included only a capsule or subsheath repair and no foveal or bony repair, and the patients with TFCC repair were splinted in 60° of supination for 3 weeks, whereas the patients who underwent ulnar shortening osteotomy were placed in removable wrist splints. The complications were quite limited for both groups, including 1 nonunion that required surgery in 1 patient in the ulnar shortening osteotomy group, and no revisions being required for the repair group. In the arthroscopic repair group, there was 1 patient with dorsal sensory branch ulnar nerve paresthesias that improved over 3 months.

Regarding other strengths of this study, this was a nice comparison of ulnar shortening osteotomy with arthroscopic repair, all performed in a similar fashion. One weakness, however, was that the patients chose their treatment after discussion with the surgeon in a nonrandomized manner and were all evaluated by the operating surgeon postoperatively.

Nonetheless, the authors have demonstrated that with a Palmer type 1B injury, without instability, there is no clear difference in the ulnar positive patient whether this is treated with ulnar shortening osteotomy or arthroscopic peripheral repair. It will remain up to the surgeon to consider which treatment is most effective and can be applied with the least morbidity. Finally, the authors did not describe whether any ulnar shortening osteotomy plates were removed and if there were any concerns for plate prominence, pain, or complications after plate removal.

D. G. Dennison, MD

Corrective Osteotomy for Isolated Malunion of the Palmar Lunate Facet in Distal Radius Fractures

Ruch DS, Wray WH III, Papadonikolakis A, et al (Duke Univ Med Ctr, Durham, NC; Wake Forest Univ-School of Medicine, Winston-Salem, NC)
J Hand Surg 35A:1779-1786, 2010

Purpose.—Malunion of the palmar lunate facet fragment of distal radius fractures is associated with both early functional impairment and late degenerative changes. The goal of this study was to describe the clinical and radiographic outcomes after corrective osteotomy for isolated malunion of the palmar lunate facet.

Methods.—Between 1995 and 2000, a retrospective review identified 13 patients with an average age of 44 years who had undergone corrective intra-articular osteotomy for isolated malunion of the palmar lunate facet. The average interval from the initial injury to the osteotomy was 5.4 months. Final evaluation was performed at 1 year. We performed statistical analysis using the Wilcoxon signed rank test.

Results.—Wrist extension improved from an average of $53°$ to $84°$ (p = .002), flexion from $46°$ to $61°$ (p < .002), supination from $38°$ to $87°$ (p = .002), and pronation from $79°$ to $87°$ (p < .001). Grip strength improved from 30% to 73% of the contralateral side (p < .002). Disabilities of the Arm, Shoulder, and Hand scores improved from an average of 50.7 to 9.7 (p < .002). Palmar tilt improved from an average of $23°$ to $11°$ (p < .002). Radial inclination improved from an average of $29°$ to $22°$ (p < .002), ulnar variance decreased from +3.9 to −0.9 mm (p = .004), and intra-articular gap decreased from 3.6 to 0.9 mm (p < .002). All patients had excellent or good results according to both the Gartland and Werley and the Fernandez scoring systems.

Conclusions.—Early intra-articular osteotomy significantly improved wrist range of motion, grip strength, Disabilities of the Arm, Shoulder, and Hand scores, and radiographic parameters. Patients reported mostly positive outcomes.

Type of Study/Level of Evidence.—Therapeutic IV.

▶ The authors presented a retrospective review of 13 patients who required corrective intra-articular osteotomy for malunion of the palmar lunate facet. Functional range of motion measurements and outcomes questionnaire assessment indicated improvement after reduction of the malunited fracture fragment at an average of 5.4 months after the initial injury. The authors indicated that because of the early presentation of these patients, contracture of the ligament between the radius and ulna has not fully established, which obviates the need for ligament release. Patients in this series achieved improved supination of the forearm from $38°$ to $87°$ and improved flexion and extension arcs. However, the narrow palmar volar plate necessary for fracture fixation needs to be placed quite distally, which required hardware removal because of complications relating to crepitus from irritating the deep flexors.

Overall, this is an interesting series that highlights the need for early malunion correction to establish anatomic reduction and avoid residual malunion complications relating to this die-punch fracture pattern.

K. Chung, MD

The Unstable Nonunited Scaphoid Waist Fracture: Results of Treatment by Open Reduction, Anterior Wedge Grafting, and Internal Fixation by Volar Buttress Plate

Ghoneim A (Suez Canal Univ, Ismailia, Egypt)
J Hand Surg 36A:17-24, 2011

Purpose.—The purpose of this study is to evaluate the results of treatment of unstable nonunited scaphoid waist fracture by anterior wedge graft and internal fixation with the use of volar buttress plate and screws.

Methods.—Fourteen adult male patients with unstable nonunited scaphoid waist fracture with a humpback deformity were treated by reduction of the collapse deformity, insertion of anterior wedge graft, and internal fixation with the use of volar buttress plate and screws. The mean patient age was 26 years, and the mean duration of the nonunion before surgery was 16.5 months. The follow-up time ranged from 9 to 19 months (mean, 11 mo). Thirteen of the fourteen nonunions healed with sound radiographic union. Pre-existing avascular necrosis was a major adverse factor for achievement of union in one patient, even after a second bone-grafting procedure.

Results.—Union was achieved in a mean of 3.8 months. Most of the patients had satisfactory correction of scaphoid deformity and the associated dorsal intercalated segment instability. Postoperatively, improvements were seen in the range of wrist flexion and extension, grip strength, and degree of dorsal intercalated segment instability.

Conclusions.—The results of the series suggest that the method of anterior wedge graft and internal fixation with the use of volar buttress plate and screws is effective for the treatment of unstable nonunited scaphoid waist fractures.

Type of Study/Level of Evidence.—Therapeutic IV.

▶ This is a well-designed retrospective review that deals with the difficult clinical problem of unstable scaphoid nonunions. The author presents an interesting alternative technique to stabilize the scaphoid after reduction and bone grafting. While I agree that Herbert screws are sometimes very difficult to place when dealing with unstable fragments, I see several disadvantages with the use of buttress plates. First, I am worried that compression is significantly less when compared with a correctly placed Herbert screw. This might contribute to the rather long period of immobilization that is reported by the author. Second, I expect that a more extensive exposure of the bone is necessary to place the implant, possibly further compromising the scarce blood supply of the scaphoid. One case with an avascular proximal pole is reported;

however, there is no information about the preoperative perfusion. Finally, I would be worried about impingement of the plate between the scaphoid and the radius. However, the postoperative range of motion averages 102° for extension/flexion movements, which is comparable to other studies.

At this point, I think that the buttress plate is rather a salvage technique, if a traditional screw cannot be placed. However, it will be interesting to follow further biomechanical and clinical studies comparing the 2 techniques.

K. Megerle, MD

Mobilizing the Stiff Hand: Combining Theory and Evidence to Improve Clinical Outcomes
Glasgow C, Tooth LR, Fleming J (EKCO Occupational Services, Brisbane, Queensland, Australia; The Univ of Queensland, Herston, Australia; The Univ of Queensland, St Lucia, Australia)
J Hand Ther 23:392-401, 2010

The purpose of this narrative review is to provide a clinically reasonable guide to intervention choices, by combining a sound understanding of theory with available research evidence. The pathology of contracture formation is presented within the context of tissue repair. The soft tissue response to stress is explained and the optimal "dose" of treatment is discussed. The evidence behind the use of exercise, joint mobilization, continuous passive motion, casting motion to mobilize stiffness, and mobilizing splinting is examined. Recommendations regarding treatment implementation and future research needs are highlighted. The importance of mobilizing splinting and exercise as treatment modalities in the management of joint contracture is demonstrated.
Level of Evidence.—5.

▶ The authors present an excellent review of the research for treatment of joint contracture in the stiff hand. The authors concluded from the literature that there is little evidence to support continuous passive motion (CPM), joint mobilization, and casting motion to mobilize stiffness (CMMS) in the treatment of the stiff hand. The authors also found that a high level of evidence exists for the use of mobilizing splinting in the management of joint contracture and a moderate level of evidence exists to support the use of active or passive exercise. In my practice, I have been known to try CPMs on stiff hands. However, CPMs are generally initiated after a patient's wounds have healed and often after we have already realized that the hand is stiff. In both cases, we may be initiating the CPM too late, beyond the initial phase of tissue healing, to offer any real benefit to the patient. More research is needed on the efficacy of hand CPMs for early phase healing. Joint mobilization is an area in which chiropractors are the experts. Since I was not trained as a chiropractor and have only witnessed conflicting consensus among therapists about how to perform a joint mobilization and the grade of the mobilization, I do not subject my patients to it. Furthermore, the risk of joint subluxation from an aggressive or poorly executed mobilization in a hand or wrist is not something I am interested in experiencing firsthand. CMMS, a protocol promoted by Colditz, is theoretically a great idea; unfortunately, I have never tried it. It appears to be similar to the upper extremity constraint-induced movement therapy programs for recovering hand function, in the hemiparetic hand, after cerebrovascular accident, in the nonflaccid hand. Mobilizing splinting, otherwise known as static progressive or dynamic splinting, is extremely effective as long as the patient is compliant in using the splint correctly. Some studies have found that up to 75% of hand patients are not likely to wear the splints we diligently fabricate. We have all experienced the patient who walks into the clinic holding his or her dynamic splint rather than wearing it. The most relevant statement from this article is: the best method of managing joint contracture is to prevent it. Active and passive exercise and early mobilization are probably the simplest methods of preventing the stiff hand and, not surprisingly, may also be the most cost-effective.

M. Outzen, MS, OTR/L, CHT

4 Hand: Carpal Tunnel Syndrome

The Effect of Transverse Carpal Ligament Lengthening on Carpal Tunnel Volumetry: A Comparison Between Four Techniques
Pavlidis L, Chalidis BE, Demiri E, et al (Orthopaedic Dept of Hippokration General Hosp, Thessaloniki, Greece)
Ann Plast Surg 65:480-484, 2010

Transverse carpal ligament (TCL) reconstruction after open carpal tunnel release has been advocated to restore wrist kinematics and grip strength. This study investigates the effect of TCL reconstruction in carpal tunnel volume (CTV). Thirty-eight cadaveric wrists were volarly approached and TCL was exposed to its proximal and distal edges. Carpal tunnel contents were removed and the CTV was measured considering that carpal tunnel resembled the shape of a truncated cone. TCL was then dissected and subsequently reconstructed by using 4 different surgical lengthening techniques. Three of these techniques were retrieved from the literature. The fourth was proposed and performed by the authors. Postreconstruction calculation of CTV was done with the same method. In 6 cadavers, a magnetic resonance imaging-based measurement of CTV was performed to assess the validity and reliability of simulation method. The average increase of CTV ranged from 31% to 44% ($P < 0.001$ for all techniques). However, no statistical significant difference was found between the 4 techniques ($P = 0.097$). Magnetic resonance imaging volumetric values were equal to simulation measured values before and after reconstruction of TCL ($P = 0.224$ and $P = 0.674$, respectively). Lengthening of TCL substantially increases the carpal tunnel capacity regardless of the applied surgical technique. The simulation model method seems to be an accurate, precise, and cost-effective approach for the evaluation of CTV.

▶ Transverse carpal ligament reconstruction following carpal tunnel release has been advocated by some surgeons. However, the need for reconstruction following release of the transverse carpal tunnel ligament is still very controversial. This cadaveric study studied 2 facets of transverse carpal ligament reconstruction following carpal tunnel release. First, the authors showed that carpal tunnel volume increased between 31% and 44% using 4 techniques of reconstruction. This suggests that all the 4 techniques may be used to effectively reconstruct the ligament while still allowing an increase in carpal tunnel volume. Second, they found that a simulation model method of measuring carpal tunnel volume did not differ from that measured by MRI. The model method could be a useful alternative technique for measuring the carpal tunnel volume. The information from this study provides a basis for further work, both cadaveric and clinical. More evidence of the benefits of transverse carpal ligament reconstruction is necessary before there will be wider acceptance of this procedure.

A. Chong, MD

An Evidence-Based Approach to Carpal Tunnel Syndrome
Shores JT, Lee WPA (Univ of Pittsburgh School of Medicine, PA)
Plast Reconstr Surg 126:2196-2204, 2010

The Maintenance of Certification module series is designed to help the clinician structure his or her study in specific areas appropriate to his or her clinical practice. This article is prepared to accompany practice-based assessment of preoperative assessment, anesthesia, surgical treatment plan, perioperative management, and outcomes. In this format, the clinician is invited to compare his or her methods of patient assessment and treatment, outcomes, and complications, with authoritative, information-based references.

This information base is then used for self-assessment and benchmarking in parts II and IV of the Maintenance of Certification process of the American Board of Plastic Surgery. This article is not intended to be an exhaustive treatise on the subject. Rather, it is designed to serve as a reference point for further in-depth study by review of the reference articles presented.

▶ Drs Shores and Lee provide us with a summary of the evidence for the treatment of carpal tunnel syndrome. They searched the literature through PubMed, Cumulative Index to Nursing and Allied Health Literature, and the Cochrane Library. From these sources, they summarize the best evidence on carpal tunnel syndrome with regard to preoperative assessment, anesthesia/analgesia, treatment, and outcomes.

In preoperative assessment, they find that the highest sensitivity and specificity among physical examination findings was the wrist flexion-carpal compression examination and the Durkan carpal compression test. The role for nerve conduction testing was complimentary in the diagnosis of carpal tunnel syndrome. Ultrasonographic testing was not as reliable as nerve conduction testing and did not offer the additional information of finding other nerve pathology.

Looking at the evidence on anesthesia, they focused on local and regional anesthetics and found that topical anesthetic, buffering of the local anesthetic, and warming all reduced the level of pain. Additionally, ropivacaine was superior to lidocaine for pain control intraoperatively and postoperatively. Ropivacaine also had less electrical effects on the cardiac cycle than bupivacaine.

In surgical treatment, they looked at comparisons among open, limited open, limited open with device assistance, and endoscopic techniques. They also reviewed suture repair techniques and postoperative management.

Endoscopic release showed accelerated improvement for 12 weeks and less scar tenderness at 3 months postoperatively versus open release. No other differences were found among the techniques. The accelerated improvement included an earlier return to work for the endoscopic release. Complication rates were the same except for transient neuropraxia being more common in endoscopic techniques in a meta-analysis.

Similarly, device-assisted carpal tunnel release showed a transient benefit over open release in some studies but no difference by 12 weeks.

Endoscopic release shows no difference in results compared with device-assisted open release.

Epineurotomy studies show no difference in adding that technique to the procedure.

Preservation of the cutaneous nerves at the incision for open carpal tunnel release demonstrates no difference.

Suture repair review shows that the material used probably makes no difference, except braided polyglactin may produce more suture granulomas and superficial infection than steel or nylon.

Postoperative management studies show that no difference is found between removing the dressing at 2 days or 2 weeks, splinting may have a detrimental effect, and supervised hand therapy for a period of 6 weeks adds no benefit over teaching the patients a home exercise program.

Postoperative pain management with oral analgesics shows no difference in using acetaminophen, naproxen, or placebo. In that single level 2 study, less than half of the placebo group required any pain medication at all.

D. J. Mastella, MD

Hand Surgery Volume and the US Economy: Is There a Statistical Correlation?
Gordon CR, Pryor L, Afifi AM, et al (Cleveland Clinic, OH)
Ann Plast Surg 65:471-474, 2010

Background.—To the best of our knowledge, there have been no previous studies evaluating the correlation of the US economy and hand surgery volume. Therefore, in light of the current recession, our objective was to study our institution's hand surgery volume over the last 17 years in relation to the nation's economy.

Methods.—A retrospective analysis of our institution's hand surgery volume, as represented by our most common procedure (ie, carpal tunnel release), was performed between January 1992 and October 2008. Liposuction and breast augmentation volumes were chosen to serve as cosmetic plastic surgery comparison groups. Pearson correlation statistics were used to estimate the relationship between the surgical volume and the US economy, as represented by the 3 market indices (Dow Jones, NASDAQ, and S&P500).

Results.—A combined total of 7884 hand surgery carpal tunnel release (open or endoscopic) patients were identified. There were 1927 (24%) and 5957 (76%) patients within the departments of plastic and orthopedic surgery, respectively. In the plastic surgery department, there was a strong negative (ie, inverse relationship) correlation between hand surgery volume and the economy ($P < 0.001$). In converse, the orthopedic department's hand surgery volume demonstrated a positive (ie, parallel) correlation ($P < 0.001$). The volumes of liposuction and breast augmentation also showed a positive correlation ($P < 0.001$).

Conclusion.—To our knowledge, we have demonstrated for the first time an inverse (ie, negative) correlation between hand surgery volumes performed by plastic surgeons in relation to the US economy, as represented by the 3 major market indices. In contrast, orthopedic hand surgery volume and cosmetic surgery show a parallel (ie, positive) correlation. This data suggests that plastic surgeons are increasing their cosmetic surgery-to-reconstructive/hand surgery ratio during strong economic times and vice versa during times of economic slowdown.

▶ Dis Gordon et al have presented their statistical analysis of the relative volume of hand surgery cases at the Cleveland Clinic over a 16-year period versus stock market indices. Their hypothesis is that during difficult economic times, as indicated by stock market index value, the number of orthopedic carpal tunnel releases (CTRs) would drop while the number of plastic surgery CTRs would rise. The proposed reason for this shift is that as the economy weakens, patients with less disposable income would not elect to have cosmetic surgery, causing a decrease in surgical volume for plastic surgeons. The resulting decrease in income for the plastic surgeon would cause him to increase the number of CTRs he performs. Meanwhile, orthopedic hand surgeons would experience a downturn in their CTR volume, presumably because of the poor economic climate and an inability to maintain their market share.

The authors' conclusions support their hypothesis, but the many weaknesses of their analysis make that conclusion questionable. The authors point out the obvious confounder of numbers of surgeons working at the Cleveland Clinic during the study period and state that "there has been a relative consistency of 2 to 3 full-time equivalents per specialty performing hand surgery at the Cleveland Clinic for the last 17 years." This statement is insufficient evidence to handle the potential effect of such a significant confounding variable. The issue of the variability in the characteristics of surgeons working in the health system studied is critical to case volume. The number of surgeons is important, but so too is their time in practice, with volume increasing usually over the first 5 to 7 years. A retiring surgeon with a well-established elective practice who is replaced by a freshly minted hand surgeon may cause a significant shift in the number of cases performed, as well as the ratio of trauma cases to elective cases. With the case numbers and surgeon numbers represented, such a change could explain the entire measured shift in cases, while the number of full-time equivalents would remain unchanged.

Another specific critique is a lack of explanation for the greater than 200% increase in orthopedic cases from 1998 to 1999 (Fig 1 in the original article). This abrupt rise is a clear outlier that requires greater in-depth analysis for explanation.

Additionally, the number of cases done in the health system during the study period may have been altered by the rise of outpatient surgery centers during that period. If one group of hand surgeons moves their CTR cases to a facility not captured in the database queried by the authors, the value of the analysis is adversely affected. This variable is never confronted.

Additional variables not accounted for in the analysis are the ratio of CTR and cosmetic surgery to total surgeon volume during the study period, the elasticity of patient flow from orthopedic hand surgeon to plastic hand surgeon that must occur to explain the changes in correlation in a theoretically closed system, and the changes in the local economy, which will have a greater effect on the patient population than the stock market indices. The list of confounding variables is long and important particularly because the study period is so long (16 years).

In conclusion, this article, while presenting an interesting hypothesis, is fundamentally flawed by a failure to analyze many important variables when considering departmental case volumes over a 16-year period. As a result, their conclusions must not be given complete credence.

D. J. Mastella, MD

Comparison of Longitudinal Open Incision and Two-Incision Techniques for Carpal Tunnel Release
Castillo TN, Yao J (Stanford Univ School of Medicine, Palo Alto, CA)
J Hand Surg 35A:1813-1819, 2010

Purpose.—This study analyzes the long-term postoperative symptoms and functional outcomes of patients who underwent either traditional open (single-incision) or 2-incision carpal tunnel release (CTR). Because 2-incision CTR preserves the superficial nerves and subcutaneous tissue between the thenar and hypothenar eminences, it may account for fewer postoperative symptoms and improved functional recovery.

Methods.—A retrospective chart review identified patients who underwent either open or 2-incision CTR for isolated carpal tunnel syndrome between 2005 and 2008 by a single surgeon. Patients with a history of hand trauma or confounding comorbidities were excluded. We mailed a Disabilities of the Arm, Shoulder, and Hand (DASH) Questionnaire and a Brigham and Women's Carpal Tunnel Questionnaire (BWCTQ) to all eligible participants. Data from the completed questionnaires were analyzed using independent t-tests and Pearson's correlation. Significance was set at p = .05.

Results.—A total of 82 patients (106 hands; 27 men and 55 women; mean age, 60.5 y) were eligible to participate. Of these, 51 patients (63 hands; 20 men and 31 women; mean age, 61.1 y) responded (62% response rate). The mean duration of follow-up was 22 months (range, 12–37 mo; SD 7.3 mo). The 2-incision group mean BWCTQ Symptom Severity Scale score (1.13, SD 0.25) was significantly lower than the open group mean Symptom Severity Scale score (1.54, SD 0.70, p = .001). The 2-incision group mean BWCTQ Functional Status Scale score (1.24, SD 0.51) was significantly lower than the open group mean Functional Status Scale score (1.71, SD 0.76, p = .008). The 2-incision group mean DASH score (5.10, SD 12.03) was significantly lower than the open group mean DASH score (16.28, SD 19.98, p = .01).

Conclusions.—Patients treated with 2-incision CTR reported statistically significantly less severe long-term postoperative symptoms and improved functional status compared with patients treated with traditional open CTR. Future prospective studies with objective measures are needed to further investigate the difference in outcomes found between these 2 CTR techniques.

▶ This retrospective level III study compared traditional open carpal tunnel release to a 2-incision nonendoscopic technique. All surgery was performed by a single surgeon, and follow-up was a minimum of 12 months. Validated outcomes tools were used, including the Disabilities of the Arm, Shoulder, and Hand (DASH) Questionnaire and the Brigham and Women's Carpal Tunnel Questionnaire (BWCTQ). The authors reported that of the 82 eligible patients, 51 patients (62%) responded to the questionnaires. The 2 groups were comparable, although there were more than twice as many patients in the open group compared with the 2-incision group (37 vs 14). All patients had electrodiagnostic confirmation of carpal tunnel syndrome prior to surgery. The authors did not mention their selection criteria, nor did they state if the 2 groups exhibited similar electrodiagnostic findings. Notable findings include a statistically significant difference in the 2 groups favoring the 2-incision technique. This was noted with both of the outcomes tools, including the BWCTQ Symptom Severity Scale and BWCTQ Functional Status Scale, as well as the DASH. Complications were not discussed.

This technique is my preferred technique for carpal tunnel release and one I have successfully used since 1993. It can be performed safely, with rapid return to function. I agree with the authors that a prospective randomized study using validated outcomes tools is warranted. It would be useful if the study looked at various time intervals following surgery, particularly because the retrospective study suffers from small sample size and contradicts prior studies that suggest no difference at longer-term follow-up.

D. S. Zelouf, MD

Median Nerve Deformation and Displacement in the Carpal Tunnel during Index Finger and Thumb Motion

van Doesburg MHM, Yoshii Y, Villarraga HR, et al (Univ Med Ctr, Utrecht, The Netherlands; Mayo Clinic, Rochester, MN)

J Orthop Res 28:1387-1390, 2010

The purpose of this study was to investigate the deformation and displacement of the normal median nerve in the carpal tunnel during index finger and thumb motion, using ultrasound. Thirty wrists from 15 asymptomatic volunteers were evaluated. Cross-sectional images during motion from full extension to flexion of the index finger and thumb were recorded. On the initial and final frames, the median nerve, flexor pollicis longus (FPL), and index finger flexor digitorum superficialis (FDS) tendons were outlined. Coordinate data were recorded and median nerve cross-sectional area, perimeter, aspect ratio of the minimal-enclosing rectangle, and circularity in extension and flexion positions were calculated. During index finger flexion, the tendon moves volarly while the nerve moves radially. With thumb flexion, the tendon moves volarly, but the median nerve moves toward the ulnar side. In both motions, the area and perimeter of the median nerve in flexion were smaller than in extension. Thus, during index finger or thumb flexion, the median nerve in a healthy human subject shifts away from the index finger FDS and FPL tendons while being compressed between the tendons and the flexor retaculumin the carpal tunnel. We are planning to compare these data with measurements in patients with carpal tunnel syndrome (CTS) and believe that these parameters may be useful tools for the assessment of CTS and carpal tunnel mechanics with ultrasound in the future.

▶ This article deals with the second investigation of the authors about the dynamic changes of the median nerve caused by the active flexion of the flexor pollicis longus (FPL) and flexor digitorum superficialis (FDS) of the index tendons within the carpal tunnel of 15 healthy individuals. To elucidate the mechanisms that lead to the development of carpal tunnel syndrome (CTS), they use a high-resolution ultrasound in an investigative setting, which they already presented in a previous article.

The finding of separately conducted investigations for the FPS and index FDS tendons is that with muscle activation, both tendons initially cause compression of the median nerve against the flexor retinaculum even in a non-diseased environment and finally displacement of the nerve. This displacement is seen as an evasion of the nerve from further compression.

It postulated that the fibrotic changes of the subsynovial connective tissue associated with CTS may render the median nerve immobile by restraining it under the flexor retinaculum, thus making it unable to laterally evade compression. This is an interesting hypothesis that may help to better understand the pathologic mechanisms that lead to chronic irritation of the median nerve in the carpal tunnel. As the authors point out, they will have to carry out further studies on CTS patients to prove their interesting hypothesis.

Although I understand the investigators' effort to keep the study setting as simple as possible, I feel that even more useful information could have been gained if they had also investigated the influence of simultaneous activation of both tendons on the median nerve, as this pattern of movement is closer to the natural use of the hand in daily life activities.

M. S. S. Choi, MD

Gliding Resistance of Flexor Tendon Associated with Carpal Tunnel Pressure: A Biomechanical Cadaver Study
Zhao C, Ettema AM, Berglund LJ, et al (Mayo Clinic, Rochester, MN)
J Orthop Res 29:58-61, 2011

The purpose of this study was to investigate the effect of carpal tunnel pressure on the gliding characteristics of flexor tendons within the carpal tunnel. Eight fresh human cadaver wrists and hands were used. A balloon was inserted into the carpal tunnel to elevate the pressure. The mean gliding resistance of the middle finger flexor digitorum superficialis tendon was measured with the following six conditions: (1) as a baseline, before balloon insertion; (2) balloon with 0 mmHg pressure; (3) 30 mmHg; (4) 60 mmHg; (5) 90 mmHg; (6) 120 mmHg. The gliding resistance of flexor tendon gradually increased as the carpal tunnel pressure was elevated. At pressures above 60 mmHg, the increase in gliding resistance became significant compared to the baseline condition. This study helps us to understand the relationship between carpal tunnel pressure, which is elevated in the patient with carpal tunnel syndrome (CTS) and tendon gliding resistance, which is a component of the work of flexion. These findings suggest that patients with CTS may have to expend more energy to accomplish specific motions, which may in turn affect symptoms of hand pain, weakness and fatigue, seen commonly in such patients.

▶ The purpose of this study was to investigate the effect of pressure changes on the gliding resistance of flexor tendons within the carpal tunnel. Establishing a link between increased carpal tunnel pressures and tendon gliding resistance will improve our understanding of the impact carpal tunnel syndrome (CTS) has on overall hand function. In this study, each cadaveric specimen acted as its own control, and the study was adequately powered. The primary outcome, mean gliding resistance (MGR), was extrapolated from a calculation of tendon excursion. The validity of this model is not discussed, and whether it accurately simulates the in vivo state is unknown. In my experience, the presence of subsynovial connective tissue does not always correlate with symptoms, and the clinical implication it has on CTS is not clear. The authors' findings suggest that increased pressures within the carpal tunnel result in reduced tendon excursion and subsequent increased MGR, which may relate to an increased work of flexion in these patients. Further research is needed to determine the role this plays in vivo.

R. Grewal, MD, MSc, FRCSC

American Academy of Orthopaedic Surgeons Clinical Practice Guideline on: The Treatment of Carpal Tunnel Syndrome
Keith MW, Masear V, Chung KC, et al
J Bone Joint Surg Am 92:218-219, 2010

Background.—The American Academy of Orthopaedic Surgeons has issued an updated clinical practice guideline on the treatment of carpal tunnel syndrome. The recommendations were developed based on systematic evidence-based processes designed to combat bias, enhance transparency, and promote reproducibility. The major recommendations were summarized.

Initial Care.—Nonoperative treatment is an early treatment option, although early surgery can be done for patients with clinical evidence of median nerve denervation or those who choose that option. Another nonoperative treatment can be tried if symptoms do not resolve within 2 to 7 weeks. Insufficient evidence exists to support specific treatment recommendations when carpal tunnel is complicated by diabetes mellitus, coexisting cervical radiculopathy, hypothyroidism, polyneuropathy, pregnancy, or rheumatoid arthritis. Carpal tunnel in the workplace has no specific treatment protocol. Before surgery is considered, patients should have local steroid injection or splinting. Oral steroids and ultrasound are also acceptable options. Heat therapy is not a recommended course of treatment. Approaches lacking support for or against their use include activity modification, acupuncture, cognitive behavioral therapy, cold laser, diuretics, exercise, electric stimulation, fitness, the graston instrument, iontophoresis, laser, stretching, massage therapy, magnet therapy, manipulation, medications (including anticonvulsants, antidepressants, and nonsteroidal anti-inflammatory drugs), nutritional supplements, phonophoresis, smoking cessation, systemic steroid injection, therapeutic touch, vitamin B6, weight reduction, and yoga.

Surgical Options.—Once surgery is chosen, carpal tunnel release is the recommended treatment. Complete division of the flexor retinaculum is the appropriate course regardless of the specific surgical technique. Procedures that are not recommended routinely include skin nerve preservation and epineurotomy. Evidence does not support or contraindicate the use of flexor retinaculum lengthening, internal neurolysis, tenosynovectomy, and ulnar bursa preservation. Preoperative antibiotics are given at the physician's discretion.

Postoperative Recommendations.—After routine carpal tunnel surgery the wrist should not be immobilized. Rehabilitation cannot be recommended or discouraged. Instruments of use in assessing patients' responses to carpal tunnel surgery include the Boston Carpal Tunnel Questionnaire;

assessment of disabilities of the arm, shoulder, and hand; the Michigan Hand Outcomes Questionnaire; the PEN; and the SF-12 or SF-36 Short Form Health Survey.

▶ This is an American Academy of Orthopaedic Surgeons clinical practice guideline on the treatment of carpal tunnel syndrome. A panel of renowned experts make 9 recommendations with grades and levels. The guidelines are also endorsed by the American Association of Neurological Surgeons and the Congress of Neurological Surgeons. The reader has the benefit of the panel having reviewed the literature and having made recommendations based on systematic evidence-based processes.

Interestingly, there is no mention of the evidence for or against electrodiagnostic testing, type of electrodiagnostic testing (full formal vs mini version done in the surgeons' office), other surgical modalities such as endoscopic or mini open carpal tunnel release, or treatment of recurrent carpal tunnel syndrome. This is unfortunate since these are questions that are relevant to the treatment of carpal tunnel syndrome. Nevertheless, this article is an important document to be aware of for the treating physician and surgeon.

S. K. Lee, MD

5 Hand: Congenital Differences

Percutaneous Release for Trigger Thumbs in Children: Improvements of the Technique and Results of 31 Thumbs
Sevencan A, İnan U, Köse N, et al (Eskisehir Osmangazi Univ, Turkey)
J Pediatr Orthop 30:705-709, 2010

Purpose.—Trigger thumb is a relatively uncommon condition in children. If it occurs or persists after 1 year of age, surgical release is the most traditional treatment method. The aim of this prospective study is to describe a technique for the percutaneous release of trigger thumb and to assess the clinical outcome of the presented technique in the pediatric age group.

Methods.—This study includes 31 thumbs of 26 consecutive children with a mean age of 2.6 years. An 18-gauge needle that was connected to 10-cc saline filled syringe was used as the surgical instrument for release. Contrary to the earlier reports, the A1 pulley was cut from distal pole of the Notta nodule towards the proximal direction.

Results.—Mean follow-up period was 2.5 years. A successful release without any complication was obtained in all (97% of thumbs) but 1 thumb. Recurrence was seen in only 1 thumb at postoperative 3 weeks.

Conclusion.—The presented minimal invasive surgical procedure has a high rate of satisfactory outcome, a minimal rate of complications, and a high rate of parent satisfaction. As percutaneous release has satisfactory and encouraging results, it can be a preferred method by the parents for trigger thumb release (Fig 1).

▶ The authors present a prospective series of 31 trigger thumbs in young children who underwent percutaneous release. The authors modified their technique during the study period of these 26 subjects, which further refines a precise incomplete release about Notta's node. Their technique uses a filled syringe and a hooded needle (Fig 1) to provide a short, stable lever arm and passive stretch of the thumb to provide tactile feedback in determining release. The technique works well in the authors' hands, and they favor it over the morbidity associated with open technique. In addition to a surgical incision, they note post-operative pain management, hospitalization, rest, and wound care as problems avoided with this method. This may be the treatment management customary in Turkey; however, congenital trigger thumb release is the

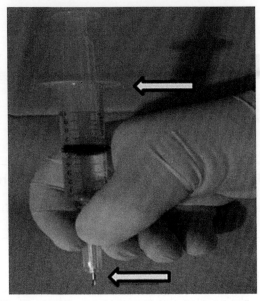

FIGURE 1.—Saline filled, guided syringe (above and below arrows), and needle with shortened cover (below arrows). (Reprinted from Sevencan A, Inan U, Köse N, et al. Percutaneous release for trigger thumbs in children: improvements of the technique and results of 31 thumbs. *J Pediatr Orthop.* 2010;30:705-709. http://lww.com).

most common procedure I perform in the pediatric age group, and none of these concerns apply. The surgical duration of this outpatient procedure is just a few minutes more than this technique; use of absorbable stitches with a waterproof bandage permits early movement and analgesia after the local anesthetic used is typically no more than pediatric ibuprofen. They provide an argument for incomplete release of the A1 pulley, and conceptually, this makes sense. However, the disparity between passive locking and active locking exists, which is occasionally evident in awake adults undergoing trigger thumb release. Therefore, open technique provides the best assurance of adequacy of release, especially in the pediatric population.

A. L. Ladd, MD

Developmental Biology and Classification of Congenital Anomalies of the Hand and Upper Extremity
Oberg KC, Feenstra JM, Manske PR, et al (Loma Linda Univ, CA; Washington Univ School of Medicine, St Louis, MO; Univ of Sydney, Australia)
J Hand Surg 35A:2066-2076, 2010

Recent investigations into the mechanism of limb development have clarified the roles of several molecules, their pathways, and interactions.

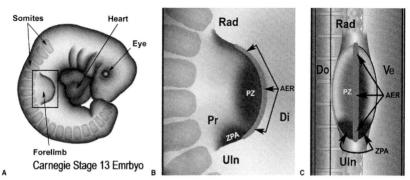

FIGURE 1.—Limb bud coordinate axes and signaling centers. A The forelimb (boxed region) of a Carnegie stage 13 embryo depicting the 3 coordinate axes—each with their own signaling center: the apical ectodermal ridge (AER—orange) coordinating proximal-distal (Pr-Di) outgrowth and differentiation; radial-ulnar asymmetry is controlled by the zone of polarizing activity (ZPA—purple). Dorsal-ventral (Do-Ve) asymmetry is regulated by dorsal ectoderm (green); within the progress zone (PZ—blue) the fate of mesodermal cells is determined by these signaling centers. The axes and signaling centers are shown in different orientations: B dorsal view and C lateral, end-on view. For interpretation of the references to color in this figure legend, the reader is referred to web version of this article. (Reprinted from Oberg KC, Feenstra JM, Manske PR, et al. Developmental biology and classification of congenital anomalies of the hand and upper extremity. *J Hand Surg.* 2010;35A:2066-2076, with permission from Elsevier.)

Characterization of the molecular pathways that orchestrate limb development has provided insight into the etiology of many limb malformations. In this review, we describe how the insights from developmental biology are related to clinically relevant anomalies and the current classification schemes used to define, categorize, and communicate patterns of upper limb malformations. We advocate an updated classification scheme for upper limb anomalies that incorporates our current molecular perspective of limb development and the pathogenetic basis for malformations using dysmorphology terminology. We anticipate that this scheme will improve the utility of a classification as a basis for diagnosis, treatment, and research (Fig 1, Table 1).

▶ The authors distill all of the most clinically relevant up-to-date research on limb formation into one readable article. The role of the apical ectodermal ridge (AER) in inciting growth of the limb bud should be familiar to most hand surgeons. Lesser known structures, such as the zone of polarizing activity (ZPA) and the dorsal ectoderm, guide radioulnar and volardorsal limb differentiation, respectively (Fig 1), through feedback loops that include sonic hedgehog, fibroblast growth factors, and wingless-type signaling factors. Disruption of the AER leads to transverse deficiencies. Duplication of the ZPA leads to a mirror hand, while loss of the ZPA results in ulnar longitudinal deficiencies. Because of the interdependence of AER and ZPA function, ulnar longitudinal deficiencies may also lead to malformations or diminution of radial-sided structures. Conversely, persistence of the ZPA with diminution of AER function leads to radial longitudinal deficiencies. The authors propose

TABLE 1.—Comparison of the IFSSH Classification Scheme and the Proposed Classification

IFSSH Classification	Proposed Classification
1. Failure of formation	1. Malformations
• Longitudinal deficiencies	A. Failure of axis formation/differentiation—entire
- Radial longitudinal deficiencies	upper limb
- Ulnar longitudinal deficiencies	1. Proximal-distal outgrowth
• Transverse deficiencies	Brachymelia with brachydactyly
• Intersegmental deficiencies	Symbrachydactyly
	Transverse deficiency
	Intersegmental deficiency
	2. Radial-ulnar (anteroposterior) axis
	Radial longitudinal deficiency
	Ulnar longitudinal deficiency
	Ulnar dimelia
	Radioulnar synostosis
	Humero-radial synostosis
	3. Dorsal-ventral axis
	Nail-patella syndrome
	B. Failure of axis formation/differentiation—handplate
	1. Radial-ulnar (anteroposterior) axis
	Radial polydactyly
	Triphalangeal thumb
	Ulnar polydactyly
	2. Dorsal-ventral axis
	Dorsal dimelia (palmar nail)
	Hypoplastic/aplastic nail
	C. Failure of handplate formation/differentiation—
	unspecified axis
	1. Soft tissue
	Syndactyly
	Camptodactyly
	2. Skeletal deficiency
	Brachydactyly
	Clinodactyly
	Kirner's deformity
	Metacarpal and carpal synostoses
	3. Complex
	Cleft hand
	Synpolydactyly
	Apert hand
2. Failure of differentiation	2. Deformations
• Soft tissue deficiency	A. Constriction ring sequence
• Skeletal deficiency	B. Arthrogryposis
	C. Trigger digits
	D. Not otherwise specified
3. Duplication	3. Dysplasias
• Radial polydactyly	A. Hypertrophy
• Ulnar polydactyly	1. Macrodactyly
• Mirror hand/ulnar dimelia	2. Upper limb
	3. Upper limb and macrodactyly
	B. Tumorous conditions
4. Overgrowth	
5. Undergrowth	
6. Constriction band syndrome	
7. Generalized skeletal disorder	

a new classification scheme based on new genetic evidence with 3 categories: malformations, deformations, and dysplasias (Table 1).

D. A. Zlotolow, MD

6 Hand: Microsurgery and Flaps

Free great toe wrap-around flap combined with second toe medial flap for reconstruction of completely degloved fingers
Rui Y, Mi J, Shi H, et al (Wuxi Hand Surgery and Orthopaedics Hosp, Jiangsu Province, China; et al)
Microsurgery 30:449-456, 2010

Surgical procedure of great toe wrap-around flap combined with second toe medial flap free transfer for reconstructing completely degloved fingers was introduced. The treatment outcomes were evaluated. 10 fingers in 7 cases were involved in this series. The great toe wrap-around flap with dorsalis pedis skin covered the dorsal and most palmar side of the injured finger. The second toe medial flap covered the proximal palmar portion of the finger. The combined flap was revascularized with nerve repair. Rehabilitation started two weeks postoperatively. All flaps survived except one was partial failure due to distal phalange necrosis. Recipient areas achieved primary wound healing in 9 fingers. Skin graft at donor site achieved primary survival except delayed healing in one case. All patients were followed-up from 34 to 76 months. The appearance of reconstructed fingers was satisfactory. Nail growth well except that one nail was the atrophic and another was defect. Range of active motion in the metacarpophalangeal joint was from 60° to 80° and the proximal interphalange joint was 40° to 70°. Two-point discrimination was between 8 mm and 12 mm. All patients walked with no interference. There was no pain and no swelling at donor site. According to the results, this procedure is recommended to reconstruct total degoling finger which has intact phalanges and tendons.

▶ Degloving injuries of the fingers are devastating injuries and represent one of the greatest reconstructive challenges for the hand surgeon. The options of completion amputation, pedicled chest or groin flap, dressing followed by skin grafting, and free tissue transfer are all viable, depending on the cultural norms and technical capabilities of the patient's local environment.

In this article, the authors from China show impressive results of a chimeric flap with a great toe wraparound flap and a second toe medial flap. From the clinical pictures presented, it is important to counsel the patients that even with this technique, fingers cannot be expected to appear normal. Furthermore, the donor site morbidity of the larger dorsal foot skin flap is considerable.

J. Chang, MD

Treatment of Thumb Tip Degloving Injury Using the Modified First Dorsal Metacarpal Artery Flap
Chen C, Zhang X, Shao X, et al (The Second Hosp of Tangshan, Hebei, China; Affiliated Hosp of North China Coal Med College, Tangshan, Hebei, China; The Second Hosp of Qinhuangdao, Changli, Hebei, China; et al)
J Hand Surg 35A:1663-1670, 2010

Purpose.—This study reports repair of a thumb tip degloving injury using the modified first dorsal metacarpal artery (FDMA) flap, including both dorsal branches of the proper digital nerve (DBPDNs).

Methods.—From May 2006 to February 2008, the modified FDMA flap was used in 11 thumbs in 11 patients. All patients suffered a degloving injury to the thumb tip, and 4 had associated bone loss ranging from 1 to 3 mm (mean, 2 mm) in length. The size of the soft tissue defects was 2.6 to 4.6 cm (mean, 3.5 cm) in length and 1.8 to 2.2 cm (mean, 2.0 cm) in width. The flaps ranged in size from 2.7 × 2.2 cm to 4.8 × 2.1 cm (mean, 3.6 × 2.1 cm). The mean pedicle length was 7.2 cm (range, 6.8−7.5 cm). Neurorrhaphy between the DBPDN and the proper digital nerve was performed in both sides in all cases. Patient follow-ups ranged from 26 to 47 months (mean, 32 mo). Sensibility of the reconstructed thumb was evaluated by static 2-point discrimination. The range of motion of the donor fingers was measured. The data were compared to those of the opposite sides.

Results.—All flaps survived completely. At the final follow-up, the mean values of static 2-point discrimination were 5 mm (range, 4−8 mm) and 6 mm (range, 4−8 mm) on the radial and ulnar sides of the distal portion of the flap, respectively. The mean values of the radial and ulnar distal portions of the flaps reached 75% and 72% of those of the opposite sides. The mean range of motion of the metacarpophalangeal, proximal interphalangeal, and distal interphalangeal joints of the donor fingers were 73°, 101°, and 70°, respectively.

Conclusions.—The modified FDMA flap, including both DBPDNs, is useful for restoration of sensation on the thumb tip and maintenance of adequate length of the thumb.

▶ Using a modification of the kite flap, the authors show excellent results as to the sensory restoration of the thumb tip after degloving. They report a mean static 2-point discrimination (PD) of 5.7 mm at the distal tip of the flap after coapting the dorsal branches of the proper digital nerves to the stumps of the palmar proper nerves of the thumb. This exceptional value is most probably even better than the discrimination on the flap's skin before transplantation. At first sight, it may be astonishing that a reinnervated flap shows a better

2-PD after the reconstructive procedure than on its original place, where it is taken from. A possible explanation for this phenomenon may be the higher axon counts of the recipient nerves.

It would have been interesting to know if this procedure was associated with any formation of symptomatic neuromas on the donor site. The article does not provide information on this possible complication.

For smaller defects, I prefer to use a free transfer of partial toe pulp skin, as reported by Lee and colleagues.[1] Using the medial digital artery and nerve with a plantar vein as a pedicle for the medial part of the second toe pulp, this method provides an excellent and fast way of reconstruction for the thumb tip with glabrous skin for defects up to 3.3 × 2.3 cm. Sometimes the use of this flap may be limited by its short pedicle.

For the record, although Coleman and Anson[2] provided us with a deep insight into the arterial anatomy of the hand, they did not introduce the first dorsal metacarpal artery flap in this article, as stated by the authors. It was Foucher and Braun[3] in 1979 who first described the so-called kite flap based on the first dorsal metacarpal artery.

M. S. S. Choi, MD

References

1. Lee DC, Kim JS, Ki SH, Roh SY, Yang JW, Chung KC. Partial second toe pulp free flap for fingertip reconstruction. *Plast Reconstr Surg.* 2008;121:899-907.
2. Coleman SS, Anson BJ. Arterial patterns in the hand based upon a study of 650 specimens. *Surg Gynecol Obstet.* 1961;113:409-424.
3. Foucher G, Braun JB. A new island flap transfer from the dorsum of the index to the thumb. *Plast Reconstr Surg.* 1979;63:344-349.

7 Hand: Peripheral Nerve

Scope-Assisted Release of the Cubital Tunnel
Mirza A, Reinhart MK, Bove J, et al (St Catherine of Siena Med Ctr, Smithtown, NY; Stony Brook Univ, NY; New York College of Osteopathic Medicine, Old Westbury)
J Hand Surg 36A:147-151, 2011

We report on a technique of endoscopic release of the cubital tunnel, which is a modification of Bruno and Tsai's technique. This article covers the history, complications, indications, and postoperative management of ulnar nerve entrapments treated endoscopically, with a special focus on our technique. This minimally invasive alternative to transposition requires no mobilization of the ulnar nerve, which could potentially reduce iatrogenic trauma to the nerve and its vascularity.

▶ This article reviews the outcome of endoscopic cubital tunnel release. The authors reported their own outcome using new cannulas and instruments to allow easier performance of the cubital tunnel release. The main advantage of their cannula is being transparent that allows direct visualization of the nerve and thus decreasing the risk of ulnar nerve injury during the endoscopic procedure. The authors reported a short-term outcome (mean 5 months) of 52 patients who underwent the procedure. Two patients had ulnar nerve anterior subluxation. One underwent medial epicondylectomy, and the second underwent anterior transposition. One patient had a hematoma that resolved without sequelae. There were no nerve injuries and no recurrent symptoms. The positive outcome and rate of complications are similar to those reported previously in the literature by Tsai et al, Hoffman and Siemionow, and Ahcan and Zorman.

B. Elhassan, MD

Regeneration and repair of peripheral nerves with different biomaterials: review

Siemionow M, Bozkurt M, Zor F (The Cleveland Clinic, OH)
Microsurgery 30:574-588, 2010

Peripheral nerve injury may cause gaps between the nerve stumps. Axonal proliferation in nerve conduits is limited to 10–15 mm. Most of the supportive research has been done on rat or mouse models which are different from humans. Herein we review autografts and biomaterials which are commonly used for nerve gap repair and their respective outcomes. Nerve autografting has been the first choice for repairing peripheral nerve gaps. However, it has been demonstrated experimentally that tissue engineered tubes can also permit lead to effective nerve repair over gaps longer than 4 cm repair that was previously thought to be restorable by means of nerve graft only. All of the discoveries in the nerve armamentarium are making their way into the clinic, where they are, showing great potential for improving both the extent and rate of functional recovery compared with alternative nerve guides.

▶ Investigations on materials proposed to bridge peripheral nerve defects (or gaps) have expanded continuously over the past few decades. A bewildering variety of materials are currently available, so clinicians and investigators are no longer surprised at reports of novel materials capable of guiding nerve regeneration. Despite the large number of materials already identified, continuing research efforts reflect the fact that satisfactory materials have not yet been found. The speed, quality, and length of nerve regeneration across a guide have not notably improved compared with those years or even decades ago.

With the current scope of investigations on this topic and wealth of materials that exhibit clinical potential, investigators should be aware that newly discovered materials deserving published reports (documentation) may have very limited values scientifically, if they had not been compared with and proven superior to available materials. Readers should not be misled by the emergence of novel materials, many of which are actually no better than or even inferior to existing materials. In this regard, investigators should emphasize comparisons with existing materials, identifying those that are superior (not simply novel).

Clinically, only a few randomized prospective studies have provided high-quality results. Interestingly, in studying 136 digital nerve transections, Weber et al[1] found improved sensation when a polyglycolic acid (PGA) conduit was used for nerve gaps of 4 mm or less, compared with a nerve graft or end-to-end nerve repair. Though those findings were questioned, it provided strong support for clinical use of PGA conduits. In 2009, Rinker and Liau[2] presented the outcomes of vein conduits and woven PGA conduits in reconstructing 76 digital nerves. They found equal sensory recovery and cost, but reoperation was required in 2 patients to remove the PGA guides because of implant extrusions.

Over the last decade, I have not made major efforts in the field of nerve regeneration; but in the early 1990s, I conducted a few clinical studies to assess the effectiveness of vein conduits to reconstruct nerve defects. I proposed to use vein conduits to reconstruct digital nerve defects as an adjunct to tendon grafting and developed methods to insert nerve slices from the proximal nerve into the conduits to enhance regeneration across an extended gap; both methods are viable, and I still use them. My colleagues are involved in testing the clinical efficacy of synthetic guides.

It is possible that decades of intense work may yield outcomes identical to those found at the start; science sometimes does move in circles. Nevertheless, I believe that future breakthroughs will eventually be built on in-depth inquiries into complex mechanisms that orchestrate the regeneration process. Such discoveries can only be expected after accumulation of abundant fundamental insights that are out of reach currently. Instead of going wider, I would suggest going deeper to uncover potential materials, to investigate the mechanisms and more elegantly design guides incorporating cells, bioactive factors, and extracellular matrix components by more sophisticated approaches.

J. B. Tang, MD

References

1. Weber RA, Breidenbach WC, Brown RE, Jabaley ME, Mass DP. A randomized prospective study of polyglycolic acid conduits for digital nerve reconstruction in humans. *Plast Reconstr Surg.* 2000;106:1036-1045.
2. Rinker BD, Liau J. A prospective randomized study comparing woven polyglycolic acid and autogenous vein conduits for reconstruction of digital nerve gaps. Presented at the 64th Annual Meeting of American Society for Surgery of the Hand; 2009; San Francisco, CA.

Muscle-in-vein Nerve Guide for Secondary Reconstruction in Digital Nerve Lesions
Ignazio M, Adolfo V (Istituto Clinico Città di Brescia—Gruppo San Donato, Italy)
J Hand Surg 35A:1418-1426, 2010

Purpose.—Although vein conduits filled with fresh skeletal muscle have been used to bridge nerve defects both experimentally and clinically with good results, this approach has never been considered a valuable tool for reconstruction of nerve defects, and the technique has been abandoned. The purpose of this study was to evaluate the application of muscle-in-vein conduits for secondary digital nerves reconstruction, with particular emphasis on the surgical technique and results.

Methods.—We present a retrospectively selected consecutive series of 21 digital nerve defects in 17 patients who were treated with vein conduits filled with fresh skeletal muscle for secondary nerve reconstruction. After a minimum follow-up of 18 months, all patients were studied with static and moving 2-point discrimination, Semmes—Weinstein monofilament testing, Visual Analog Scale, and Disabilities of the Arm, Shoulder, and Hand questionnaire. Outcome data were stratified according to the

American Society for Surgery of the Hand guidelines, the modified Highet and Sander's criteria, and the Logic Tree.

Results.—The average nerve gap bridged with the muscle-in-vein conduit was 2.2 cm (range, 1—3.5 cm). We classified 14 of 22 reconstructed nerves as excellent or good according to American Society for Surgery of the Hand guidelines, whereas 17 were between S4 and S3 using modified Highet and Sander's criteria. The Logic Tree yielded results between S4 and S3 in 14 of 21 reconstructed nerves. The average Disabilities of the Arm, Shoulder, and Hand survey scores were 22.5 for the disability/symptoms module and 21.4 and 17 for the sports/music and work subcomponents, respectively.

Conclusions.—Use of muscle-in-vein conduits should be considered and promoted for sensory nerve reconstruction for a number of reasons: the encouraging results with the technique; the abundant availability of both donor tissues; the flexibility of the conduit resulting from the combination of muscle and vein; the simplicity with which tubes can be fashioned; immunological compatibility; and the absence of adjunctive costs.

Type of Study/Level of Evidence.—Therapeutic IV.

▶ A biological conduit made of an autologous vein graft filled with a muscle strip yields better results than if the single components are used alone, as one tissue can compensate for the limitations of the other, if used together. The multitude of conduit materials and their combinations and the many different methods of outcome assessment used in different publications make it difficult to compare the results. The strength of this study lies in a thorough assessment of the results by using multiple tests. This allows for a comparison with other studies.

The authors achieved good results with the combination of autologous vein and muscle grafts that compare favorably with the gold standard autologous nerve grafts. They show that this combination can provide a reliable, inexpensive, and almost unlimited source of nerve substitute. A limitation with this method, as with many other conduits as well, is the limited defect length that can safely be reconstructed. The average grafted length in this study was 2.2 cm. Before more evidence is provided for the safe use with defects longer than 3 cm, autologous nerve grafting will remain the treatment of choice for long reconstructions. The potential side effects of sural nerve harvesting can well be minimized with proper harvesting technique.

For short defects, however, one should definitely consider using this technique, as there is enough evidence also from other studies that it may functionally be even better than autologous nerve grafting without the donor site problems of the latter.[1,2]

Like many researchers before them, the authors of this study mistakenly cite Gluck's publication from 1880 as the first report of nerve reconstruction with a conduit.[3] While it was indeed Gluck who first reported about bridging nerve defects with Danish leather, bone drains, catgut, and muscle in animals, he actually did so in a separate publication in 1881.[4]

M. S. S. Choi, MD

References

1. Weber RA, Breidenbach WC, Brown RE, Jabaley ME, Mass DP. A randomized prospective study of polyglycolic acid conduits for digital nerve reconstruction in humans. *Plast Reconstr Surg.* 2000;106:1036-1045.
2. Meek MF, Coert JH. Clinical use of nerve conduits in peripheral-nerve repair: review of the literature. *J Reconstr Microsurg.* 2002;18:97-109.
3. Gluck T. Ueber Neuroplastik auf dem Wege der Transplantation. *Arch Klin Chir.* 1880;25:606-616.
4. Gluck T. Ueber Transplantation, Regeneration und entzündliche Neubildung. *Arch Klin Chir.* 1881;26:896-915.

8 Hand: Tendon

Augmentation of Zone II Flexor Tendon Repair Using Growth Differentiation Factor 5 in a Rabbit Model
Henn RF III, Kuo CE, Kessler MW, et al (Hosp for Special Surgery, NY; North Shore and Long Island Jewish Hosps, Manhasset, NY)
J Hand Surg 35A:1825-1832, 2010

Purpose.—Modulation of zone II flexor tendon repair healing using growth factors may reduce the incidence of complications, such as rupture and fibrosis. We hypothesized that sutures coated with growth differentiation factor 5 (GDF5) will stimulate the healing of zone II flexor tendon repairs.

Methods.—We created and immediately repaired zone II flexor tendon lacerations in the second and fourth toe of the right forepaw of 44 New Zealand White rabbits. One tendon was repaired with suture coated with GDF5, whereas the other tendon was repaired with suture without GDF5 (control). We randomized the allocation of GDF5 and control suture to either toe. A proximal tenotomy of the flexor digitorum profundus at the level of the wrist was performed to relieve tension on the more distal repairs. Rabbits were euthanized at 21 or 42 days after repair. Four rabbits (8 tendons) underwent histological analysis at each time point; the remaining repairs were tested biomechanically in a blinded fashion.

Results.—Control tendons demonstrated distinct borders at the transection site and less endogenous repair at 3 weeks. The Soslowsky histological score for collagen was better in the GDF5 group at both time points (p≤.003). All tendons failed at the repair site. The maximum load was significantly greater (p=.04) in the GDF5 group (11.6 ± 3.5 N) compared with control tendons (8.6 ± 3.0 N) at 3 weeks. The maximum load was not significantly different (p=.12) at 6 weeks. We observed no significant differences in stiffness at either time point (p>.11).

Conclusions.—The results demonstrate that GDF5 has an early beneficial effect on tendon healing in zone II flexor tendon repairs in a rabbit flexor tendon injury model (Fig 3).

▶ Biological modulation of flexor tendon healing is the new frontier in the management of flexor tendon injuries. The results of this study show that growth factors have great promise to enhance the rehabilitation and clinical outcome following flexor tendon injuries.

This work builds on previously published work demonstrating the potential of growth differentiation factor 5 (GDF5) to positively influence tendon

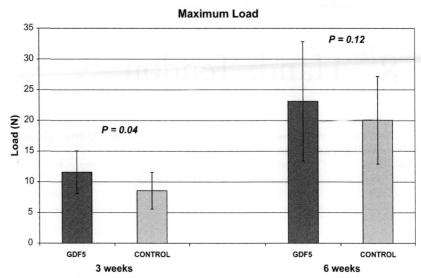

FIGURE 3.—Maximum load. Mean ± standard deviation is shown for each group. p Values comparing the control and GDF5 groups are given for each time point. (Reprinted from Henn RF III, Kuo CE, Kessler MW, et al. Augmentation of zone II flexor tendon repair using growth differentiation factor 5 in a rabbit model. *J Hand Surg*. 2010;35A:1825-1832. Copyright 2010, with permission from the American Society for Surgery of the Hand.)

healing. Using a widely accepted model of flexor tendon injury and repair in the rabbit, the authors demonstrate that GDF5 can positively increase the maximum load of the repaired tendon at 3 weeks. However, no difference was noted at 6 weeks.

This study provides more evidence for the potential of GDF5 as a biological modulator of flexor tendon healing. There are several points worth taking note of in this experimental work. First, polyglactin 910 was chosen as the suture material because of its known delivery kinetics for GDF5. However, this material is not usually used for human flexor tendon repair. Suture material commonly used in flexor tendon repair may not be suitable for GDF5 or other growth factor delivery and needs to be assessed. Second, the average maximum load at 3 weeks was 11.6 N (see Fig 3), compared with 93.3 N for normal rabbit flexor tendons. The biological effect in humans may not be sufficient to reduce the risk of repair rupture in the first few weeks following repair. Experiments using higher order larger animals would provide more insight into the viability of this technique in humans. Finally, the effects of mobilization and adhesion formation were not assessed in this study.

A. Chong, MD

Trigger Thumb in Children: Results of Surgical Treatment in Children Above 5 Years of Age

Han SH, Yoon HK, Shin DE, et al (CHA Univ, Seongnam, Korea)
J Pediatr Orthop 30:710-714, 2010

Background.—There have been debates about the results of surgical treatment in older children, even though many studies showed excellent results in pediatric trigger thumb. The objective of this study was to identify the possible problems or complications related to the delayed surgery for trigger thumb in children. Authors clinically reexamined the patients who had undergone A1 pulley release above the age of 5 years and analyzed the results of surgical treatment.

Methods.—A retrospective study of 31 trigger thumbs was performed on 23 consecutive children treated using a standardized surgical technique. The mean age at the operation was 7.46 years and average period of clinical follow-up was 2 years and 3 months. We investigated the presence or absence of interphalangeal joint flexion contracture, triggering, recovery of active range of motion, postoperative period that the patients get more than 0 degree interphalangeal joint extension, and complications.

Results.—Flexion contracture and painful triggering were successfully relieved after surgery in all cases. Patients showed variable periods in improving temporary extension weakness of interphalangeal joint, but there was no statistical difference in the final result between early and delayed improvement or between symptom duration and healing time. None of these patients had any postoperative complications.

Conclusions.—Surgical treatment with A1 pulley release for over 5 years of age resulted in successful resolution of trigger thumb and satisfactory clinical outcome in all our cases regardless the age at the time of surgery. From the author's findings, we can expect satisfactory results of surgical treatment in pediatric trigger thumb even in the case of delayed diagnosis or late treatment.

▶ The results of this study lend further evidence to the opinion that trigger thumb releases in children may be delayed even after the age of 3 years with no consequences in long-term motion or function. The 23 patients in this study averaged 7 years of age and were able to recover the range of motion of their thumb interphalangeal joint by final follow-up. Some patients did, however, experience a temporary extensor lag. When counseling parents of children with trigger thumbs, it is important to stress the lack of urgency of surgical release. Although the risks of both the procedure and the anesthesia are minimal, complications may occur. Given the relatively benign natural history of trigger thumbs in children, parents should feel that they have time to make an informed decision regarding their child's care.

D. A. Zlotolow, MD

Complications of Open Trigger Finger Release
Will R, Lubahn J (Hamot Med Ctr, Erie, PA)
J Hand Surg 35A:594-596, 2010

Purpose.—Open release of A1 pulleys for trigger finger has been thought of as a relatively benign procedure with a low complication rate. Few studies have examined the rate of complications in trigger finger release. The objective of this study was to retrospectively review the complications documented for a cohort of patients who received open trigger finger releases.

Methods.—We conducted a retrospective chart review of 43 patients who had had 78 open trigger finger releases by a single surgeon. Any postoperative complications that were documented were recorded. Complications were then divided into major and minor. Major complications required further surgery or resulted in significant limitations of activities of daily living; minor complications hindered recovery, responded to treatment (if applicable), and either resolved or had little impact on function.

Results.—Two major complications were noted: a synovial fistula that required excision, and proximal interphalangeal joint arthrofibrosis that required cast application for pain relief. The major complication rate was 3% per trigger release (2/78). Twenty-seven minor complications in 22 digits were documented for these cases, including decreased range of motion, scar tenderness, pain, and wound erythema. The minor complication rate was 28% (22/78). The overall, combined complication rate for these primary interventions was 31% (24/78).

Conclusions.—Open trigger finger release is thought to be a low-risk procedure by most practitioners. In this study, we found that major complications do occur infrequently; however, the rate of minor complications was surprisingly high and related mostly to wound complications or loss of finger range of motion. The surgeon performing open trigger finger releases should inform the patient of the likelihood of having these minor complications.

▶ Will and Lubahn present a single-surgeon retrospective chart review of consecutive open trigger releases. They find complication rates perhaps higher than anticipated for what is considered a simple procedure. The major complication rate (ones that result in difficulty with activities of daily living) in their series was 3% (2/78). There were an unusual synovial fistula and significant arthrofibrosis.

The minor complication rate (hindered recovery with little or no residual issues) was higher at 28% (22/78).

Overall, they show that something less than a completely benign postoperative course may be expected up to 30% of the time. These findings are significant. The major limitation of the study is a low power with a total of 78 open trigger releases over a 6.5-year span. This number corresponds to a rate of open trigger releases of 12 per year or 1 per month. While trigger release is a simple surgical procedure requiring little postoperative therapy, 1 procedure per month may be too low a rate of occurrence for a robust system of care to be developed and may therefore contribute to a higher rate of minor complications.

D. J. Mastella, MD

Zone-II Flexor Tendon Repair: A Randomized Prospective Trial of Active Place-and-Hold Therapy Compared with Passive Motion Therapy
Trumble TE, Vedder NB, Seiler JG III, et al (Univ of Washington Med Ctr, Seattle; Georgia Hand and Microsurgery PC, Atlanta, GA; et al)
J Bone Joint Surg Am 92:1381-1389, 2010

Background.—In order to improve digit motion after zone-II flexor tendon repair, rehabilitation programs have promoted either passive motion or active motion therapy. To our knowledge, no prospective randomized trial has compared the two techniques. Our objective was to compare the results of patients treated with an active therapy program and those treated with a passive motion protocol following zone-II flexor tendon repair.

Methods.—Between January 1996 and December 2002, 103 patients (119 digits) with zone-II flexor tendon repairs were randomized to either early active motion with place and hold or a passive motion protocol. Range of motion was measured at six, twelve, twenty-six, and fifty-two weeks following repair. Dexterity tests were performed, and the Disabilities of the Arm, Shoulder, and Hand (DASH) outcome questionnaire and a satisfaction score were completed at fifty-two weeks by ninety-three patients (106 injured digits).

Results.—At all time points, patients treated with the active motion program had greater interphalangeal joint motion. At the time of the final follow-up, the interphalangeal joint motion in the active place-and-hold group was a mean (and standard deviation) of $156° \pm 25°$ compared with $128° \pm 22°$ ($p < 0.05$) in the passive motion group. The active motion group had both significantly smaller flexion contractures and greater satisfaction scores ($p < 0.05$). We could identify no difference between the groups in terms of the DASH scores or dexterity tests. When the groups were stratified, those who were smokers or had a concomitant nerve injury or multiple digit injuries had less range of motion, larger flexion contractures, and decreased satisfaction scores compared with patients without these comorbidities. Treatment by a certified hand therapist resulted in better range of motion with smaller flexion contractures. Two digits in each group had tendon ruptures following repair.

Conclusions.—Active motion therapy provides greater active finger motion than passive motion therapy after zone-II flexor tendon repair without increasing the risk of tendon rupture. Concomitant nerve injuries, multiple digit injuries, and a history of smoking negatively impact the final outcome of tendon repairs.

▶ This randomized prospective study of flexor tendon therapy protocols evaluated an active versus passive program following 4-stranded flexor tendon repairs within zone II. The results indicated that the active program exhibited better overall range of motion with lesser flexion contractures and greater patient satisfaction scores than the passive program. Patients treated by a certified hand therapist exhibited improved motion and greater satisfaction. An increased rupture rate was not found when using the active program. Although 16 surgeons performed the repairs, all were experienced, fellowship-trained hand surgeons, and all flexor profundus repairs were 4-stranded. Disabilities of the Arm, Shoulder, and Hand (DASH) scores did not differ between the 2 groups. A patient-rated wrist and hand evaluation might have provided more meaningful information when compared with the DASH outcome measure. The study did demonstrate improved results in both groups when treatment was administered by a certified hand therapist, with worse results in those with multiple digit injuries. Smoking also influenced results, with less motion, greater joint contractures, and lower satisfaction scores. In summary, this is a valuable study that supports the use of an early active range of motion protocol following 4-stranded flexor tendon repairs administered by a certified hand therapist, demonstrating improved results over the traditional passive program with no apparent increase in rupture rate.

D. S. Zelouf, MD

Anatomic Outcome of Percutaneous Release Among Patients With Trigger Finger

Calleja H, Tanchuling A, Alagar D, et al (St Luke's Med Ctr, Quezon City, Philippines)
J Hand Surg 35A:1671-1674, 2010

Purpose.—To investigate the adequacy and safety of percutaneous trigger finger release on symptomatic patients.

Methods.—Two orthopedic non-hand surgeons performed percutaneous A1 pulley release on the thumb, index, middle, and ring fingers with the use of a 19-gauge needle in 25 fingers of 24 patients. Open inspection was then performed to determine the extent of release and any injury to the surrounding anatomic structures.

Results.—Triggering was eliminated in all fingers. Of the 25 A1 pulleys, 19 were partially released; only 6 were completely released. Noted injury included only superficial abrasions in 15 tendons. None of the patients had injury to the digital artery or nerve.

Conclusions.—In the percutaneous release of trigger fingers, complete anatomic release of the A1 pulley is not always adequately achieved, even though clinically patients experience relief of triggering. It is a safe procedure for the thumb, index, middle, and ring fingers as long as the recommended technique is observed.

▶ Calleja and his coauthors explored the efficacy and safety of percutaneous trigger finger release on symptomatic patients using a 19-gauge needle. Twenty-five fingers in 24 patients were treated percutaneously in this case series. These patients were then opened to explore the release and identify any areas of iatrogenic injury to the surrounding soft tissues. They found that only 6 of the 25 A1 pulleys were completely released using the percutaneous technique, though triggering was clinically resolved in all fingers. Superficial abrasions were identified in 15 tendons with no other adverse effects.

In this study, the authors found that the distal segment of the A1 pulley was more frequently intact in those that were incompletely released. They attributed this finding to their technique of starting the percutaneous release at the proximal-most portion of the A1 pulley. Because all patients in this study demonstrated intraoperative resolution of their triggering despite an incomplete release, the authors suggested that a complete release of the A1 pulley may not be necessary. Clearly, greater patient volumes would lend strength to this conclusion: only 25 fingers were studied for a condition that is frequently seen in most hand surgeons' practices. In reading this article, I was also curious to know how much experience the authors had with percutaneous release prior to the study's initiation. Do the data represent an early part of the learning curve for the authors? The authors explicitly report that all releases were performed by 2 orthopedic nonhand surgeons.

E. K. Shin, MD

Zone II Combined Flexor Digitorum Superficialis and Flexor Digitorum Profundus Repair Distal to the A2 Pulley

Pike JM, Gelberman RH (Washington Univ School of Medicine, St Louis, MO)
J Hand Surg Am 35:1523-1527, 2010

Combined transection of both the flexor digitorum superficialis (FDS) and the flexor digitorum profundus (FDP) tendons distal to the A2 pulley is challenging due to the intimacy of the FDS—FDP relationship at that level. This report describes our surgical technique for repair of combined FDS and FDP transections following decussation of the FDS tendon. Each slip of the FDS is repaired using 5-0 or 6-0 polypropylene sutures in a Becker configuration, creating a 4-strand repair for each slip. Repair of the FDP tendon is performed using Winters' core-suture technique with looped 4-0 pseudomonofilament nylon suture, modified to achieve a locking loop and an 8-strand repair. The suture is placed with 1.2 cm of the lacerated end of the tendon, and a single knot is placed inside the repair site. We use a peripheral suture of 6-0 polypropylene for a running, nonlocked configuration to strengthen and tidy the repair. The suture is placed 2 mm from the lacerated edges of the apposed tendon ends and at least 2 mm deep into the substance of the tendon (rather than only within the epitenon). An early passive mobilization rehabilitation is preferred, with the aim to maximize intrasynovial excursion and minimize applied musculotendinous force.

The surgical technique of repair of intrasynovial lacerations of the digital flexor tendons aims to (1) minimize secondary iatrogenic trauma to the tendon and the surrounding gliding surface during repair, (2) coapt tendon ends with sufficient strength to resist physiological tensile loads applied during early postoperative rehabilitation, and (3) achieve a smooth, nonbulbous repair site to minimize the work required for digital flexion. Combined transection of both the flexor digitorum superficialis (FDS) and the flexor digitorum profundus (FDP) tendons distal to the A2 pulley is particularly challenging due to the FDS—FDP relationship at that level.

Different techniques are required to repair distal FDS tendon transections due to the structure of the 2 slips in the region of the proximal interphalangeal joint (PIP). This report describes our surgical technique for repair of combined FDS and FDP transections following decussation of the FDS tendon (Figs 2 and 3).

▶ Combined transection of the flexor digitorum superficialis (FDS) and flexor digitorum profundus (FDP) tendons distal to the A2 pulley presents a special challenge to the operating surgeon. Though numerous techniques have been described for repair of the FDS slips and the FDP tendon in no-man's-land, the authors present their surgical approach for addressing lacerations specifically distal to the FDS decussation.

The authors describe repair of the FDS slips using 5-0 Prolene suture in a Becker configuration (Fig 2). The FDP tendon is repaired using the core suture technique described by Winters with looped 4-0 nylon suture, modified to achieve a locking loop and an 8-strand repair (Fig 3). The suture is placed

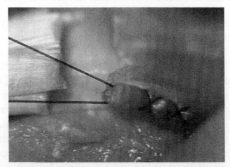

FIGURE 2.—Flexor digitorum superficialis repair. Becker suture of the ulnar half of an FDS slip using 5-0 Prolene (Ethicon Inc.). This is repeated for each half of the FDS slips on both sides of the laceration, providing a 4-strand repair of each slip. (Reprinted from Pike JM, Gelberman RH. Zone II combined flexor digitorum superficialis and flexor digitorum profundus repair distal to the A2 pulley. *J Hand Surg Am.* 2010;35:1523-1527. Copyright 2010, with permission from the American Society for Surgery of the Hand.)

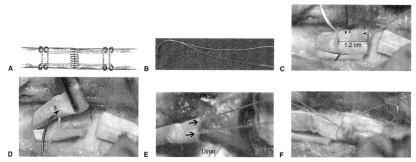

FIGURE 3.—Flexor digitorum profundus repair. **A** Diagram depicting final repair and suture configuration. **B** The 4-0 looped pseudomonofilament nylon suture (Supramid Extra; S. Jackson Inc.). **C** The initial pass is placed with a purchase length of 1.2 cm (arrowhead 1); the transverse pass is placed closer to the lacerated tendon end to create a locking loop (arrowhead 2). **D** The third pass enters farther from the lacerated end than the transverse pass to create a second locking loop (arrowhead 3). The same passes are performed on the opposite tendon end to complete the first sequence of passes (4 strands now cross the repair site). **E** The suture limbs are exiting the radial and ulnar bundles of the tendon from their radial aspects (arrows); the second sequence of passes will use the ulnar half of the bundles to complete the 8-strand repair. **F** After the first sequence of passes is completed for the other tendon end, the ends are gently approximated to avoid locking the ends apart before the knots are tied. (Reprinted from Pike JM, Gelberman RH. Zone II combined flexor digitorum superficialis and flexor digitorum profundus repair distal to the A2 pulley. *J Hand Surg Am.* 2010;35:1523-1527. Copyright 2010, with permission from the American Society for Surgery of the Hand.)

with 1.2 cm of purchase from the lacerated end of the tendon, and a single knot is placed inside the repair site. The postoperative care of these patients is also discussed.

This article provides excellent intraoperative images and associated figures to clarify the authors' surgical techniques. While much of the content may represent a review for the veteran surgeon, pearls and pitfalls are presented to guide the surgical novice.

E. K. Shin, MD

A Biomechanical Study of Extensor Tendon Repair Methods: Introduction to the Running-Interlocking Horizontal Mattress Extensor Tendon Repair Technique

Lee SK, Dubey A, Kim BH, et al (New York Univ School of Medicine)
J Hand Surg 35A:19-23, 2010

Purpose.—Extensor tendon injuries are common; however, relatively few studies have evaluated extensor tendon repair methods. The purpose of this study was to investigate the properties of the running-interlocking horizontal mattress repair method with regard to tendon shortening, stiffness, strength, and time needed to perform the repair, compared with the modified Bunnell method and the augmented Becker method.

Methods.—Twenty-four extensor tendons from 8 fresh-frozen cadaveric hands were harvested from zone 6. The harvested tendons were randomly assigned into 1 of 3 repair groups: augmented Becker, modified Bunnell, and running-interlocking horizontal mattress repair methods. The running-interlocking horizontal mattress repair combines a running suture with an interlocking horizontal mattress suture. Each repaired tendon was measured for length before and after repair and tested for stiffness, ultimate load to failure, and time required to perform the repair.

Results.—The running-interlocking horizontal mattress repair was significantly stiffer (8,506 N/m) than the augmented Becker (5,971 N/m) and the modified Bunnell (6,719 N/m) repairs. The running-interlocking horizontal mattress repair resulted in significantly less shortening (1.7 mm) than the augmented Becker (6.2 mm) and modified Bunnell (6.3 mm) repairs. The running-interlocking horizontal mattress repair took significantly less time to perform without a significant difference in the ultimate load to failure (running-interlocking horizontal mattress repair, 51 N; augmented Becker, 53 N; modified Bunnell, 48 N).

Conclusions.—The running-interlocking horizontal mattress repair is significantly stiffer and faster to perform than either the augmented Becker or the modified Bunnell repairs, and it results in less shortening than either of these methods. The running-interlocking horizontal mattress repair should be strong enough to withstand some early motion.

▶ Compared with the vast number of investigations devoted to flexor tendon repairs, there is indeed a paucity of work evaluating extensor tendon repairs. Extensor tendons require much smaller gliding amplitude and have better tolerance of adhesions. However, because of its complex structural and mechanical interdependence, the extensor apparatus cannot endure shortening or loss of structures. The authors compared mechanical performance of 3 repair methods and determined that the running-interlocking horizontal mattress suture provides good strength but leads to little tendon shortening. This method is a valuable addition to the existing methods and appears to have merits. I am unsure how the tension was set in executing the repair, which could affect the shortening and stiffness documented. How to standardize surgical repair tension in studying the extensor tendon poses an important technical question. Unfortunately, this point was neither clear nor discussed. Clinically, I use relatively simple methods, such as a running-locking peripheral suture, a 4-strand repair, or a looped suture repair. Kessler-type repairs are also used if they are unlikely to twist the tendons. I do not have a preference for one particular method and use different methods to accommodate repairs at different locations. Repair strength is not a priority to consider, but restoring near-normal structural integrity is of critical importance in the digits. For more proximal injuries, stronger repairs are preferred. Postsurgery, either a controlled early active motion regimen or dynamic splinting equally favors recovery of tendon gliding with little chance of repair rupture.

J. B. Tang, MD

Carbodiimide-Derivatized Hyaluronic Acid Surface Modification of Lyophilized Flexor Tendon: A Biomechanical Study in a Canine in Vitro Model

Ikeda J, Zhao C, Sun Y-L, et al (Mayo Clinic, Rochester, MN)
J Bone Joint Surg Am 92:388-395, 2010

Background.—Intrasynovial grafts are the ideal solution to replace defects in intrasynovial flexor tendons, but autologous graft sources are rarely available. The purpose of the present study was to test the hypotheses that an intrasynovial tendon prepared with repetitive freeze-thaw cycles and lyophilization (as a means of reducing immunogenicity) has increased frictional force (gliding resistance) in comparison with fresh intrasynovial tendons and that a lyophilized intrasynovial flexor tendon that is modified with carbodiimide-derivatized hyaluronic acid and gelatin has decreased frictional force in comparison with untreated lyophilized tendons.

Methods.—Thirty-six flexor digitorum profundus tendons from the second and fifth digits of canine hind paws were randomly assigned to three groups. Twelve tendons were immediately assessed both mechanically and morphologically and served as the normal tendon group. The other twenty-four tendons were prepared with repetitive freeze-thaw cycles and lyophilization and were randomly assigned to two groups, including one group in which the tendons were treated with carbodiimide-derivatized hyaluronic acid and gelatin and one group in which the tendons were not treated. The frictional force was measured during 1000 cycles of simulated flexion-extension motion in all tendons, and the mean frictional forces were compared. The tendons were then observed with use of transmitted light microscopy for residual hyaluronic acid on the tendon surface, and the smoothness of the surface was evaluated with use of scanning electron microscopy.

Results.—The frictional force after lyophilization was significantly increased by 104.9% after the first cycle and by 99.5% after 1000 cycles in comparison with the normal tendon ($p < 0.05$). The frictional force of the lyophilized tendons after treatment with carbodiimide-derivatized hyaluronic acid and gelatin was not significantly different from that of normal tendons. The untreated lyophilized tendon surfaces were observed on scanning electron microscopy to be rough in appearance, whereas the normal surface and the surface treated with carbodiimide-derivatized hyaluronic acid and gelatin were smooth, with residual hyaluronic acid present on the gliding surface.

Conclusions.—Lyophilization alters tendon surface morphology and increases tendon frictional force. Surface modification with carbodiimide-derivatized hyaluronic acid and gelatin can mitigate this adverse effect.

Clinical Relevance.—Tendon surface modification with carbodiimide-derivatized hyaluronic acid and gelatin can improve the gliding ability of lyophilized flexor tendons and therefore may improve the utility of lyophilized tendon allografts as a tendon graft substitute.

▶ Chemical modification of the surface of tendon allografts is a novel addition to the continuing efforts of the decade-long work in chemical modifications of tendon surfaces to lessen resistance to tendon gliding. Minimizing resistance to tendon movement holds great significance for secondary tendon grafting; easily movable grafts will reduce the chance of adhesion formation, hence improving amplitude of tendon movement. As the operative field of tendon grafting is broad and, in some cases, an extensive portion of the sheath is lost, adhesions are frequent.

In interpreting findings, one should be aware that the in vitro test setting creates angular tendon gliding against one pulley, which actually is different from in vivo situations, where most of the sheath pulley is preserved and tendons move along a rather smooth gliding curve. When a sharply angulated tendon glides against the pulley edge, changes in gliding resistance tend to be increased. Therefore, the effectiveness of such modifications will need to be tested in an in vivo setting more physiologically in the sheath environment and with tendons assuming close-to-normal curvature.

My efforts have been directed at reducing tendon gliding resistance after primary end-to-end repair, rather than secondary tendon grafting. After years of search, partial venting of the major pulleys (such as A2 or the entire A4) stood out as a simple yet efficient surgical option; narrowed or restrictive portions of annular pulleys are a major cause of resistance to tendon gliding. Our recent study indicates that restrictive annular pulleys increase resistance even more than digital tissue edema. It is thus clear to me that venting the restrictive portions of the pulley greatly eases resistance to tendon gliding after primary end-to-end tenorrhaphy.

J. B. Tang, MD

Effects of a Lubricin-Containing Compound on the Results of Flexor Tendon Repair in a Canine Model in Vivo
Zhao C, Sun Y-L, Kirk RL, et al (Mayo Clinic, Rochester, MN; et al)
J Bone Joint Surg Am 92:1453-1461, 2010

Background.—Tendon surface modification with a synthetic biopolymer, carbodiimide-derivatized hyaluronic acid and gelatin with the addition of lubricin (CHL), has been shown to reduce gliding resistance after tendon repair in an in vitro model. The purpose of the study was to investigate whether CHL would reduce adhesion formation and improve digital function after flexor tendon repair in a canine model in vivo.

Methods.—Sixty dogs were randomly assigned to either a biopolymer-treated group (n = 30) or an untreated control group (n = 30). The second and fifth flexor digitorum profundus tendons from each dog were lacerated fully at the zone-II area and then repaired. Passive synergistic motion therapy was started on the fifth postoperative day and continued until the dogs were killed on day 10, day 21, or day 42. The repaired tendons were evaluated for adhesions, normalized work of flexion, gliding resistance, repair strength, stiffness, and histological characteristics.

Results.—The normalized work of flexion of the repaired tendons treated with CHL was significantly lower than that of the non-CHL-treated repaired tendons at all time points (p < 0.05), and the prevalence of severe adhesions was also significantly decreased in the CHL-treated tendons at day 42 (p < 0.05). However, the repair failure strength and stiffness of the CHL-treated group were also significantly reduced compared with those of the control group at days 21 and 42 (p < 0.05) and the rate of tendon rupture was significantly higher in the treated group than in the control group at day 42 (p < 0.05).

Conclusions.—Treatment with the lubricin-containing gel CHL appears to be an effective means of decreasing postoperative flexor tendon adhesions, but it is also associated with some impairment of tendon healing. Future studies will be necessary to determine if the positive effects of CHL on adhesion formation can be maintained while reducing its adverse effect on the structural integrity of the repaired tendon.

▶ This is a nicely executed in vivo experimental study on the effectiveness of a novel lubricin-containing component for surface modification of tendons, using a primary flexor tendon repair model in dogs. Similar to the findings of previous reports, use of these compounds decreases the degree of adhesions, but at the cost of increasing the rate of repair ruptures and gapping. The adverse effect is actually striking: 13 (22%) of 60 treated tendons ruptured, but only 2 (3%) of 60 nontreated tendons ruptured. The findings corroborate the extensively documented detrimental effects of direct application of chemicals to the site of primary repairs.

Limitation of adhesions has long been a theme of discussion and impetus for investigations. The proven methods to decrease adhesion formation remain (1) early motion of the repaired tendons and (2) meticulous surgery that ensures smooth and strong tendon connection. I suggest that medications including this novel lubricin-containing compound, or its modified version, be tested in conjunction with tendon grafting in vivo where we may expect beneficial effects of reduced adhesions as well, but do not have concerns about tendon strength.

Over the years, my colleagues and I have worked to improve healing strength, aiming to increase the vigor and the safety margin of tendon motion. In a chicken model, after adeno-associated virus 2—mediated transfer of basic fibroblast growth factor or vascular endothelial growth factor genes into the healing tendons, the healing strength increased substantially at weeks 2 to 4. We expect that more vigorous tendon motion consequently decreases the chances of adhesions. More recently, we have introduced engineered microRNA to the healing tendons to downregulate the activity of transforming growth factor β, attempting to modify adhesion formation from a molecular perspective. Our efforts in both areas are ongoing.

J. B. Tang, MD

Biomechanical Properties of a New Multilocking Loop Peripheral Suture Technique for the Repair of Flexor Tendons: A Comparative Experimental Study

Turk YC, Guney A, Oner M, et al (Erciyes Univ Med Faculty, Kayseri, Turkey)
Ann Plast Surg 65:425-429, 2010

We aimed to evaluate the biomechanical properties of a new multilocking loop peripheral suture technique. For this aim, 40-deep digital flexor tendons of adult male sheep front limb were divided and then repaired using one of the following methods: simple peripheral suture plus 2- or 4-strand Kessler core suture or a new multilocking loop peripheral suture combined with either 2- or 4-strand Kessler core suture. Intact tendons were used as controls. The following biomechanical parameters were tested: ultimate tensile strength, energy to failure, 2-mm gap formation force, stiffness, and mechanism of failure. Regardless of the number of core suture strands, the new technique resulted in greater ultimate tensile strength, energy to failure, 2-mm gap formation force, and stiffness values, compared with simple running peripheral suture. In conclusion, the new multilocking loop peripheral suture technique represents a biomechanically strong and technically suitable method for flexor tendon repair.

▶ The search for the perfect flexor tendon suture technique continues. In this sheep tendon study, the authors found that their new multilocking peripheral suture was stronger than a simple peripheral suture. It was also interesting that this effect made the need for a second pair of core sutures unnecessary. The ultimate strength and other assays of strength of repair were higher for a 2-strand repair plus multilocking peripheral suture than for a 4-strand repair plus simple peripheral suture.

While technically possible in an individual sheep tendon, it is harder to perform clinically with intact pulleys and in tight confines. My concern is that this repair may be too complex to teach to all trainees. Therefore, we continue to advocate a 4-strand repair with at least 1 cm of purchase, locking technique, and a running epitendinous suture, followed by early active motion.

J. Chang, MD

Swan Neck Deformity after Distal Interphalangeal Joint Flexion Contractures: A Biomechanical Analysis

Chinchalkar SJ, Lanting BA, Ross D (St Joseph's Health Care, London, Ontario, Canada; Univ of Western Ontario, London, Ontario, Canada)
J Hand Ther 23:420-425, 2010

The relationship between the flexor and extensor systems of the digits is both intricate and balanced, such that disruption of one system can affect the entire dynamics of the finger. The imbalance may be obvious, whereas the precipitating factor may be less obvious. These authors describe a case and provide a detailed biomechanical analysis of how a flexion contracture of the distal interphalangeal joint led to a swan neck deformity in one of their patients.

▶ The authors present a thorough review of the complex biomechanics leading to the formation of the swan neck deformity after a zone II flexor tendon repair in the ring finger. As interesting and complex as the explanation of the biomechanics of this phenomenon may be, the simple question remains: could the deformity to the patient's finger, which required additional surgery and rehabilitation, been avoided? Kleinert splints notoriously maintain the digits in flexion at rest, ultimately leading to complications with flexion contractures, which is why they are rarely used anymore, at least on the West Coast. We will never know whether a stronger repair (4 to 6 strand), some version of an early active motion program, and a dorsal block splint, which maintains the interphalangeal joints in extension at rest, would have proved to have been a better plan for this patient, but we may conjecture.

M. Outzen, MS, OTR/L, CHT

Diagnosis and localisation of flexor tendon injuries by surgeon-performed ultrasound: A cadaveric study
Ravnic DJ, Galiano RD, Bodavula V, et al (Indiana Univ School of Medicine, Indianapolis; Northwestern Univ Feinberg School of Medicine, Chicago, IL; New York Univ Med Centre; et al)
J Plast Reconstr Aesthet Surg 64:234-239, 2011

Background.—Flexor tendon injuries are common problems faced by hand surgeons. To minimise the surgical trauma associated with localisation and retrieval of the proximal tendon end, we investigated the use of surgeon-performed ultrasound in the evaluation of injured flexor tendons in a cadaver model. Our goal was to use surgeon-performed ultrasound: (1) to correctly diagnose flexor tendon injuries and (2) to correctly localise the proximal tendon ends within 1 cm.

Methods.—Flexor tendon injuries with varying degrees of retraction were randomly created in individual digits of cadaver upper extremities, with a number of tendons left uninjured. A surgeon, blinded to the injury status of each digit, imaged each tendon by ultrasound. Predicted injury status of each tendon and localisation of the proximal stump was recorded. A total of 81 tendons were studied.

Findings.—Correct diagnosis of flexor tendon injury was made in 78 of 81 tendons (96.2% success). Correct localisation of the proximal tendon stump was made in 39 of 50 lacerated tendons (78% success). Small finger injuries were most difficult to assess (66.7% success). With the small finger excluded from our analysis, the localisation success rate increased to 86.8%. The average time taken to image each digit was just under 2.5 min.

Conclusions.—Surgeon-performed ultrasound evaluation of the hand is a reliable means to diagnose flexor tendon injuries and to accurately localise the proximal tendon ends. This imaging modality may limit the need for extensive surgical exploration during flexor tendon repair. We do not recommend using this technique to image flexor tendon injuries of the small finger at this time.

▶ The authors present a cadaveric study assessing the accuracy of ultrasound in the diagnosis of tendon laceration in the finger. They demonstrated a 96.2% accuracy in diagnosing a laceration and a 78% accuracy in locating the proximal tendon point of retraction. Results became less reliable in the small finger. This is an interesting use of a rapidly expanding technology. Ultrasound is an inexpensive noninvasive imaging modality that is being used more and more often to aid in orthopedic diagnosis. This study demonstrates both the advantages and insufficiencies of the technique. The authors suggest that the ultrasound could prevent unnecessary dissection when attempting to find the proximally retracted tendon after a laceration. However, in some cases, the surgeon inaccurately identified the site of retraction as proximal to the actual tendon's location. This would have subjected this patient to a more extensive dissection.

Probably the greatest limitation to the study was that it was performed by a single surgeon and there was no formal training in the ultrasound technique. Therefore, it's unclear how transferable this technique is to the general practicing population. A more extensive study testing interobserver reliability and with a more controlled instruction of the technique of digital ultrasound would be useful.

As of yet, I have not had any experience with ultrasound for the diagnosis of finger tendon lacerations. We have used it more frequently for evaluation of the rotator cuff and some in my group have done percutaneous trigger release with ultrasound guidance, so it is likely just a matter of time and experience before it may be used to aid in the diagnosis and localization of tendon injuries.

T. B. Hughes, MD

9 Dupuytren's Contracture

Dupuytren's Fibroblast Contractility by Sphingosine-1-Phosphate Is Mediated Through Non-Muscle Myosin II
Komatsu I, Bond J, Selim A, et al (Duke Univ Med Ctr, Durham, NC; Univ of Pennsylvania School of Medicine, Philadelphia; Univ of Oklahoma-Health Sciences Ctr, Oklahoma City)
J Hand Surg 35A:1580-1588, 2010

Purpose.—Previous studies suggest that Dupuytren's disease is caused by fibroblast and myofibroblast contractility within Dupuytren's nodules; however, the stimulus for cell contractility is unknown. Sphingosine-1-phosphate (S1P) is a serum-derived lysophospholipid mediator that enhances cell contractility by activating the S1P receptor, $S1P_2$. It is hypothesized that S1P stimulates Dupuytren's fibroblast contractility through $S1P_2$ activation of non-muscle myosin II (NMMII). This investigation examined the role of S1P and NMMII activation in Dupuytren's disease progression and suggests potential targets for treatment.

Methods.—We enmeshed Dupuytren's fibroblasts into fibroblast-populated collagen lattices (FPCLs) and assayed S1P-stimulated FPCL contraction in the presence of the $S1P_2$ receptor inhibitor JTE-013, the Rho kinase inhibitor Y-27632, the myosin light chain kinase inhibitor ML-7, and the NMMII inhibitor blebbistatin. Tissues from Dupuytren's fascia (n = 10) and normal palmar fascia (n = 10) were immunostained for NMMIIA and NMMIIB.

Results.—Sphingosine-1-phosphate stimulated FPCL contraction in a dose-dependent manner. Inhibition of $S1P_2$ and NMMII prevented S1P-stimulated FPCL contraction. Rho kinase and myosin light chain kinase inhibited both S1P and control FPCL contraction. Dupuytren's nodule fibroblasts robustly expressed NMMIIA and NMMIIB, compared with quiescent-appearing cords and normal palmar fascia.

Conclusions.—Sphingosine-1-phosphate promotes Dupuytren's fibroblast contractility through $S1P_2$, which stimulates activation of NMMII. NMMII isoforms are ubiquitously expressed throughout Dupuytren's nodules, which suggests that nodule fibroblasts are primed to respond to

S1P stimulation to cause contracture formation. S1P-promoted activation of NMMII may be a target for disease treatment.

▶ The clinical aspects of Dupuytren's disease are well described and understood. However, the biological mechanisms by which the contractures occur are still poorly understood. This in vitro study using Dupuytren's fibroblasts suggests that sphingosine-1-phosphate (S1P) may be involved in the pathological contracture process. Downstream effectors of S1P may be potential targets to modify the biology and natural history of the disease.

One important aspect of the work is the findings that the Dupuytren's cell lines behaved the same in vitro as with normal palmar fascia fibroblasts. This underscores the limitations of the in vitro experimental environment, which does not replicate the true microenvironment in Dupuytren's disease. More work is necessary to confirm and validate these interesting and potentially important findings.

A. Chong, MD

Injectable Collagenase Clostridium Histolyticum: A New Nonsurgical Treatment for Dupuytren's Disease
Gilpin D, Coleman S, Hall S, et al (Brisbane Hand and Upper Limb Clinic, Queensland; Rivercity Private Hosp, Auchenflower, Queensland; Emeritus Res, Malvern, Victoria, Australia; et al)
J Hand Surg 35A:2027-2038, 2010

Purpose.—The Collagenase Option for the Reduction of Dupuytren's (CORD) II study investigated the efficacy and safety of injectable Xiaflex (collagenase clostridium histolyticum), in patients with Dupuytren's contracture.

Methods.—This was a prospective, randomized, placebo-controlled trial with 90-day double-blind and 9-month open-label phases. We randomized patients with contractures affecting metacarpophalangeal (MCP) or proximal interphalangeal (PIP) joints 2 to 1 to collagenase (0.58 mg) or placebo. Cords received a maximum of 3 injections. Cord disruption was attempted the day after injection using a standardized finger extension procedure. Primary end point was reduction in contracture to 0° to 5° of normal 30 days after the last injection.

Results.—We enrolled 66 patients; 45 cords (20 MCP to 25 PIP joints) received collagenase and 21 cords (11 MCP to 10 PIP joints) received placebo in the double-blind phase. Statistically significantly more cords injected with collagenase than placebo met the primary end point (44.4% vs 4.8%; p <. 001). The mean percentage decrease in degree of joint contracture from baseline to 30 days after last injection was 70.5% ± 29.2% in the collagenase group and 13.6% ± 26.1% in the placebo group (p < .001). The mean increase in range of motion was significantly greater in the collagenase (35.4° ± 17.8°) than in the placebo (7.6° ± 14.9°; p < .001) group. Efficacy after open-label treatment was similar to that after the double-blind phase: 50.7% of all joints achieved 0° to 5° of normal. More patients were satisfied with collagenase (p < .001). No joint had recurrence of contracture. One patient had a flexion pulley rupture and one patient underwent routine fasciectomy to address cord proliferation and sensory abnormality. No tendon ruptures or systemic allergic reactions were reported. Most adverse events were related to the injection or finger extension procedure.

Conclusions.—Collagenase clostridium histolyticum is the first Food and Drug Administration—approved, nonsurgical treatment option for adult Dupuytren's contracture patients with a palpable cord that is highly effective and well tolerated.

Type of Study/Level of Evidence.—Therapeutic I.

▶ This study evaluated the efficacy of collagenase versus placebo in a population of Australians with Dupuytren's disease over a 12-month period. Labeled the Collagenase Option for the Reduction of Dupuytren's (CORD) II, the study consisted of a prospective, randomized, placebo-controlled trial, along with an open-label phase. In the initial phase, 45 cords received collagenase, while 21 cords received placebo. The results showed that collagenase-injected cords demonstrated a statistically significant improvement in the contracture when compared with the placebo group (70.5% vs 13.6%). Efficacy in the open-label portion of the study was similar, but only 50.7% of all joints achieved full extension. A number of patients required more than 1 injection to achieve full extension. Joints with low baseline contracture severity did respond better to injection than those with high baseline contracture severity. Of note is that prior surgery did not affect attainment of the primary end point. Not surprisingly, the results also demonstrated that full correction was much more likely in the setting of metacarpophalangeal disease when compared with proximal interphalangeal disease (65% vs 28%). There were also no recurrences at 12 months. Significant complications were rare, with only 1 patient experiencing a pulley rupture. Most patients did exhibit transient swelling and pain.

This well-performed level I study affirms the findings of the CORD I study and echoes my early personal experience with this technique. Used properly, collagenase can be a safe, effective, less invasive option for our patients with Dupuytren's disease. Based on the available literature, this treatment option should be in the armamentarium of the hand surgeon for the treatment of Dupuytren's contracture.

D. S. Zelouf, MD

Collagenase Injection as Nonsurgical Treatment of Dupuytren's Disease: 8-Year Follow-Up

Watt AJ, Curtin CM, Hentz VR (Stanford Univ Hosps and Clinics, Palo Alto, CA)

J Hand Surg 35A:534-539, 2010

Purpose.—Collagenase has been investigated in phase II and phase III clinical trials for the treatment of Dupuytren's disease. The purpose of this study is to report 8-year follow-up results in a subset of patients who had collagenase injection for the treatment of Dupuytren's contracture.

Methods.—Twenty-three patients who participated in the phase II clinical trial of injectable collagenase were contacted by letter and phone. Eight patients were enrolled, completed a Dupuytren's disease questionnaire, and had independent examination of joint motion by a single examiner.

Results.—Eight patients completed the 8-year follow-up study: 6 had been treated for isolated metacarpophalangeal (MCP) joint contracture, and 2 had been treated for isolated proximal interphalangeal (PIP) joint contracture. Average preinjection contracture was 57° in the MCP group. Average contracture was 9° at 1 week, 11° at 1 year, and 23° at 8-year follow-up. Four of 6 patients experienced recurrence, and 2 of 6 had no evidence of disease recurrence at 8-year follow-up. Average preinjection contracture was 45° in the PIP group. Average contracture was 8° at 1 weeks, 15° at 1 year, and 60° at 8-year follow-up. Both patients experienced recurrence at 8-year follow-up. No patients had had further intervention on the treated finger in either the MCP or the PIP group. Patients subjectively rated the overall clinical success at 60%, and 88% of patients stated that they would pursue further injection for the treatment of their recurrent or progressive Dupuytren's disease.

Conclusions.—Enzymatic fasciotomy is safe and efficacious, with initial response to injection resulting in reduction of joint contracture to within 0°−5° of normal in 72 out of 80 patients. Initial evaluation of long-term recurrence rates suggests disease recurrence or progression in 4 out of 6 patients with MCP contractures and 2 patients with PIP contractures; however, recurrence was generally less severe than the initial contracture in the MCP group. In addition, patient satisfaction was high.

▶ This is an important article that reports long-term follow-up after collagenase injection for Dupuytren's disease. It demonstrates good efficacy for the metacarpophalangeal (MP) joint and questionable efficacy for the proximal interphalangeal (PIP) joint. The MP joints maintained fairly good correction; the 2 PIP joints recurred to a worse degree than the preinjection level.

There were several limitations. Different doses (2500-10 000 U) were used; however, the doses do not seem to correlate with the recurrence rate. As is the case with any study attempting to obtain long-term follow-up, there was a relatively high loss of follow-up (only followed 8 of 23 for the entire 8 years). This would potentially introduce bias. Relative to high loss of follow-up, the overall number of the study is small (n = 8) with only 2 PIP joints followed. These PIP joints fared poorly, but how did the other ones do?

I could not agree more with the authors that the hand surgery community needs a prospective randomized trial of surgical fasciectomy versus collagenase injection versus needle aponeurotomy with long-term follow-up. What are the potential complications of such procedures, what is the recurrence rate, and how do the patients fare if they have repeated treatments? I applaud the authors for reporting to the best of their ability early long-term results of a new treatment method of a common and vexing hand disorder.

S. K. Lee, MD

10 Carpus

Intercarpal ligamentous laxity in cadaveric wrists
Rimington TR, Edwards SG, Lynch TS, et al (Georgetown Univ Hosp, Washington, DC)
J Bone Joint Surg [Br] 92-B:1600-1605, 2010

The purposes of this study were to define the range of laxity of the interosseous ligaments in cadaveric wrists and to determine whether this correlated with age, the morphology of the lunate, the scapholunate (SL) gap or the SL angle. We evaluated 83 fresh-frozen cadaveric wrists and recorded the SL gap and SL angle. Standard arthroscopy of the wrist was then performed and the grades of laxity of the scapholunate interosseous ligament (SLIL) and the lunotriquetral interosseous ligament (LTIL) and the morphology of the lunate were recorded. Arthroscopic evaluation of the SLIL revealed four (5%) grade I specimens, 28 (34%) grade II, 40 (48%) grade III and 11 (13%) grade IV. Evaluation of the LTIL showed 17 (20%) grade I specimens, 40 (48%) grade II, 28 (30%) grade III and one (1%) grade IV.

On both bivariate and multivariate analysis, the grade of both the SLIL and LTIL increased with age, but decreased with female gender. The grades of SLIL or LTIL did not correlate with the morphology of the lunate, the SL gap or the SL angle. The physiological range of laxity at the SL and lunotriquetral joints is wider than originally described. The intercarpal ligaments demonstrate an age-related progression of laxity of the SL and lunotriquetral joints. There is no correlation between the grades of laxity of the SLIL or LTIL and the morphology of the lunate, the SL gap or the SL grade. Based on our results, we believe that the Geissler classification has a role in describing intercarpal laxity, but if used alone it cannot adequately diagnose pathological instability.

We suggest a modified classification with a mechanism that may distinguish physiological laxity from pathological instability.

▶ Carpal instability presents a challenge to practicing hand consultants in the office and the operating room. In a cadaveric model, the authors have studied ligament laxity and bone morphology changes in the scaphoid and the lunate. The scapholunate interosseous and the lunotriquetral ligaments were studied, and the laxity was correlated with arthroscopic findings. The study supports use of the Geissler classification but advises that it cannot adequately diagnose pathologic sensitivity on its own. The modifications suggested by the authors require clinical correlation. The article further evaluates physiologic laxity and instability. The age-related changes can be possibly expected, and clear delineation of laxity versus instability warrants further consideration. The full article warrants review by the practicing hand surgeon who treats these difficult problems.

C. Carroll IV, MD

Analysis of Carpal Malalignment Caused by Scaphoid Nonunion and Evaluation of Corrective Bone Graft on Carpal Alignment

Watanabe K (Nagoya Ekisaikai Hosp, Nakagawa-ku, Japan)
J Hand Surg 36A:10-16, 2011

Purpose.—To clarify the correlation between a scaphoid deformity and carpal malalignment in patients with scaphoid waist nonunion and to investigate how accurately a corrective bone graft improves carpal malalignment according to the preoperative plan.

Methods.—A total of 38 patients were analyzed retrospectively. Surgery was performed according to the anterior wedge bone graft method described by Fernandez. The scaphoid deformity and carpal malalignment were evaluated by the changes in the intrascaphoid angle (ISA) and axial length (AL) and by the changes in the radiolunate angle (RLA) and scapholunate angle (SLA), respectively, compared with the uninjured side by using standardized x-rays. Each variable was measured at 1 year after surgery. By performing multiple regression analysis, the correlation between the scaphoid deformity and carpal malalignment and between the correction of the scaphoid deformity and the change in carpal alignment were analyzed.

Results.—Compared with the uninjured side, the mean respective changes in the ISA, AL, RLA, and SLA were 11°, −1.3 mm, 14°, and 11°, preoperatively. The changes in the RLA and SLA correlated with the change in the ISA, but not with the change in the AL. The mean postoperative corrections of the ISA and AL were 15° from full extension and 1.7 mm, and the changes in the RLA and SLA were 18° and 12° from full extension, respectively. The change in the RLA correlated with the corrections of the ISA and AL. Although the change in the SLA did not correlate with either of them, the mean postoperative SLA was not significantly different from the mean value of the uninjured side.

Conclusions.—The degree of humpback deformity of the scaphoid correlated with the degree of carpal malalignment. The corrective bone graft resulted in the expected recovery of carpal alignment according to the preoperative plan.

Type of Study/Level of Evidence.—Prognostic IV (Fig 1).

▶ This article is a thorough radiographic analysis of the changes that occur with scaphoid nonunion and subsequent correction of the humpback deformity associated with this condition. While it is somewhat difficult to follow the comparisons being made, when analyzed carefully, the author proves what we all likely currently believe to be true: correction of the humpback deformity

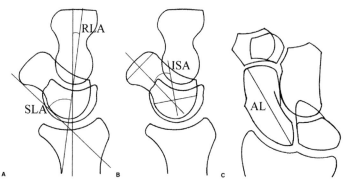

FIGURE 1.—Illustrations of variables. A RLA, radiolunate angle; SLA, scapholunate angle. B ISA, intrascaphoid angle. C AL, axial length. (Reprinted from Watanabe K. Analysis of carpal malalignment caused by scaphoid nonunion and evaluation of corrective bone graft on carpal alignment. *J Hand Surg.* 2011;36A:10-16, Copyright (2011), with permission from the American Society for Surgery of the Hand.)

of a scaphoid fracture leads to correction of the dorsal intercalated segment instability (DISI) deformity seen in scaphoid nonunions.

The author carefully analyzes 4 variables: the intrascaphoid angle (ISA), the axial length of the scaphoid, the radiolunate angle (RLA), and the scapholunate angle (Fig 1). The author finds that the degree of deformity of the scaphoid, as measured by the ISA, correlates preoperatively with the DISI deformity noted compared to the contralateral side (ie, if the scaphoid is more flexed compared to normal, the DISI deformity is greater compared to normal).

Also interesting was the observation by the author that there were 2 clusters of data points when comparing changes in ISA with changes in RLA. He suggests that those with long-standing nonunions (compared with those with more recent trauma) will have greater soft-tissue contractures and greater fixed deformities that will not be as correctable by changing the ISA. Unfortunately, the author did not follow this suggestion with an analysis of the time from injury, so this is purely supposition.

I do feel that correction of the humpback deformity is critical to correction of carpal malalignment and prevention of long-term problems from scaphoid nonunions. However, in some cases, I feel that this correction can be completed without the use of a structural bone graft. Stable screw fixation, cancellous grafting, and deformity correction are what is needed for a successful outcome.

T. B. Hughes, MD

11 Carpal Tunnel Syndrome and Compressive Neuropathies

Individual Finger Sensibility in Carpal Tunnel Syndrome
Elfar JC, Yaseen Z, Stern PJ, et al (Univ of Rochester, NY; Univ of Cincinnati, OH)
J Hand Surg 35A:1807-1812, 2010

Purpose.—Sensibility testing plays a role in the diagnosis of carpal tunnel syndrome (CTS). No single physical examination test has proven to be of critical value in the diagnosis, especially when compared with electrodiagnostic testing (EDX). The purpose of this study was to define which digits are most affected by CTS, both subjectively and with objective sensibility testing.

Methods.—A prospective series of 35 patients (40 hands) with EDX-positive, isolated CTS were evaluated preoperatively using 2 objective sensibility tests: static 2-point discrimination (2PD) and abbreviated Semmes-Weinstein monofilament (SWMF) testing. Detailed surveys of subjective symptoms were also collected.

Results.—Patients identified the middle finger as the most symptomatic over all others (51%). Objective 2PD results of each digit mirrored the subjective data, with higher values for the middle finger (mean 6.07 mm, (p < .0001). Values for the index finger failed to show a significant difference from the ulnar-innervated small finger. The most symptomatic finger matched 2PD results in over two thirds of patients. The SWMF testing showed similar, statistically significant results (middle > thumb > index > small). Correlations failed between EDX, symptoms, and SWMF results or 2PD in the index finger. Positive but weak correlation (p = .002, r = .42) was found between EDX and 2PD only in the middle fingers.

Conclusions.—The middle finger is the most likely to show changes in 2PD in patients with positive EDX findings for CTS. Middle finger 2PD is best able to correlate with EDX when compared with 2PD of other

digits. The SWMF testing also shows the middle digit testing as more sensitive, but this finding may be difficult to use clinically.
Type of Study/Level of Evidence.—Diagnostic I.

▶ Carpal tunnel syndrome continues to be a common problem in the physician's and hand surgeon's office and operating room. Collectively, we continue to look for the best way to diagnose and treat this common hand disorder. The authors have carefully analyzed the relationship between sensory testing and electrodiagnostic testing. The middle finger is the most commonly reported digit in patients with the disease. The authors found that changes in 2-point discrimination sensation in the middle finger weakly correlated with findings on electrodiagnostic testing. The study warrants review as we continue to search for the most accurate way to diagnose carpal tunnel syndrome, as surgical indications will rely on the testing and the accuracy of the chosen testing. Further study will be necessary as we search for the optimal method of accurately diagnosing this common problem.

C. Carroll IV, MD

Accuracy of In-Office Nerve Conduction Studies for Median Neuropathy: A Meta-Analysis
Strickland JW, Gozani SN (Reconstructive Hand Surgeons of Indiana, Carmel; Indiana Univ School of Medicine, Indianapolis)
J Hand Surg 36A:52-60, 2011

Purpose.—Carpal tunnel syndrome is the most common focal neuropathy. It is typically diagnosed clinically and confirmed by abnormal median nerve conduction across the wrist (median neuropathy [MN]). In-office nerve conduction testing devices facilitate performance of nerve conduction studies (NCS) and are used by hand surgeons in the evaluation of patients with upper extremity symptoms. The purpose of this meta-analysis was to determine the diagnostic accuracy of this testing method for MN in symptomatic patients.

Methods.—We searched the MEDLINE database for prospective cohort studies that evaluated the diagnostic accuracy of in-office NCS for MN in symptomatic patients with traditional electrodiagnostic laboratories as reference standards. We assessed included studies for quality and heterogeneity in diagnostic performance and determined pooled statistical outcome measures when appropriate.

Results.—We identified 5 studies with a total of 448 symptomatic hands. The pooled sensitivity and specificity were 0.88 (95% confidence interval [CI], 0.83−0.91) and 0.93 (95% CI, 0.88−0.96), respectively. Specificities exhibited heterogeneity. The diagnostic odds ratios were homogeneous, with a pooled value of 62.0 (95% CI, 30.1−127).

Conclusions.—This meta-analysis showed that in-office NCS detects MN with clinically relevant accuracy. Performance was similar to interexaminer agreement for MN within a traditional electrodiagnostic laboratory. There was some variation in diagnostic operating characteristics. Therefore, physicians using this technology should interpret test results within a clinical context and with attention to the pretest probability of MN, rather than in absolute terms.

▶ The authors performed a meta-analysis of previously published studies that compared the use of in-office nerve conduction velocity (NCV) with those electrodiagnostic (EDX) studies performed in a neurologist's laboratory. There were only 5 articles included in the final analysis, but they were deemed, using some objective criteria, to be high-quality studies. The sensitivity and specificity of the tests were 0.88 and 0.93, respectively. The authors do an excellent review of their techniques and detail how they determine the number of articles to be included.

Probably the greatest limitation to the results was that the comparison was made between in-office studies and formal EDX studies. However, clinical parameters were not used in the comparison, and therefore, while it shows good correlation between electrical testing techniques, it does not necessarily correlate to the diagnosis of carpal tunnel syndrome (CTS). The authors point out that, as with all EDX testing, whether done in office or in a neurologist's EDX laboratory, their results are only useful with a clinical framework. I still find that a great number of EDX and in-office NCV studies demonstrate median neuropathy in patients who do not have classic CTS symptoms. This has frequently led to an inaccurate diagnosis and possibly inappropriate treatment. It is critical when treating patients with hand complaints to detail specific history and physical examination findings of CTS and then use EDX studies to confirm a diagnosis as well as provide some prognostic information regarding treatment. It is my practice to use the presence of numbness in the classic median nerve distribution (especially with provocative maneuvers such as the carpal compression test) as the best diagnostic criteria for CTS.

T. B. Hughes, MD

Determinants of Pain in Patients with Carpal Tunnel Syndrome
Nunez F, Vranceanu A-M, Ring D (Massachusetts General Hosp/Harvard Med School, Boston)
Clin Orthop Relat Res 468:3328-3332, 2010

Background.—Carpal tunnel syndrome causes numbness, weakness, and atrophy. Pain without numbness is not characteristic of this disease.

Questions/Purposes.—We tested the hypothesis that among patients with carpal tunnel syndrome confirmed by electrophysiologic testing, pain catastrophizing and/or depression would be good predictors of pain intensity at the time of diagnosis, whereas nerve conduction velocity would not.

Patients and Methods.—Fifty-four patients completed a measure of tendency to misinterpret pain, a measure of depressive symptoms, anxiety about pain, self-efficacy in response to pain, and a five-point Likert measure of pain intensity. One-tailed Spearman correlation was performed to find a correlation between pain and continuous variables. One-way ANOVA was performed to assess differences between categorical variables. For each group, all variables with significant correlations with pain intensity were included in a multiple linear regression analysis.

Results.—Sex, age, and electrophysiologic measures did not correlate with pain intensity. All measures of illness behavior correlated with pain intensity and were entered in a multiple linear regression model; only misinterpretation of nociception and depression were significantly associated and accounted for 39% of the variation in pain intensity.

Conclusions.—Illness behavior (specifically depression and misinterpretation of nociception) predicts pain intensity in patients with carpal tunnel syndrome.

▶ This is another study by Nunez and associates that looks at the psychological aspects of disease in the upper limb. The authors found that depression and misinterpretation of pain were correlated with pain symptoms, not with severity of carpal tunnel syndrome (CTS) based on electromyogram results. They quantify what most practitioners already know, which is that the patients' perception of pain and disability will affect their disease experience as much as their pathophysiologic diagnosis.

The authors remind us that CTS is primarily numbness and that when there is pain, it is associated with that numbness. Pain without numbness is not CTS, and these symptoms will not be relieved by surgery. Also, the presence of psychological dysfunction may be more important to the complaints of pain and disability than the amount of nerve dysfunction.

In my experience, the number 1 cause of failed CTS is misdiagnosis, and this article's conclusions suggest why this is so. The article points out the common misconception by the lay public that hand pain is caused by CTS. This misconception leads to the diagnosis and surgical treatment of this hand pain as CTS. Unfortunately, what the authors fail to mention is that while electrodiagnostic testing can objectively measure nerve function, this testing can also demonstrate dysfunction when no CTS is present. This, combined with activity-related hand pain, can lead to carpal tunnel surgery that leads to mild or no improvement in symptoms. It is my practice to use the presence of numbness in the classic median nerve distribution (especially with provocative maneuvers such as the carpal compression test) as the best diagnostic criteria for CTS.

T. B. Hughes, MD

12 Carpus: Trauma

Surgical Compared with Conservative Treatment for Acute Nondisplaced or Minimally Displaced Scaphoid Fractures: A Systematic Review and Meta-Analysis of Randomized Controlled Trials
Buijze GA, Doornberg JN, Ham JS, et al (Academic Med Centre, Amsterdam, The Netherlands; Onze Lieve Vrouwe Gasthuis, Amsterdam, The Netherlands; et al)
J Bone Joint Surg Am 92:1534-1544, 2010

Background.—There is a current trend in orthopaedic practice to treat nondisplaced or minimally displaced fractures with early open reduction and internal fixation instead of cast immobilization. This trend is not evidence-based. In this systematic review and meta-analysis, we pool data from trials comparing surgical and conservative treatment for acute nondisplaced and minimally displaced scaphoid fractures, thus aiming to summarize the best available evidence.

Methods.—A systematic literature search of the medical literature from 1966 to 2009 was performed. We selected eight randomized controlled trials comparing surgical with conservative treatment for acute nondisplaced or minimally displaced scaphoid fractures in adults. Data from included studies were pooled with use of fixed-effects and random-effects models with standard mean differences and risk ratios for continuous and dichotomous variables, respectively. Heterogeneity across studies was assessed with calculation of the I^2 statistic.

Results.—Four hundred and nineteen patients from eight trials were included. Two hundred and seven patients were treated surgically, and 212 were treated conservatively. Most trials lacked scientific rigor. Our primary outcome parameter, standardized functional outcome, which was assessed for 247 patients enrolled in four trials, significantly favored surgical treatment (p < 0.01). With regard to our secondary parameters, we found heterogeneous results that favored surgical treatment in terms of satisfaction (assessed in one study), grip strength (six studies), time to union (three studies), and time off work (five studies). In contrast, we found no significant differences between surgical and conservative treatment with regard to pain (two studies), range of motion (six studies), the rates of nonunion (six studies) and malunion (seven studies), and total treatment costs (two studies). The rate of complications was higher in the surgical treatment group (23.7%) than in the conservative group (9.1%), although this difference was not significant (p = 0.13). There was a nearly

73

74 / Hand and Upper Limb Surgery

significantly higher rate of scaphotrapezial osteoarthritis in the surgical treatment group (p = 0.05).

Conclusions.—Based on primary studies with limited methodological quality, this study suggests that surgical treatment is favorable for acute nondisplaced and minimally displaced scaphoid fractures with regard to functional outcome and time off work; however, surgical treatment engenders more complications. Thus, the long-term risks and short-term benefits of surgery should be carefully weighed in clinical decision-making.

▶ This article represents a meta-analysis of 8 randomized controlled trials comparing surgical and conservative management for either acute nondisplaced or minimally displaced fractures of the scaphoid in adults. Pooled data allowed for the comparison of roughly 200 patients with each treatment. The authors state in their discussion that surgical treatment results in significantly better patient-reported functional outcome, greater patient satisfaction, better grip strength, shorter time to union, and earlier return to work. However, there are no significant differences between surgical and conservative treatment with regard to pain, range of motion, rates of nonunion, malunion, infection, complications, or total treatment cost. Most of the included studies did not assess total treatment costs and overall patient satisfaction, and complication rates favored the conservative management group by a factor of 2 to 1.

The impression that this article gives is that surgical treatment may provide a more expeditious, albeit possibly complicated, recovery after scaphoid treatment. Nonoperative treatment, although less often complicated, seems to yield poorer results with regard to outcome parameters and patient satisfaction.

The authors admit a number of limitations. Although all the included studies were randomized trials, there was heterogeneity with regard to secondary outcomes measures used and low-quality evidence overall in the included studies.

It is hard to actually translate the results of this meta-analysis directly into one's clinical decision making. On the one hand, there seems to be short-term benefits owed to the faster return to function overall in the surgical treatment group; however, these benefits may, in the treating surgeon's opinion, be transient and therefore be less important than the increased risk of osteoarthritis with surgical treatment. Arthritis was noted in 2 of the studies to be significantly greater in the surgical treatment group by a factor of 4 to 1. It seems like the results of this study may be used to justify either approach for the management of nondisplaced or minimally displaced scaphoid fractures. In all cases, this study notes the importance of randomized control studies using validated outcomes measures as a way to best lead to a definitive recommendation regarding this injury.

J. C. Elfar, MD

Functional Outcomes of Nonunion Scaphoid Fracture Treated by Pronator Quadratus Pedicled Bone Graft

Noaman HH, Shiha AE, Ibrahim AKH (Sohag Univ, Egypt; Assiut Univ, Egypt)
Ann Plast Surg 66:47-52, 2011

Between 1998 and 2007, a pronator quadratus pedicled bone graft was performed for 45 patients of ununited scaphoid fracture. One of them had bilateral ununited scaphoid fracture. There were 29 men and 16 women with a median age at operation of 24 (16–32) years. The affected side was the right side (dominant hand) in 32 patients whereas 13 patients had fracture of the nondominant left side. There had been 32 proximal pseudoarthrosis (through or proximal to the junction of the proximal and middle thirds of the bone) and 14 of the middle third of the scaphoid. The original fractures were caused by motor cycle accidents in 23 patients, falling on outstretched hand in 15 patients, and sport injuries in the remaining 7 patients. Surgery was indicated from 5 months to 6 years after injury (average 43 months) because of complaints of pain on heavy work. The fracture has been missed at the initial examination in 23 patients whereas cast immobilization was done for 6 weeks and 3 months in 15 and 7 cases, respectively, that had failed to result in union. There were no preoperative osteoarthritic changes, but in 25 cases, there were avascular necrosis of the proximal fragment of the scaphoid. Forty-three patients showed radiographic union after an average of 14 weeks (12–16 weeks). One patient had dislodgement of the graft and refused to do it again. The average range of movement of wrist improved after operation. Taken as a percentage of the normal range, dorsiflexion increased from 69% to 80%, palmar flexion from 66% to 76%, radial deviation from 45% to 70%, and ulnar deviation from 67% to 84%. Grip strength improved from 82% to 92% of normal. All the patients have been able to return to their former activities with no pain.

▶ Although applying current treatment guidelines to fresh scaphoid fractures diagnosed in a timely manner can achieve bone union in almost all patients, nonunion of the fractured scaphoid, especially when accompanied with avascular necrosis (AVN) of the proximal pole, sclerosis or bony absorption, a hump-back deformity, and long duration (greater than 3-5 years), remains a frustrating problem. The rate of success in treating nonunions in long-standing and troublesome cases may be no greater than 50%. Vascularized bone grafts—from either distal radius or medial femoral condyle—proved to be more efficacious than conventional treatments, but their effectiveness has not been universal in those hard-to-treat cases.

Pronator quadratus pedicle bone grafts were introduced in the 1980s. Surprisingly, not many reports have specifically documented outcomes of this procedure, despite the decades elapsed. In this report, union was achieved in 44 among 45 cases. Twenty-five cases had AVN of the proximal pole; 5 had nonunion over 3 years. This procedure appears to yield outcomes comparable to a vascularized radial bone graft or a vascularized medial femoral condyle graft. Nevertheless, the authors did not state whether they presented a consecutive or a well-selected case series; neither did they describe the degree of associated bone absorption and severity of AVN. Assuming they had a moderate degree of AVN and considering the duration of bone nonunion, the overall good and excellent rate and union rate are much greater than I would have expected. The good and excellent rate by loosely defined and subjective criteria (Herbert and Fisher's score) could be inflated, which must be taken with a grain of salt. The exceedingly high excellent rate (41 of 45 patients) is higher than what I see in practice.

The true challenge is the nonunion in the proximal pole with AVN, to which I have found no good solution. In addition, collapse of the scaphoid may present as a lasting problem. I found it difficult to agree with the final concluding remarks, in which the authors consider this method a solution for scaphoid nonunions, especially with proximal pole fragments. The authors' conclusions may be partly due in the cases without severe AVN or scaphoid collapse but unlikely to be proven true in cases with above signs. In my experience, treatment of such serious cases can be very disappointing. Over the past 10 years, my colleagues and I have used either pedicle pronator quadratus graft or vascularized distal radial bone graft (based on the 1, 2 intercompartmental suprareticacular artery), but we have not been lucky enough to obtain results as positive as the authors describe here. The pedicle may be entrapped or compromised after transfer; we actually do not know the fate of such grafts—whether they indeed obtain sufficient blood supply. Clinically, limitation of wrist motion and a certain degree of pain (and hence patient dissatisfaction) are not uncommon. Nevertheless, we believe that for cases with lasting nonunion and AVN, a vascularized graft is more beneficial than other options, but this is not a solution in all cases!

J. B. Tang, MD

Arthroscopically Assisted Use of Injectable Bone Graft Substitutes for Management of Scaphoid Nonunions
Chu P-J, Shih J-T (Taoyuan Armed Forces General Hosp, Taiwan)
Arthroscopy 27:31-37, 2011

Purpose.—The purpose of this study was to analyze the clinical follow-up results (minimum, 2 years) in patients with nonunions of the scaphoid with minimal sclerosis treated with arthroscopically assisted percutaneous internal fixation augmented by injection of a bone graft substitute.

Methods.—From January 2006 through November 2007, a consecutive series of 15 patients with fibrous union or nonunion of a carpal scaphoid fracture with minimal sclerosis or resorption at the nonunion site were treated with arthroscopically assisted percutaneous internal fixation combined with the use of injectable bone graft substitute. Preoperative and postoperative evaluations included measurement of clinical (grip strength and range of motion), radiographic, and functional (Mayo Modified Wrist Score) parameters, as well as satisfaction. The sample included

13 men and 2 women with a mean age of 31 years (range, 20 to 45 years). We recorded union and return to activity and analyzed data with regular clinical follow-up at a mean of 33 months (range, 24 to 46 months).

Results.—We confirmed union in 14 of 15 patients (93%) at a mean of 15.4 weeks according to clinical examinations and standard radiography. For the Mayo Modified Wrist Score, there were 10 excellent and 4 good results. A total of 14 of 15 patients (93%) returned to work or sports activities at their preinjury level.

Conclusions.—Arthroscopically assisted treatment with percutaneous internal fixation with injectable bone graft substitute is a reliable and minimally invasive method to achieve union and scaphoid healing.

Level of Evidence.—Level IV, therapeutic case series.

▶ The authors present an interesting approach to the treatment of scaphoid nonunions. Although the concept of minimally invasive scaphoid reconstruction seems intriguing, still some questions remain unanswered in this study. Most importantly, the nonunions are not adequately characterized. It is well established that neither the degree of scaphoid deformity nor the vascularity of the fragments can be reliably assessed by conventional X-ray studies. However, neither CT scans nor MRI studies are reported. Even the authors state that their technique is not suitable for all patients, but it remains unclear what their selection criteria were. An arthroscopic approach might be suitable for minimally displaced fractures or very early nonunions, in which no considerable debridement and reduction is necessary. As soon as a significant amount of osseous substance is missing, the scaphoid will inevitably be shortened (and most likely deformed) by the use of a compression screw, because the filler material will probably not be able to maintain the length of the bone. I would also expect that the arthroscopic reduction of a displaced nonunion is very challenging. Unfortunately, the authors fail to report postoperative carpal angles and do not include lateral views of the reconstructed scaphoid in their case example, so proper reduction of the fragments cannot be assessed. Because for one-third of patients healing times of 18 weeks or more are reported, it seems questionable why the authors claim "early rehabilitation and return of function" for their technique.

Nevertheless, I think that arthroscopy might be a helpful tool for a subset of scaphoid fractures and nonunions. However, these cases should be carefully selected, and I am not sure whether bone grafting can or should be replaced by filler materials. Further studies are warranted.

K. Megerle, MD

Radiographic Evaluation of the Modified Brunelli Technique Versus the Blatt Capsulodesis for Scapholunate Dissociation in a Cadaver Model

Pollock PJ, Sieg RN, Baechler MF, et al (William Beaumont Army Med Ctr, El Paso, TX; Walter Reed Natl Military Med Ctr, Washington, DC; Union Memorial Hosp, Baltimore, MD)
J Hand Surg 35A:1589-1598, 2010

Purpose.—A variety of soft tissue surgical procedures have been developed for treatment of scapholunate (SL) dissociation. The purpose of this study was to compare the degree of correction obtained (as measured on preoperative and postoperative radiographs) when performing the modified Brunelli technique (MBT) with that of the more commonly performed Blatt capsulodesis (BC) and to evaluate each technique after simulated wrist motion.

Methods.—Five cadaver wrists were used for this study. The SL interval, SL angle, and radiolunate angle were recorded radiographically, with the SL ligament intact, for each wrist in several loaded positions: neutral, flexion, extension, radial deviation, ulnar deviation, and clenched fist. The SL interosseous ligament was then completely incised, and the radiographic measurements were repeated to demonstrate SL instability. The radiographic measurements were then repeated after MBT reconstruction and after BC reconstruction. Additional radiographic measurements were taken after simulated wrist motion.

Results.—Sectioning of the SL ligament resulted in radiographic evidence of SL dissociation. Use of the MBT demonstrated improved correction of the SL interval and the SL angle in the clenched fist position, which was statistically significant when compared with BC. The correction for the SL angle was maintained on the MBT specimens with simulated wrist motion.

Conclusions.—The results demonstrate that in this cadaver model, the MBT better restores the normal carpal relationship of the SL interval and SL angle when compared to the BC, as measured on radiographs. This correction might correlate with improved carpal dynamics and improved clinical outcomes.

▶ This is a biomechanical cadaveric study comparing Blatt capsulodesis (BC) with modified Brunelli technique (MBT) for scapholunate (SL) instability. They conclude that the MBT gives superior results. MBT better restores the normal carpal relationship of the SL interval and SL angle when compared with the BC, as measured on radiographs. The study is clinically relevant in that it addresses a common problem of SL instability. The methods within the confines of a cadaveric study were sound; the authors simulated dynamic wrist motion by hanging weights on select tendons. The limitation of the study is the same with any cadaveric study in that it is uncertain how this will translate to the clinical scenario, particularly with regard to healing and long-term follow-up.

In particular to these 2 reconstructions, the BC does not address the coronal plane instability, so it would be predicted to underperform the MBT with regard to the SL interval. Although the MBT outperforms the BC and mostly normalizes the radiographic parameters of SL interval and SL angle, I am uncertain in the long term how the MBT will perform with regard to maintaining the SL interval, given that its ulnar attachment is the dorsum of the lunate via a bone suture anchor and the dorsal radiocarpal ligament. This reconstruction attempts to reconstruct only the dorsal portion of the SL interosseous ligament, and its fixation points may be suboptimal. Will the reconstruction attenuate over time?

In the end, this article is an important one for the surgeon to know who treats wrist ligament disorders. The MBT seems to be gaining traction in the surgical community; this article gives further support to this trend.

S. K. Lee, MD

Clinical prediction rule for suspected scaphoid fractures: A Prospective Cohort Study
Rhemrev SJ, Beeres FJP, van Leerdam RH, et al (Medisch Centrum Haaglanden, The Hague, The Netherlands; et al)
Injury 41:1026-1030, 2010

Background.—The low prevalence of true fractures amongst suspected fractures magnifies the shortcomings of the diagnostic tests used to triage suspected scaphoid fractures.

Purpose.—The objective was to develop a clinical prediction rule that would yield a subset of patients who were more likely to have a scaphoid fracture than others who lacked the subset criteria.

Methods.—Seventy-eight consecutive patients diagnosed with a suspected scaphoid fracture were included. Standardised patient history, physical examination, range of motion (ROM) and strength measurements were studied. The reference standard for a true fracture was based on the results of magnetic resonance imaging, bone scintigraphy, follow-up radiographs and examination.

Results.—Analysis revealed three significant independent predictors: extension <50%, supination strength ≤10% and the presence of a previous fracture.

Conclusion.—Clinical prediction rules have the potential to increase the prevalence of true fractures amongst patients with suspected scaphoid fractures, which can increase the diagnostic performance characteristics of radiological diagnostic tests used for triage.

▶ This article's significance lies in the authors' attempt to devise a more accurate way of diagnosing patients with suspected scaphoid fractures based on clinical criteria rather than diagnostic tests. They state that the usefulness of diagnostic tests is decreased because of the low prevalence of true scaphoid fractures among suspected fractures. We have all seen this in our own practices, where a relatively small percentage of patients clinically suspected of having a scaphoid fracture actually turn out having the fracture (confirmed MRI, CT, or bone scan).

Strengths of this article are its prospective nature, appropriate inclusion and exclusion criteria, and attention to detail in the methods. The 3 significant predictors of scaphoid fracture in this study are wrist extension < 50%, supination strength ≥10%, and the presence of a previous hand fracture of either the involved or uninvolved hand or wrist. There were no weaknesses that this reviewer could appreciate in the execution of this study. However, one way the study design might have been improved is if other patient variables, such as preexisting medical conditions or current medications, were considered as potentially significant factors in the clinical prediction of suspected scaphoid fractures.

As the authors note, further study is required before these 3 independent predictors can be used clinically for the diagnosis of scaphoid fractures. A larger number of subjects across a larger geographic region would be helpful in this regard. However, this was a very well thought-out and executed study and an excellent step in helping the clinician get back to basics, ie, use his or her clinical acumen to increase diagnostic accuracy, rather than becoming more and more dependent on advanced imaging modalities.

In my own practice, if a patient presents with a clinically suspected scaphoid fracture and negative initial radiographs, I will offer the patient the option of getting an advanced imaging study (such as an MRI) right away to get a faster diagnosic or to be fitted with a short-arm thumb spica cast as if there were a fracture and be reevaluated in 2 weeks with plain radiography. If at that time the radiographs are still negative and the patient still displays signs and symptoms consistent with a scaphoid fracture, then I will order the MRI. If a scaphoid fracture is still not seen on the follow-up radiographs and I am no longer clinically suspicious for a scaphoid fracture, the cast is discontinued.

S. S. Shin, MD, MMS

Open Reduction for Perilunate Injuries—Clinical Outcome and Patient Satisfaction
Kremer T, Wendt M, Riedel K, et al (The Univ of Heidelberg, Ludwigshafen, Germany)
J Hand Surg 35A:1599-1606, 2010

Purpose.—Perilunate injuries cause severe carpal malalignment. Open reduction and internal fixation of these injuries has become the treatment of choice. This study evaluated clinical outcome and the patients' perception of disability in activities of daily living after open reduction, ligament reconstruction, and/or internal fixation of the scaphoid. In addition, potential prognostic factors for functional outcome and individual perceptions of disability were analyzed and compared with radiologic findings.

Methods.—This study consisted of a retrospective analysis of patients with perilunate dislocations or fracture dislocations (Mayfield stage 3/4) who were treated in a single institution from 1995 to 2004. Evaluation focused on postoperative radiologic results, range of motion, pain, sensitivity, grip strength, Mayo and Krimmer wrist scores, arthrosis, and the patients' disability in performing activities of daily living (according to the Disabilities of the Arm, Shoulder, and Hand score).

Results.—Of the 72 patients treated in the study period, 39 patients (all men) were available for complete follow-up (average, 65.5 mo). Thirty injuries were fracture dislocations; the dominant hand was injured in 14 cases. Normal scapholunate (SL) angles and Gilula arcs were achieved intraoperatively in 34 and 25 cases, respectively. At follow-up, 18 patients had larger than normal SL angles, and 6 patients had ulnar shifting of the carpus. Twenty patients were diagnosed with radiocarpal arthrosis. According to the Visual Analog Scale, pain was 1.8 at rest and 4.8 with activities. Average extension/flexion was 77°; radial/ulnar abduction was reduced to 42°. Average grip strength was reduced to an average of 36.6 kg (compared with 51.6 kg on the opposite side). Twenty-seven patients returned to their former occupations. Average Mayo and Krimmer wrist scores were both 70. The average Disabilities of the Arm, Shoulder, and Hand score was 23.

Conclusions.—Satisfactory results can be achieved with open reduction for perilunate injuries. However, despite this treatment, loss of reduction and arthrosis are frequent findings. Radiologic results do not necessarily correlate with functional outcome; high patient satisfaction was observed in this study.

▶ This article is significant in that it presents longer term data in regard to the clinical outcome of perilunate injuries treated with open reduction and repair, with an average follow-up of 5.5 years. Although there are numerous studies describing clinical outcome following the treatment of perilunate injuries, these studies are generally short term in follow-up (less than 4 years) and vary in the manner in which these injuries were treated, for example, closed versus open reduction and type(s) of repair.

Although this study is retrospective in nature, its strengths lie in the presentation and careful analysis of the data. The authors conclude, and this is supported by other longer term studies on this subject, that although clinical measurements and radiologic results worsen over time, functional results and patient satisfaction do not necessarily do the same. Multiple scores for function (Mayo and Krimmer) and patient satisfaction (Disability of the Arm, Shoulder, and Hand) were used in this study to evaluate outcome.

The findings in this study are important for both hand surgeons and patients alike, particularly when discussing expectations in regard to what happens in the long term after such a severe injury and its treatment. It must be stressed to the patient that although his or her radiographs or clinical measurements may worsen over time, this does not necessarily mean that he or she will be any less satisfied or will require further treatment, such as a salvage procedure for arthrosis.

In my personal experience with these injuries, I also agree with the authors that the standard of care is an open reduction of the carpal malalignment through a dorsal approach (and then volar, if necessary), a carpal tunnel release if median nerve symptoms are present, repair of the scaphoid fracture (if present) with a headless compression screw, repair of the scapholunate ligament tear (if present) with sutures or suture anchors, and pinning of the intercarpal and midcarpal joints for stability. Our knowledge of the long-term outcome of this injury has definitely been enhanced by this study.

S. S. Shin, MD, MMS

13 Carpus: Kienböck's Disease

Lunate Revascularization After Capitate Shortening Osteotomy in Kienböck's Disease

Afshar A (Urmia Univ of Med Sciences, Iran)

J Hand Surg 35A:1943-1946, 2010

Purpose.—The aim of surgical treatment in the early stages of Kienböck's disease is to decrease compressive loading of the lunate to promote revascularization. Capitate shortening osteotomy is one technique that has been advocated in Kienböck's disease with ulnar neutral or positive variance and Lichtman stage I to IIIA. The purpose of this study was to examine the revascularization process of the lunate after capitate shortening osteotomy.

Methods.—This was a retrospective study of 9 patients with Kienböck's disease with Lichtman stage II or IIIA and ulnar neutral or positive variance. I confirmed avascular necrosis of the lunate in all the patients by magnetic resonance imaging preoperatively. Capitate shortening osteotomy was performed through a dorsal approach and fixed with K-wires. I used magnetic resonance images with fat suppression to detect the revascularization of the lunate after surgery.

Results.—The mean follow-up was 12 months (range, 8–16 mo). All patients demonstrated partial revascularization of the lunate and the mean revascularization time was 4.7 months (range, 3–7 mo), which was interpreted as the beginning of the revascularization process.

Conclusions.—Capitate shortening osteotomy is an efficient technique to induce the revascularization process in the early stages of Kienböck's disease.

Type of Study/Level of Evidence.—Therapeutic IV.

▶ The author presents a case series of 9 patients who had undergone capitate shortening osteotomy for Lichtman stage II or IIIA Kienböck's disease. In this retrospective analysis, MRI was performed both preoperatively and postoperatively. Unfortunately, the time frame for imaging after surgery was poorly defined and spanned from 3 to 7 months postoperatively; all patients were advised to obtain an MRI approximately 3 months following surgery. A second MRI was performed 3 months after the first MRI in 4 patients and was ordered when the first study was negative for revascularization. The capitate shortening osteotomy was performed through a dorsal approach using Kirschner wires for fixation. The mean follow-up was 12 months, and the mean revascularization time was 4.7 months.

Based on the radiographic outcomes, the author concluded that capitate shortening osteotomy "is an efficient technique to induce the revascularization process in the early stages of Kienböck's disease." However, he points out that this technique is best reserved for patients who are ulnar neutral or ulnar positive. It would be difficult to compare the results of this study with any other techniques reported for treatment of Kienböck's disease. Revascularization of the lunate is not well correlated with clinical outcomes. No clinical outcome scores were measured in this study. The follow-up period was also relatively brief. Because Kienböck's disease is a rare entity, it may be useful to explore the efficacy of various surgical techniques with a multicenter research trial.

E. Shin, MD

Joint Leveling for Advanced Kienböck's Disease
Calfee RP, Van Steyn MO, Gyuricza C, et al (Washington Univ School of Medicine at Barnes-Jewish Hosp, St Louis, MO; Hosp for Special Surgery, NY)
J Hand Surg 35A:1947-1954, 2010

Purpose.—The use of joint leveling procedures to treat Kienböck's disease have been limited by the degree of disease advancement. This study was designed to compare clinical and radiographic outcomes of wrists with more advanced (stage IIIB) Kienböck's disease with those of wrists with less advanced (stage II/IIIA) disease following radius-shortening osteotomy.

Methods.—This retrospective study enrolled 31 adult wrists (30 patients; mean age, 39 y), treated with radius-shortening osteotomy at 2 institutions for either stage IIIB (n = 14) or stage II/IIIA (n = 17) disease. Evaluation was performed at a mean of 74 months (IIIB, 77 mo; II/IIIA, 72 mo). Radiographic assessment determined disease progression. Clinical outcomes were determined by validated patient-based and objective measures.

Results.—Patient-based outcome ratings of wrists treated for stage IIIB were similar to those with stage II/IIIA (shortened Disabilities of the Arm, Shoulder, and Hand score, 15 vs 12; modified Mayo wrist score, 84 vs 87; visual analog scale pain score, 1.2 vs 1.7; visual analog scale function score, 2.6 vs 2.1). The average flexion/extension arc was 102° for wrists with stage IIIB and 106° for wrists with stage II/IIIA Kienböck's. Grip strength was 77% of the opposite side for stage IIIB wrists versus 85% for stage II/IIIA. Postoperative carpal height ratio and radioscaphoid angle were worse for wrists treated for stage IIIB (0.46 and 65°, respectively) than stage II/IIIA (0.53 and 53°, respectively) disease. Radiographic disease progression occurred in 7 wrists (6 stage II/IIIA, 1 stage IIIB). The one stage IIIB wrist that progressed underwent wrist arthrodesis.

Conclusions.—In this limited series, clinical outcomes of radius shortening using validated, patient-based assessment instruments and objective measures failed to demonstrate predicted clinically relevant differences between stage II/IIIA and IIIB Kienböck's disease. Given the high percentage of successful clinical outcomes in this case series of 14 stage IIIB wrists, we believe that static carpal malalignment does not preclude radius-shortening osteotomy.

Type of Study/Level of Evidence.—Therapeutic IV.

▶ This article is a retrospective study that includes 30 patients and 31 wrists with Kienböck's disease. The study compares 2 groups of patients all treated with a radial shortening osteotomy. The first group involves intermediate stage disease with no carpal collapse (II/IIIA). The second group involves patients with more advanced collapse (IIIB). The results show that pain relief is reliably found in both groups independent of the stage of the disease and independent of the advancement of radiographic deterioration of the wrist.

What is perhaps most attractive about this study is the idea that a treatment that works for Kienböck's disease before carpal collapse may also be reasonable in Kienböck's disease after collapse. The mainstays of treatment of advanced Kienböck's disease (IIIB or greater) include reliable procedures, such as proximal row carpectomy, which has a good outcome both radiographically and clinically. Perhaps the best role for this study is underlining the fact that the clinical results actually bear out reasonable outcomes, even when radial shortening osteotomy is attempted in a patient with some carpal collapse for whatever reason.

J. C. Elfar, MD

14 Distal Radius

Ethnic Disparities in Recovery Following Distal Radial Fracture
Walsh M, Davidovitch RI, Egol KA (NYU Hosp for Joint Diseases)
J Bone Joint Surg Am 92:1082-1087, 2010

Background.—Ethnic disparities have been demonstrated in the treatment of chronic diseases, such as diabetes and heart disease. It is unclear if similar ethnic disparities appear with respect to recovery following fracture care.

Methods.—We retrospectively reviewed 496 individuals (253 whites, 100 blacks, and 143 Latinos) with a fracture of the distal part of the radius. Assessment of physical function and pain was conducted at three, six, and twelve months following treatment. The Disabilities of the Arm, Shoulder and Hand (DASH) score was used to assess physical function, and a visual analog scale was used to assess pain. Multiple linear regression was used to model physical function and pain across ethnicity while controlling for age, sex, mechanism of injury, level of education, type of fracture, type of treatment (operative or nonoperative), and Workers' Compensation status.

Results.—Both blacks and Latinos exhibited poorer physical function and greater pain than whites did at most follow-up points. Latinos reported more pain at each follow-up point in comparison with blacks and whites ($p < 0.001$ at three, six, and twelve months). These significant differences remained after controlling for Workers' Compensation status, which was also strongly associated with both pain and function.

Conclusions.—These findings suggest that recovery is different between ethnic groups following a fracture of the distal part of the radius. These ethnic disparities may result from multifactorial sociodemographic factors that are present both before and after fracture treatment.

▶ This retrospective review of patients described as white, black, and Latinos examines the disparity in response to treatment of almost 500 patients over a 3-year period. How ethnicity information was obtained is not described; in most studies, as is with the US Census, this information is volunteered rather than relied upon with any specific genetic testing or family history description. Thus, some inaccuracies are inherent. Also, all fractures were, for this study, viewed as one homogeneous representation of a fracture, rather than fracture pattern or fragility fracture, and approximately 25% of patients were lost to follow-up. However, the authors report a compelling difference between the Latinos' perception of pain, as well as better pain and function overall in whites.

Two surprising findings: (1) Blacks had the best function at 1 year, with impressive gains in the preceding 6 months. The average patient's postfracture therapy visits ranged from 34 (Latino) to 50 (blacks) per year; the higher number in blacks may support the better function noted. (2) The number of therapy visits overall is quite high: The numbers represented are much higher than my average patient receives over the duration of fracture care, and thus suggests a bias of the study in general. An alternative study with no therapy provided to any patient other than instruction for home exercise may tease out or refine the role ethnic disparities have on fracture management.

A. L. Ladd, MD

Synergistic Effect of Statins and Postmenopausal Hormone Therapy in the Prevention of Skeletal Fractures in Elderly Women

Bakhireva LN, Shainline MR, Carter S, et al (Univ of New Mexico, Albuquerque; Lovelace Clinic Foundation, Albuquerque, NM)
Pharmacotherapy 30:879-887, 2010

Study Objective.—To examine the role of concurrent 3-hydroxy-3-methylglutaryl coenzyme A reductase inhibitor (statin) use and postmenopausal hormone therapy on osteoporosis-related fractures.

Design.—Case-control study.

Data Source.—Large integrated health plan in New Mexico.

Patients.—Case patients were 1001 women with incident fractures of the hip, wrist, forearm, or spine that occurred between January 1, 2000, and December 31, 2005, and controls were 2607 women without fractures during the same time frame; both groups were selected from the same population of women aged 50 years or older who utilized health plan services during the study time frame.

Measurements and Main Results.—Postmenopausal hormone therapy use was classified as "current" (12 mo before index date) or "never or past." The risk of fractures was ascertained among continuous ($\geq 80\%$ medication possession ratio during 12 mo before the index date) and current (3 mo before index date) statin users relative to patients without hyperlipidemia who did not use lipid-lowering drugs. The interaction between statins and hormone therapy was examined in multivariable logistic regression. The association between statin use and fractures was examined separately among current and never or past hormone therapy users after controlling for other risk factors. Nineteen percent of the study participants were current hormone therapy users; 9.5% were current and 4.8% were continuous statin users. No association between continuous statin use and fractures was observed among never or past hormone therapy users (odds ratio [OR] 0.80, 95% confidence interval [CI] 0.53–1.22). In contrast, a strong protective effect (OR 0.19, 95% CI 0.04–0.87) was observed among women who concurrently used statins and hormone therapy for 1 year, independent of age; corticosteroid, bisphosphonate, thiazide diuretic, calcitonin, methotrexate, or antiepileptic drug use; chronic kidney disease; and Charlson comorbidity index. *Conclusion.*—Concurrent statin use and hormone therapy may have a synergistic protective effect on skeletal fractures beyond the additive effect of each individual therapy.

▶ The article was refreshing to read—finally some real evidence-based medicine in our own literature! This multivariate analysis reveals a potential protective effect for women who have high cholesterol and have recently taken/are taking statins and who are simultaneously on some (not well-described) hormone replacement. Also helpful is the use of the Charlson comorbidity index,[1] which provides a severity score assessing general risk factors based on comorbidity. What is not known from this study is if people who don't require statins, that is, who are in potentially better health, may have an even more protective role. Regardless, this is useful information in understanding a patient's potential response to treatment—a treatment that will likely be one of our own choosing because we like it or trained with it and, by the very nature of what we do, can never be measured with such systematic rigor.

A. L. Ladd, MD

Reference

1. Charlson ME, Pompei P, Ales KL, MacKenzie CR. A new method of classifying prognostic comorbidity in longitudinal studies: development and validation. *J Chronic Dis.* 1987;40:373-383.

The Role of Bone Grafting in Distal Radius Fractures

Tosti R, Ilyas AM (Thomas Jefferson Univ Hosp, Philadelphia, PA)
J Hand Surg Am 35:2082-2084, 2010

Background.—The distal radius nearly always heals but union can include a deformity that compromises function. Bone grafts may fill bone voids and maintain alignment, but the use of bone grafts and graft substitutes varies substantially no matter which surgical approach is used. A case was presented and evidence reviewed to determine the best approach.

Case Report.—Woman, 55, who was right hand dominant complained of right wrist pain, swelling, and deformity after a fall. On radiographs she had an extra-articular distal radius fracture with 40° dorsal angulation and extensive dorsal metaphyseal comminution. A 10° dorsal angulation and large residual dorsal defect of at least 1 cm remained after manipulative reduction and splint immobilization in the emergency department. There was no cortical contact. Surgery was chosen.

Evidence.—Most of the evidence concerning the management of dorsal voids after reduction of a dorsally displaced and comminuted fracture of the distal radius comes from uncontrolled case studies. The variations in fracture patterns, graft types, adjuncts, surgical approaches, fixation devices, and postoperative protocols make it difficult to compare. However, even in controlled studies only short-term or radiographic benefits have been identified. Long-term outcomes do not differ between the use and avoidance of grafts. Bone graft and bone graft substitutes that use volar locking plate fixation have not been the topic of any controlled studies. The use of bone grafts is determined by tradition, training, experience, or personal preference rather than evidence. Bone grafts and bone graft substitutes entail considerable risks and expenses and should be used only if better evidence can be obtained.

Conclusions.—For the patient in question, volar locked plating is preferred. The use of bone grafts or graft substitutes or both will not offer sufficient benefits to justify the higher costs, donor site morbidity, and increased surgical time. Routine rehabilitation and active use of the arm despite the dorsal metaphyseal defect would be considered appropriate follow-up. If plates or locking technology were either unavailable or too expensive, the preference would be to use closed, or possibly open, reduction and percutaneous pinning with no bone graft. If addition support was desired, open bone grafting might reinforce fracture reduction and fixation, but the only clinical benefits would be short term.

▶ This article is in the section "Evidence-Based Medicine" of *Journal of Hand Surgery*. Yet no real evidence-based medicine exists associated with bone grafting, especially with bone graft substitutes. Too many variables exist: type of fracture, fixation methodologies, and industry pushing a variety of products all contribute to the lack of sound evidence. Never will come a time when case-controlled studies, funded by government or nonrelated party, are carried out that can help us determine the role of grafting. Until then, experience and hard luck will prevail, the ex cathedra dictum that has guided surgery throughout its formative years, and likely for many to come.

A. L. Ladd, MD

Should an Ulnar Styloid Fracture Be Fixed Following Volar Plate Fixation of a Distal Radial Fracture?
Kim JK, Koh Y-D, Do N-H (Ewha Womans Univ Mokdong Hosp, Seoul, South Korea)
J Bone Joint Surg Am 92:1-6, 2010

Background.—Ulnar styloid fractures often occur in association with distal radial fractures. The purpose of this study was to determine whether an associated ulnar styloid fracture following stable fixation of a distal radial fracture has any effect on wrist function or on the development of chronic distal radioulnar joint instability.

Methods.—One hundred and thirty-eight consecutive patients who underwent surgical treatment of an unstable distal radial fracture were included in this study. During surgery, none of the accompanying ulnar styloid fractures were internally fixed. Patients were divided into nonfracture, nonbase fracture, and base fracture groups, on the basis of the location of the ulnar styloid fracture, and into nonfracture, minimally displaced (≤2 mm), and considerably displaced (>2 mm) groups, according to the amount of ulnar styloid fracture displacement at the time of injury. Postoperative evaluation included measurement of grip strength and wrist range of motion; calculation of the modified Mayo wrist score and Disabilities of the Arm, Shoulder and Hand score; as well as testing for instability of the distal radioulnar joint at a mean of nineteen months postoperatively.

Results.—Ulnar styloid fractures were present in seventy-six (55%) of the 138 patients. Forty-seven (62%) involved the nonbase portion of the ulnar styloid and twenty-nine (38%) involved the base of the ulnar styloid. Thirty-four (45%) were minimally displaced, and forty-two (55%) were considerably (>2 mm) displaced. We did not find a significant relationship between wrist functional outcomes and ulnar styloid fracture level or the amount of displacement. Chronic instability of the distal radioulnar joint occurred in two wrists (1.4%).

Conclusions.—An accompanying ulnar styloid fracture in patients with stable fixation of a distal radial fracture has no apparent adverse effect on wrist function or stability of the distal radioulnar joint.

▶ The authors have described their results after treating 138 distal radius fractures. These distal radius fractures were treated with locked volar plating, with patients being divided into ulnar styloid without fracture, nonbase fracture, or base fracture. The ulnar styloid fractures were also described with displacement being less than or greater than 2 mm. The findings included 76 ulnar styloid fractures of the 138 patients, and 62% of those fractures were nonbase ulnar styloid fractures and 38% involved the base of the ulnar styloid. Forty-five percent of the ulnar styloid fractures were minimally displaced, and 55% were displaced greater than 2 mm. They found no significant relationship between wrist functional outcome and ulnar styloid fracture level or displacement. They concluded that an accompanying ulnar styloid fracture in the setting of a distal radius fracture with stable fixation has no significant adverse effect. They did, however, warn that chronic instability did result in 2 of the wrists.

All the patients had their distal radius fractures treated with a 2.5-mm volar locking compression plate. Function and outcome scores included grip strength, range of motion, modified Mayo wrist score, and the disabilities of the arm, shoulder, and hand score. Regarding the patients who did develop chronic instability of the distal radioulnar joint (DRUJ), these occurred in 2 patients, both of whom had an association for osteosynthesis type C fracture. One occurred in a patient without an ulnar styloid fracture and the other in a patient with a significantly displaced ulnar styloid fracture, which was of a nonbase type, and both of these patients had known intraoperative laxity of the DRUJ at the time of surgery. The authors also comment that the patients with DRUJ laxity declined any additional treatment despite the instability, because their symptoms were not viewed as troublesome.

Of the 76 ulnar styloid fractures, 41% or 31 ulnar styloid fractures appeared united at the time of follow-up; 18 of the 47 ulnar styloid nonbase fractures and 13 of the 29 ulnar styloid base fractures were united. They also described that 15 of the 34 minimally displaced ulnar styloid fractures and 16 of the 42 considerably displaced ulnar styloid fractures were united. The authors report that there was no correlation with ulnar styloid union rate and ulnar styloid fracture level or displacement.

The treatment of an ulnar styloid fracture that accompanies a distal radius fracture is continuing to evolve. With the variability in the literature regarding the outcome of ulnar styloid fractures and DRUJ instability, treatment of these injuries can be puzzling at times. It is also unknown if the advent of locked volar plating itself has improved the outcome of these combined injuries compared with some older studies that reported on these styloid fractures in the setting of perhaps less stable internal fixation or external fixation of the distal radius. There are also other factors that may affect DRUJ stability, such as the distal oblique bundle of the interosseous ligament that may be present in approximately 40% of patients.[1]

Fortunately, this study does give further support to the approach of observation in the setting of a stable DRUJ after volar plating of the distal radius fracture. Interestingly, the 2 patients who did wind up with chronic instability were identified to have the instability at the time of surgery. This finding does highlight the importance of careful inspection of the DRUJ after volar plate fixation. My personal approach would be to address the instability if it is identified intraoperatively.

D. G. Dennison, MD

Reference

1. Noda K, Goto A, Murase T, Sugamoto K, Yoshikawa H, Moritomo H. Interosseous membrane of the forearm: an anatomical study of ligament attachment locations. *J Hand Surg Am.* 2009;34:415-422.

Should an Ulnar Styloid Fracture Be Fixed Following Volar Plate Fixation of a Distal Radial Fracture?

Kim JK, Koh Y-D, Do N-H (Ewha Womans Univ Mokdong Hosp, Seoul, South Korea)
J Bone Joint Surg Am 92:1-6, 2010

Background.—Ulnar styloid fractures often occur in association with distal radial fractures. The purpose of this study was to determine whether an associated ulnar styloid fracture following stable fixation of a distal radial fracture has any effect on wrist function or on the development of chronic distal radioulnar joint instability.

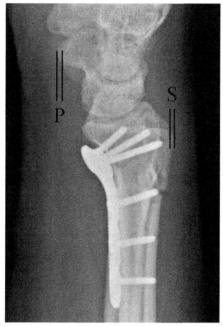

FIGURE 2.—The pisoscaphoid distance (P) and the radioulnar distance (S) were measured on a lateral radiograph of the wrist. The pisoscaphoid distance indicates the distance between the volar end of the pisiform and the volar end of the scaphoid, and the radioulnar distance represents the distance between the dorsal cortices of the radius and ulna at the distal radioulnar joint. (Reprinted with permission from The Journal of Bone and Joint Surgery, Inc., Kim JK, Koh Y-D, Do N-H. Should an ulnar styloid fracture be fixed following volar plate fixation of a distal radial fracture? *J Bone Joint Surg Am.* 2010;92:1-6, with permission from the Journal of Bone and Joint Surgery.)

Methods.—One hundred and thirty-eight consecutive patients who underwent surgical treatment of an unstable distal radial fracture were included in this study. During surgery, none of the accompanying ulnar styloid fractures were internally fixed. Patients were divided into nonfracture, nonbase fracture, and base fracture groups, on the basis of the location of the ulnar styloid fracture, and into nonfracture, minimally displaced (≤2 mm), and considerably displaced (>2 mm) groups, according to the amount of ulnar styloid fracture displacement at the time of injury. Postoperative evaluation included measurement of grip strength and wrist range of motion; calculation of the modified Mayo wrist score and Disabilities of the Arm, Shoulder and Hand score; as well as testing for instability of the distal radioulnar joint at a mean of nineteen months postoperatively.

Results.—Ulnar styloid fractures were present in seventy-six (55%) of the 138 patients. Forty-seven (62%) involved the nonbase portion of the ulnar styloid and twenty-nine (38%) involved the base of the ulnar styloid. Thirty-four (45%) were minimally displaced, and forty-two (55%) were considerably (>2 mm) displaced. We did not find a significant relationship between wrist functional outcomes and ulnar styloid fracture level or the amount of displacement. Chronic instability of the distal radioulnar joint occurred in two wrists (1.4%).

Conclusions.—An accompanying ulnar styloid fracture in patients with stable fixation of a distal radial fracture has no apparent adverse effect on wrist function or stability of the distal radioulnar joint (Fig 2).

▶ Kim et al present us with a thoughtful and thorough examination of a large number of distal radius fractures to clarify the potential importance of the associated ulnar styloid fracture. Their hypothesis is that the ulnar styloid involvement has no impact on wrist function after stable fixation of a distal radius fracture. The impetus for their study is the advent of volar locked plating of distal radius fractures, which provides a uniformity of treatment for distal radius fractures not seen in previous studies. Their methods are clear and rigorous, and their conclusions are well supported. They follow clinical function and define radiographic parameters (the pisoscaphoid and radioulnar distances) that can be measured on plain films to support the clinical findings. They find that the ulnar styloid fracture does not impact the wrist's final functional outcome. This study is well done and helpful in that it clarifies that ulnar styloid fractures do not need to be surgically addressed to provide the patient a stable well-functioning wrist. However, it is still advisable to assess the stability of the distal radioulnar joint (DRUJ) following fixation of the radius, and if there is any residual instability, then either fixation of the ulnar styloid or repair of the triangular fibrocartilage complex or both is advisable with pinning of the DRUJ in supination.

D. J. Mastella, MD

Volar Fixed-Angle Plating of Extra-Articular Distal Radius Fractures—A Biomechanical Analysis Comparing Threaded Screws and Smooth Pegs
Weninger P, Dall'Ara E, Leixnering M, et al (Lorenz Boehler Trauma Hosp, Vienna, Austria; Vienna Univ of Technology, Austria; et al)
J Trauma 69:E46-E55, 2010

Background.—Distal radius fractures represent the most common fractures in adult individuals. Volar fixed-angle plating has become a popular modality for treating unstable distal radius fractures. Most of the plates allow insertion of either threaded locking screws or smooth locking pegs. To date, no biomechanical studies compare locking screws and pegs under axial and torsional loading.

Methods.—Ten Sawbones radii were used to simulate an AO/OTA A3 fracture. Volar fixed-angle plates (Aptus Radius 2.5, Medartis, Switzerland) with threaded locking screws (n = 5) or smooth locking pegs (n = 5) were used to fix the distal metaphyseal fragment. Each specimen was tested under axial compression and under torsional load with a servohydraulic testing machine. Qualitative parameters were recorded as well as axial and torsional stiffness, torsion strength, energy absorbed during monotonic loading and energy absorbed in one cycle.

Results.—Axial stiffness was comparable between both groups ($p = 0.818$). If smooth pegs were used, a 17% reduction of torsional stiffness ($p = 0.017$) and a 12% reduction of minimum torque ($p = 0.012$) were recorded. A 12% reduction of energy absorbed ($p = 0.013$) during monotonic loading and unloading was recorded if smooth pegs were used. A 34% reduction of energy absorbed in one cycle ($p < 0.007$) was recorded if threaded screws were used. Sliding of the pegs out of the distal radius metaphyses of the synthetic bones was recorded at a mean torque of 3.80 Nm ± 0.19 Nm. No sliding was recorded if threaded screws were used.

Conclusions.—According to the results of this study using Sawbones, volar fixed-angle plates with threaded locking screws alone are mechanically superior to volar fixed-angle plates with smooth locking pegs alone under torsional loading.

▶ The authors present a biomechanical analysis of volar plates used for distal radius fracture fixation with either all locking threaded screws or all locking smooth pegs in a Sawbones model. The design of the study is quite good because the implants studied are controlled for all factors (core diameter, locking mechanism, plate thickness, and insertion angle of pegs/screws), except whether the distal fixation was with all locked threaded screws or all locked smooth pegs. Also, the design studied forces on these constructs in both axial compression and torsion, whereas most of the other studies looking at distal radius fixation with volar plates study only axial compression. In fact, the authors of this study found no difference in axial compression, which is consistent with previous studies by Martineau et al[1] as well as our own group (unpublished). However, the authors found a decrease in torsional stability in the smooth peg constructs. The caveat to this finding is that these results were found in one specific volar plate (Medartis) and that these findings may not be applicable to all plates in which the patterns of the distal screw/peg trajectory are different. Nevertheless, the implications of this finding would be concerning for rotational motion of the forearm during rehabilitation following fixation of these fractures. However, all smooth peg constructs do not appear to fail under torsion in the clinical scenario, as I have not seen the loss of the plate-bone interface in my practice, nor have there been any published cases of this phenomenon. Nevertheless, the finding is interesting, and hand surgeons should consider these results when considering placement of only smooth pegs in a locked volar plate and starting early rehabilitation including forearm rotation.

J. Yao, MD

Reference

1. Martineau PA, Waitayawinyu T, Malone KJ, Hanel DP, Trumble TE. Volar plating of AO C3 distal radius fractures: biomechanical evaluation of locking screw and locking smooth peg configurations. *J Hand Surg Am.* 2008;33:827-834.

Fracture of the Distal Radius: Risk Factors for Complications After Locked Volar Plate Fixation

Soong M, van Leerdam R, Guitton TG, et al (Lahey Clinic, Burlington, MA; Massachusetts General Hosp, Boston; Rhode Island Hosp, Providence)
J Hand Surg 36A:3-9, 2011

Purpose.—To identify risk factors for complications after volar locking plate fixation of distal radius fractures.

Methods.—We assessed early postoperative complications in 594 patients with fracture of the distal radius repaired with a volar locking plate and a minimum 1-month evaluation in the medical record. Later complications were assessed among 321 patients as a subset of the original cohort with a minimum 6 months' evaluation. We compared patient demographics, fracture characteristics, and aspects of management between patients with and without complications in bivariate analysis. Multivariable logistic regression analysis was applied to identify the factors independently associated with complications.

Results.—A total of 47 complications were documented in the medical record. Early complications occurred in 24 of 594, including 8 intra-articular screws and 7 patients with loss of fixation. Late complications occurred in 23 of 321, including 14 patients diagnosed with tendon irritation (one rupture of the flexor pollicis longus tendon) and 5 patients who had subsequent surgery to address dysfunction of the distal radioulnar joint (malunion, synostosis, and arthrofibrosis). Of the 47 complications, 26 were attributed to the plate, of which 9 were considered major (intra-articular screws and tendon rupture; 1.3% (8 out of 594) and less than 1% (1 out of 321) of the early and late groups, respectively). In the logistic regression models, fall from a height and an ipsilateral elbow injury were positive independent predictors of early complications, whereas high-volume surgeons and plates other than the most commonly used plate were positive independent predictors of later complications.

Conclusions.—Volar locking plate fixation of distal radius fractures was associated with relatively few plate-related complications in our institutions. Factors indicating higher energy or complexity predicted early complications. The most common late complication was tendon irritation, which is less discrete and perhaps variably diagnosed. Further study is warranted regarding plate design and familiarity, which may help reduce complications.

Type of Study/Level of Evidence.—Prognostic IV.

▶ The authors address the very interesting topic of complications after volar plate fixation by performing a retrospective analysis of a large series of patients. However, the value of their study is limited by several methodological problems. Most importantly, the authors only performed a chart review of their study population instead of inviting the patients for follow-up visits or following them through telephone interviews. It is therefore very questionable if any calculations concerning the frequency of complications should be performed under these circumstances, as patients might have sought care at different institutions or were not bothered enough to return to their original surgeon. In addition, by exclusively relying on the charts, almost half of the patients were lost to follow-up within the first 6 months. The authors themselves question the quality of their routine follow-up examinations, as one of their findings is a significantly higher rate for late complications for high-volume surgeons. Unfortunately, several variables have been defined quite arbitrarily; for example, the authors defined surgeons as high volume, if they operated on more than 20 wrists within the 6-year study period.

Their extensive statistical analysis results in only one other finding: patients with more severe accidents (fall from height and concomitant injuries to the elbow) are more likely to have early complications.

I appreciate the authors' effort to investigate this interesting topic because it is my impression that there are an increasing number of patients with tendon-related complications after volar plate fixation has widely gained popularity. However, I think that further studies are necessary to address this problem.

K. Megerle, MD

Evaluation of Early Postoperative Pain and the Effectiveness of Perifracture Site Injections Following Volar Plating for Distal Radius Fractures

Chung MS, Roh YH, Baek GH, et al (Seoul Natl Univ Bundang Hosp, Seongnam, Korea)
J Hand Surg 35A:1787-1794, 2010

Purpose.—Few studies have investigated the effectiveness of early post-operative pain control regimens after volar plating for distal radius fractures. This study evaluated postoperative levels of pain after volar plating of distal radius fractures under axillary nerve block in patients with and without injections of local anesthetics, narcotics, and epinephrine around the fracture site.

Methods.—Perioperative pain levels were prospectively assessed in 44 consecutive patients who had had volar plating for a distal radius fracture under axillary nerve block at a mean time of 2.8 days after trauma. Intravenous, patient-controlled analgesia and prescheduled analgesic medications were administered to all patients. In addition, patients were randomly allocated to 2 groups: perifracture site injection (PI; n = 22) and no perifracture site injection (no-PI; n = 22). At the end of surgery, PI group patients were administered perifracture site injections and blocks of the superficial radial and interosseous nerves with a local anesthetic mixture consisting of ropivacaine, morphine, and epinephrine. During the first 48 hours after surgery, pain visual analog scale (VAS) scores (0 to 100), total amount of narcotic consumption, incidences of additional narcotic requirement, and opioid-related side effects were assessed.

Results.—The overall mean pain VAS scores among all 44 study subjects were 29 before surgery, and 58, 47, 40, and 27 at 4, 8, 24, and 48 hours after surgery, respectively. Thirteen patients needed additional pain rescue despite the multimodal analgesic approach used. No intergroup differences were observed between the PI and no-PI groups in terms of VAS pain scores, total narcotic consumption, adjuvant pain rescue incidence, and opioid-related side effects.

Conclusions.—Postoperative mean pain VAS scores after volar plating of distal radius fractures were found to be 58 at 4 hours and 47 at 8 hours. Perifracture site injections were not found to provide any additional pain control benefit.

Type of Study/Level of Evidence.—Therapeutic II.

▶ This article is a well-designed, prospective, randomized trial on postoperative pain after volar plating of distal radius fractures investigating the effects of injection of local anesthetics and opiate. Postoperative pain relief has been demonstrated in some but not all of the investigations on similar injections in other clinical scenarios. All of the patients were operated on under regional anesthesia with a brachial plexus block using lidocaine with an expected duration of 3 hours of anesthesia. The patients were all admitted and maintained on intravenous patient-controlled analgesia for 48 hours postoperatively. This study revealed no statistical difference in patients' pain levels or use of narcotics after surgery with injection. In fact, the postoperative visual analog scale (VAS) pain scores were higher at 8 and 24 hours after surgery in the patients who received local anesthetic injections. This finding emphasizes the rebound pain phenomenon that occurs with worsening pain after the block wore off. Furthermore, this group of patients reported relatively high VAS scores compared with many other procedures, which at first glance seem to be more painful interventions (eg, joint replacement surgery). It is interesting to wonder what effect the same injection regimen would have had in patients undergoing this same surgery under general anesthesia. In our practice, in an urban US setting, about 90% of our patients with this surgery are done as outpatients. We prefer longer-acting local anesthetic agents when regional anesthesia is used for some of these reasons, and the anesthesiologists, nurses, and surgeons all caution our patients about prevention and management of the rebound pain phenomenon.

P. Blazar, MD

Physical Activity Slows Femoral Bone Loss but Promotes Wrist Fractures in Postmenopausal Women: A 15-Year Follow-up of the OSTPRE Study
Rikkonen T, Salovaara K, Sirola J, et al (Univ of Kuopio, Finland; Kuopio Univ Hosp, Finland)
J Bone Miner Res 25:2332-2340, 2010

Results on fracture risk among physically active persons are contradictory. The aim of this study was to investigate the long-term association between the self-reported physical activity (PA), the risk of fractures, and bone loss among peri- and postmenopausal women. The association between PA and fracture risk was examined during 15 years of follow-up in the population-based Osteoporosis Risk Factor and Prevention (OSTPRE) Study among 8560 women with a mean age of 52.2 years (range 47 to 56 years) at baseline. The amount and type of PA, as well as the types and mechanisms of fractures, were registered with self-administered questionnaires at 5-year intervals (ie, 1989, 1994, 1999, and 2004). A total of 2641 follow-up fractures were verified in 2073 women (24.2%). The study cohort was divided into quartiles by average hours of reported PA during the whole follow-up. Areal bone mineral density (aBMD) at the proximal femur ($n = 2050$) and lumbar spine (L_2–L_4; $n = 1417$) was followed at 5-year intervals from a random stratified subsample with dual X-ray absorptiometry (DXA). Risk of fracture was estimated by using the Cox proportional hazards model with a mean follow-up time of 15.2 years. Weekly average time spent on leisure-time PA was 0.4, 1.7, 3.3, and 7.0 hours from the least to the most active quartiles, respectively. The risk of wrist fracture was higher in the active quartiles (II to IV) than in the most inactive quartile (I), with hazard ratios (HRs) of 1.3 [95% confidence interval (CI) 1.05–1.57, $p = .014$] for the second (II), 1.2 (95% CI 1.01–1.51, $p = .045$) for the third (III), and 1.4 (95% CI 1.14–1.69, $p = .001$) for the fourth (IV) quartile, respectively. Overall, most of the fractures were reported as a result of a fall (69.0%), with a 2.1 times higher rate of wrist fractures during the winter (November to April) than during summer season. There were no significant associations of PA with any other fracture types. Bone loss at the femoral neck, trochanter, and Ward's triangle was significantly associated with long-term PA (ANCOVA $p < .05$), whereas no associations of bone loss and PA in lumbar spine were seen. PA is associated with a moderate rise in wrist fracture risk, which might be explained in part by a higher number of outdoor activities. Regular PA of at least 1½ hours per week does not seem to increase the risk of other fractures and might significantly decrease proximal femur bone loss among peri- and postmenopausal women.

▶ This prospective observational study investigated the long-term association between physical activity (PA), fracture risk, and bone loss among perimenopausal and postmenopausal women. PA was found to moderately increase the risk of wrist fractures. However, regular PA of at least 1 hour to 1 hour and 30 minutes per week did not increase the risk of other fractures.

This study has a large sample size and an excellent long-term follow-up. The population was fairly homogenous, consisting of participants from the same geographical region and a similar age. The cohort was largely active, with only 23% reported to have no regular PA. Perhaps if a more inactive subset was included, a more striking difference would have been seen between the groups. The bone density data may also have been subject to underlying selection bias, as it is not clear whether this cohort included the randomly selected (14.5%) and/or the high-risk (8.5%) subjects from the original study (23%, 3220/14220) who received bone density scans.

The moderate increase in wrist fractures seen with PA in this study must not overshadow its health benefits. The increased fracture risk may have been related to seasonal outdoor conditions, and it was reported that the strongest predictors for any fracture were a positive family history, baseline menopause, and baseline body mass index. This study emphasizes the importance of long-term weight-bearing activities, as there was a correlation between low activity levels and a loss of femoral bone mass. This study also raises issues of other fracture prevention strategies that should be investigated in future studies, such as the role of balance training and other safety measures for fall prevention that should be incorporated in fracture care for the elderly. Because of the age of this cohort (range, 47-56 years), they are not yet at risk of more serious fragility fractures (ie, hip), and further follow-up will be valuable for improving our understanding of the role of PA and fracture risk.

R. Grewal, MD, MSc, FRCSC

Quality of Life After Volar Plate Fixation of Articular Fractures of the Distal Part of the Radius
Gruber G, Zacherl M, Giessauf C, et al (Med Univ of Graz, Austria; District Hosp of Weiz, Austria; et al)
J Bone Joint Surg Am 92:1170-1178, 2010

Background.—Outcome measurement following surgery is increasingly the focus of attention in current health-care debates because of the rising costs of medical care and the large variety of operative options. The purpose of the present study was to correlate quality of life after volar locked plate fixation of unstable intra-articular distal radial fractures with functional and radiographic results as well as with quality-of-life data from population norms.

Methods.—Fifty-four consecutive patients with intra-articular distal radial fractures and a mean age of sixty-three years were managed with a volar locked plate system. Range of motion, grip strength, and radiographs were assessed at a mean of six years postoperatively. The wrist-scoring systems of Gartland and Werley and Castaing were adopted for the assessment of objective outcomes. The Disabilities of the Arm, Shoulder and Hand and Short Form-36 questionnaires were completed as subjective outcome measures, and the results were compared with United States and Austrian population norms.

Results.—Functional improvement continued for two years postoperatively. At the time of the latest follow-up, >90% of all patients had achieved good or excellent results according to the scoring systems of Gartland and Werley and Castaing. The results of the Short Form-36 questionnaire were similar to the United States and Austrian population norms. The mean Disabilities of the Arm, Shoulder and Hand score was 5 points at two years, and it increased to 13 points at six years. The twenty patients with radiocarpal arthritis had significantly poorer results in the physical component summary measure of the Short Form-36 questionnaire (p = 0.012).

Conclusions.—The results of the present single-center study show that, following distal radial fracture fixation, wrist arthritis may affect the patient's subjective well-being, as documented with the Short Form-36, without influencing the functional outcome. Well-designed longitudinal clinical trials are needed to confirm the findings of the present investigation in terms of quality of life after surgical treatment of intra-articular distal radial fractures.

▶ This is one of the few articles in the orthopedic literature to report on the long-term outcomes of distal radius fractures and correlate functional and radiographic results with quality of life. The authors report that although post-traumatic arthritis seen radiographically following intra-articular distal radius fractures may not influence objective results, subjective assessments of pain, function, and quality of life may be adversely affected.

The strengths of this study include its prospective design, the homogeneity of the study cohort, and excellent long-term follow-up (83.1% at 6 years). The authors used a valid, reliable, region-specific outcome measure to quantify patient-rated pain and disability (the disabilities of the arm, shoulder, and hand [DASH] score), and a general health survey (36-Item Short Form Health Survey [SF-36]) to represent quality of life. A major limitation of this study is the lack of a comparative group and small sample size (n = 54). The use of a wrist-specific questionnaire[1,2] may have been useful as comorbid upper extremity pathology, as may be seen in an elderly cohort, may negatively influence scores. The Gartland and Werley score, a physician-rated scale, was used to calculate function, but there have not been any validity studies on this questionnaire to date.[3]

This study demonstrates that quality of life (based on SF-36 scores) was not related to either radiographic or functional results but did correlate with the DASH scores, a patient-rated pain and disability scale. It is important to recognize that as physicians, our traditional method of assessing outcomes (range of motion, grip strength, and radiographic findings) may not correlate with the patient's subjective pain and disability or reflect the impact it is having on their quality of life. Future studies should focus on patient-rated rather than physician-rated outcomes to fully capture the impact of disease.

R. Grewal, MD, MSc, FRCSC

References

1. Kotsis SV, Lau FH, Chung KC. Responsiveness of the Michigan Hand Outcomes Questionnaire and physical measurements in outcome studies of distal radius fracture treatment. *J Hand Surg Am.* 2007;32.84-90.
2. MacDermid JC, Turgeon T, Richards RS, Beadle M, Roth JH. Patient rating of wrist pain and disability: a reliable and valid measurement tool. *J Orthop Trauma.* 1998; 12:577-586.
3. Changulani M, Okonkwo U, Keswani T, Kalairajah Y. Outcome evaluation measures for wrist and hand: which one to choose? *Int Orthop.* 2008;32:1-6.

Management of distal radius fractures: Treatment protocol and functional results

Cherubino P, Bini A, Marcolli D (Univ of Insubria, Varese, Italy)
Injury 41:1120-1126, 2010

Distal radius fractures are the most frequent lesions encountered during clinical practice. The treatment is controversial and still debated in the literature. For a correct management of these lesions many authors recently emphasised the importance of anatomical reduction, a stable fixation and early joint mobilisation.

We report our experience in the daily management of these lesions. The fractures are evaluated considering fracture type, fracture reduction criteria, adequacy of reduction criteria and overall fracture stability. The best treatment option must be decided in accordance to the type of fracture, the extent of metaphyseal comminution, the quality of the bone and the medical condition of the patient.

▶ The purpose of this article was for the authors to report on their experience in the daily management of distal radius fractures, with a focus on a variety of fixation methods and surgical approaches. Based on recent American Academy of Orthopaedic Surgeons recommendations[1] and a Cochrane review[2] there is insufficient evidence to support the use of one fixation method over another.

Current trends are shifting toward increased use of volar locking plates (VLP), but as the authors have clearly outlined, this may not always be the optimal strategy. Good results are reported with more traditional techniques such as external fixation, pins, and plaster. This report represents level 5 evidence (expert opinion) and does not include any comparative data or a methodological description of data collection. The authors draw our attention to focusing on the goals of distal radius fracture treatment, a focus on stable fixation to allow for anatomic union and early joint motion and remind us that all fixation options should be considered. The final choice should depend on the fracture pattern, patient factors, surgeon skill, and cost.

I have seen many referred cases where surgeons go to extreme lengths to use a VLP, at times compromising the treatment goals discussed above. As their use is increasing, reports of complications are emerging, and it is becoming clear that the VLP is not a panacea. I would reiterate the authors' comments and encourage all surgeons to consider which method of fixation is best in their hands to ensure a predictable result. To obtain an answer to the long-standing debate over which fixation method is best, a large multicenter randomized controlled trial is needed.

R. Grewal, MD, MSc, FRCSC

References

1. Handoll HH, Madhok R. Surgical interventions for treating distal radial fractures in adults. *Cochrane Database Syst Rev.* 2003;(3). CD003209.

2. Surgeons AAOS. *Evidence Based Clinical Practice Guidelines for the Treatment of Distal Radius Fractures*, http://www.aaos.org/research/guidelines/drfguideline.pdf; 2009. Accessed April 25, 2011.

Rotational Fluoroscopy Assists in Detection of Intra-Articular Screw Penetration During Volar Plating of the Distal Radius

Tweet ML, Calfee RP, Stern PJ (Univ of Cincinnati College of Medicine, OH)
J Hand Surg 35A:619-627, 2010

Purpose.—Intra-articular screw penetration is one complication of volar plate fixation of distal radius fractures. This study was designed to determine the most commonly used imaging techniques and views during volar plating of distal radius fractures and to evaluate surgeons' ability to detect intra-articular screw placement on static fluoroscopic images and rotational fluoroscopy.

Methods.—Active members of the American Society for Surgery of the Hand were polled regarding preferred imaging techniques (fluoroscopic vs cassette radiographs) and views (rotational fluoroscopy or static orthogonal/anatomic tilt/semipronated imaging) during volar plating of distal radius fractures. After the survey, volar locking plates were applied to 30 cadaveric distal radiuses. We intentionally penetrated a single screw into the radiocarpal joint in half of the specimens (15 arms) and intentionally did not penetrate the radiocarpal joint in the other half. Imaging (standard posteroanterior [PA] and lateral views, 11° tilt PA and 22° tilt lateral views, and two 360° fluoroscopy movies) was performed using a custom jig. Five surgeons blinded to results reviewed randomized image sets evaluating for intra-articular screw placement. Receiver operating characteristic curves were constructed to compare the reliability of each fluoroscopic projection or movie.

Results.—Among 696 survey respondents, 606 exclusively used fluoroscopic imaging (without cassette radiographs) and over 450 preferred either tilt images or rotational fluoroscopy to detect intra-articular screw penetration. In our cadaveric model, rotational fluoroscopy provided the highest sensitivity (93%) and specificity (96%) for the detection of intra-articular screw penetration. Rotational fluoroscopy was significantly more reliable (p<.01) than most images (standard lateral, 11° PA, 22° lateral, paired PA/lateral) and trended strongly toward better reliability for all remaining images (standard PA [p=.07], paired 11° PA/22° lateral [p=.08], and 22° tilt fluoroscopy movie [p=.11]).

Conclusions.—Rotational fluoroscopy improves the surgeon's ability to detect intra-articular screw penetration during volar plating of the distal radius. No combination of imaging allowed detection of all intra-articular screws. A high level of suspicion for intra-articular screw penetration should be maintained during volar plating of distal radial fractures.

▶ This is an excellent study demonstrating how the surgeon can better detect intra-articular penetration of screws during volar plating of distal radius fractures. The question and methods are sound, and the conclusion is one that helps the surgeon's practice. The authors report that 360° rotational fluoroscopy improves the surgeon's ability to detect intra-articular screw penetration. This message is essential for the surgeon who regularly treats distal radius fractures with volar plating. I currently use a 360° fluoroscopic evaluation in my clinical practice.

Interestingly, only 11% of respondents use the 45° pronated oblique view. This view is essential for evaluating 2 key issues: penetration of the distal plate screws/pegs out the dorsoulnar cortex and adequacy of dorsoulnar fragment intra-articular reduction (if there is that fragment). In addition, the 45° supinated oblique view demonstrates the dorsoradial cortical area for screw penetration. Lister's tubercle is the apex of the triangular shape of the dorsal radial cortex. Screws that have penetrated the dorsal cortex may appear all within the distal radius on a true lateral film but may be out dorsoradially or dorsoulnarly. 360° rotational fluoroscopy that incorporate oblique views will also help elucidate these issues.

S. K. Lee, MD

Dynamic Compared with Static External Fixation of Unstable Fractures of the Distal Part of the Radius: A Prospective, Randomized Multicenter Study
Hove LM, Krukhaug Y, Revheim K, et al (Investigation performed at Haukelaud Univ Hosp, Bergen; Norway; Stavanger Univ Hosp, Norway; St Olav's Univ Hosp, Trondheim, Norway)
J Bone Joint Surg Am 92:1687-1696, 2010

Background.—External fixation is an established method of treating certain types of distal radial fractures. We have designed a dynamic external fixator to treat these fractures. The purpose of the present study was to compare this device with current static bridging external fixators in terms of anatomical and functional results.

Methods.—We conducted a prospective randomized study to compare the radiographic and clinical results of dynamic external fixation with those of static external fixation for the treatment of seventy unstable distal radial fractures. Mobilization of the wrist was begun in the dynamic fixator group on the day after surgery. The external fixation frames were kept in place for a mean of six weeks. The patients were assessed clinically and radiographically at the time of removal of the fixator and at three, six, and twelve months.

Results.—Dynamic fixation resulted in a significantly better restoration of radial length at all follow-up visits in comparison with static fixation. There were no significant differences in radial tilt or radial inclination between the two groups. Wrist flexion, radial deviation, and pronation-supination were regained significantly faster in the dynamic fixator group. Wrist extension was significantly better in the dynamic fixator group in comparison with the static fixator group at all follow-up times. Self-evaluation with use of the Disabilities of the Arm, Shoulder and Hand score and a visual analog pain score demonstrated no significant differences between the two groups at the time of the latest follow-up. Superficial pin-track infections were significantly more common in the dynamic external fixator group than in the static fixator group.

Conclusions.—Continuous dynamic traction with a dynamic external fixator compares favorably with the use of static external fixators for the treatment of unstable fractures of the distal part of the radius.

▶ This study is significant in that it prospectively compares the results of distal radius fractures treated with either a static bridging external fixator or a novel dynamic bridging external fixator. Strengths of the study include its prospective randomized nature and thorough analysis of clinical and radiographic parameters postoperatively. One particular weakness of the study, which the authors also mention in their discussion, is that AO type-A and AO type-C fractures were not evaluated separately but together in this study. Any differences or similarities in the results of treatment of these two groups would certainly be interesting to the reader. In Table III in the original article, the authors state that the only significant difference clinically at 1 year is in wrist extension (65° vs 54°); there were no significant differences at 1 year for any of the other parameters, that is, wrist flexion, radial deviation, ulnar deviation, forearm pronation, and forearm supination. I am uncertain as to why this was the only parameter that demonstrated any significant difference and also whether the reader would determine this 11° difference in wrist extension at 1 year would be enough for him to change from a traditional static bridging fixator to a dynamic one. It would be interesting to see what the clinical results would be at longer term follow-up, for example, at least 2 years. The use of the external fixator for distal radius fractures has gone by the wayside for me in my practice, although I do not deny their importance and necessity in some clinical situations. I have no personal experience with the dynamic fixator as described in this study, only the static bridging one. However, were I ever to use a fixator again, the results of this study would not change my preference to a dynamic fixator.

S. S. Shin, MD, MMS

Ultrasound-guided reduction of distal radius fractures
Ang S-H, Lee S-W, Lam K-Y (Changi General Hosp, Singapore)
Am J Emerg Med 28:1002-1008, 2010

Introduction.—In our local emergency departments (EDs), manipulation and reduction (M&R) of distal radius fractures are performed by emergency doctors, with blind manual palpation, using postreduction x-rays to assess adequacy. We sought to study the effectiveness of ultrasound guidance in the reduction of distal radius fractures in adult patients presenting to a regional ED.

Methods.—This was a before-and-after study. Eligible patients were adults older than 21 years who presented to the ED with distal radius fractures that required M&R. Sixty-two patients were prospectively enrolled from October 2007 until June 2008, and they underwent ultrasound-guided M&R. The control group was a retrospective cohort of 102 patients who presented from January to June 2007. They had M&R done using the blind manual palpation method. All M&R procedures were performed by doctors within the ED, and supervision was provided by senior emergency physicians. Ultrasound guidance was performed by the senior emergency physicians.

Results.—Baseline characteristics between the ultrasound and control groups were similar. The rate of repeat M&R was reduced in the ultrasound group (1.6% vs 8.8%; $P = .056$). The postreduction radiographic indices were similar between the 2 groups, although the ultrasound group had improved volar tilt (mean, 5.93° vs 2.61°; $P = .048$). An incidental finding of a reduced operative rate was also found between the ultrasound and control groups (4.9% vs 16.7%; $P = .02$).

Conclusion.—Ultrasound guidance is effective and recommended for routine use in the reduction of distal radius fractures.

▶ This study reports a decrease in repeat manipulation among patients with distal radius fractures undergoing ultrasound-guided reductions when compared with traditional techniques.

The study is well designed and demonstrates how ultrasound can be used to improve patient outcomes in the acute setting: patients underwent fewer attempts at reduction and, as a result, were less likely to obtain serial radiographs. Although ultrasound technology is highly user dependent, the authors seem to indicate that the technique was easy to learn. I would be interested in obtaining more details regarding the learning curve for the procedure. In addition, it is not clear whether an additional person was required to perform the ultrasound or whether the ultrasound and reduction could be done by the same physician. The study's main weakness is that it does not address the cost associated with this intervention. The results, however, seem to indicate that the ultrasound guidance is a safe and effective technique to improve accuracy of reduction following displaced distal radius fractures.

T. D. Rozental, MD

Biomechanical Comparison of Locking Versus Nonlocking Volar and Dorsal T-Plates for Fixation of Dorsally Comminuted Distal Radius Fractures
Gondusky JS, Carney J, Erpenbach J, et al (Balboa Naval Med Ctr—San Diego, CA; et al)
J Orthop Trauma 25:44-50, 2011

Objectives.—The purpose of this study was to gain insight into the effect of plate location and screw type for fixation of extra-articular distal radius fractures with dorsal comminution (Orthopaedic Trauma Association Type 23-A3.2).

Methods.—Sixteen pairs of cadaver radii were randomized to four plating configurations: dorsal locking, dorsal nonlocking, volar locking, and volar nonlocking. A standard 1-cm dorsal wedge osteotomy was used. Cyclic axial loads were applied for 5000 cycles. Stiffness and fragment displacement were recorded at 500 cycle-intervals. Pre- and post-cyclic loading radiographs were analyzed. An axial load to failure test followed and construct stiffness and failure strength recorded. Biomechanical data were analyzed using a two-way analysis of variance ($P < 0.05$). Failure modes were descriptively interpreted.

Results.—Cyclic testing data revealed no difference between constructs at any interval. Within all construct groups, displacement that occurred did so within the first 500 cycles of testing. Pre- and postcyclic loading radiographic analysis showed no differences in construct deformation. Load to failure testing revealed no differences between groups, whereas volar constructs approached significance ($P = 0.08$) for increased failure strength. Dorsal constructs failed primarily by fragment subsidence and fragmentation, whereas volar constructs failed by plate bending.

Conclusions.—No difference in all measured biomechanical parameters supports equivalence between constructs and surgeon discretion in determining operative method. Minimal fragment displacement and construct deformation during physiological testing support previous data that early postoperative motion can be recommended. Fragment displacement that occurs does so in the early periods of motion (Figs 1 and 6B1).

▶ The authors describe a cadaver model to assess the strength of various plating constructs for the treatment of distal radius fractures. They compared 4 groups: volar and dorsal plate placement, each with locked or unlocked screws. They do control for implant differences by using simple T-plates (Fig 1). This allows the comparison to analyze the position or screw type rather than differences in the hardware. However, as with other similar biomechanical studies comparing locked and nonlocked distal radius plates, I think the biomechanical model they use fails to reproduce the clinical situation. The model involves bicortical fixation of the distal radius metaphysis. In the cadaver model, plates were placed 1.5 cm proximal to the nadir of the lunate facet. This means that there is a large metaphyseal portion of bone in which good bicortical fixation may be achieved (Fig 6B1). Therefore, unlocked screws do provide good stability in this model and the strength of the construct is equivalent to the locked construct. In most

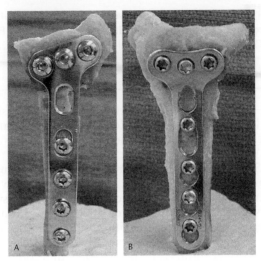

FIGURE 1.—Representative photographs illustrating two of the four plating constructs tested in the study. (A—B) Synthes 3.5-mm stainless steel T-plates (Synthes, Paoli, PA) dorsal nonlocking and volar locking, respectively. (Reprinted from Gondusky JS, Carney J, Erpenbach J, et al. Biomechanical comparison of locking versus nonlocking volar and dorsal T-plates for fixation of dorsally comminuted distal radius fractures. *J Orthop Trauma*. 2011;25:44-50, with permission from Lippincott Williams & Wilkins.)

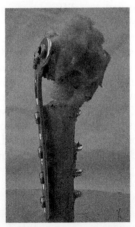

FIGURE 6.—Failure mode. (Reprinted from Gondusky JS, Carney J, Erpenbach J, et al. Biomechanical comparison of locking versus nonlocking volar and dorsal T-plates for fixation of dorsally comminuted distal radius fractures. *J Orthop Trauma*. 2011;25:44-50, with permission from Lippincott Williams & Wilkins.)

clinical scenarios, however, there is more dorsal comminution opposite the screw holes and there is concern of placing screws through the dorsal cortex for fear of tendon injury. In these scenarios, it seems unlikely that unlocked screws would provide the same stability as a locked construct. Certainly in situations in which sturdy bicortical fixation can be achieved, such as in a radial shaft fractures, there is little need for locking fixation.

I typically use volar locking plates for the operative treatment of distal radius fractures, as I feel the stability is greater than that which I can obtain with non-locked plates. I typically use dorsal plates for dorsal lip fractures that may be best stabilized by the buttress of the plate, therefore making locking screw fixation less critical.

T. B. Hughes, MD

15 Distal Radius, Distal Radioulnar Joint and Forearm

A New Total Distal Radioulnar Joint Prosthesis: Functional Outcome
Schuurman AH, Teunis T (Univ Med Centre Utrecht, the Netherlands)
J Hand Surg 35A:1614-1619, 2010

Purpose.—To present the evolution of design and the short-term functional outcome of our distal radioulnar joint (DRUJ) prosthesis. This total DRUJ prosthesis differs from others in that it consists of 2 parts and attains bony fixation by its hydroxyapatite coating.

Methods.—Nineteen patients received a DRUJ prosthesis after a failed Darrach procedure (n = 10), Sauvé-Kapandji procedure (n = 7), trauma (n = 1), or DRUJ synovitis (n = 1). Indications for the placement were decreased grip, decreased forearm motion, and pain due to ulnar impingement syndrome and instability of the distal ulna. Seven prostheses were removed, 5 due to loosening, 1 due to continuing pain, and 1 at the request of the patient. The 5 prostheses that loosened were an intermediate prototype no longer in use. In 12 remaining cases, range of motion, grip strength, and pinch strength were measured, and patients completed the Disabilities of the Arm, Shoulder, and Hand (DASH) questionnaire. Pain was assessed with the visual analog scale (range, 0−10). A paired *t*-test was performed to assess the significance of the difference between pre-operative and postoperative measurements.

Results.—Statistically significant improvements were seen in forearm pronation, from an average of 79° to 88°; grip strength, from an average of 10 kg to an average of 16 kg; and visual analog scale score, decreased from a mean of 5.3 to a mean of 3.5. The distal ulna was clinically stable in all 12 patients who retained the prosthesis.

Conclusions.—The intermediate prototype had a high failure rate, 5 out of 5. The early results for the current prosthesis prototype show clinical improvement. Based on these results, we conclude that this prosthesis offers a new treatment option for ulnar instability after distal ulnar resection.

111

Type of Study/Level of Evidence.—Therapeutic IV.

▶ The authors describe their results of 19 patients treated with a total distal radio-ulnar joint arthroplasty. In particular, they have noted improvement in forearm pronation, grip strength, and visual analog scale (VAS) scores. Of the 19 patients, the main results are based on 12 patients with a mean follow-up of just over 4 years. The implant that they are reporting about is a hydroxyapatite-coated implant with a polyethylene ring on the radial component and a tapered ulnar stem component that goes through the polyethylene ring in the radial component, allowing for pistoning and rotation. The authors very cautiously report that some of the earlier implants, 5 of them in particular, were all loosening, possibly because of too tight of a tolerance between the ulnar stem and the polyethylene ring. The subsequent 12 patients who had better outcome were thought to be related to an increased tolerance between the distal ulnar component and the polyethylene cylinder. Of the 3 types of implants that were used, A, B, and C types, the C type (which had better associated results) also included a small pin at the base of the radial component that was thought to also improve the stability within the radial metaphysis.

They have demonstrated a moderate improvement in VAS scores, pronation, and grip strength at a mean of approximately 4 years from surgery. The study is difficult to compare directly with other distal radioulnar joint (DRUJ) implant studies because of the heterogeneity of the existing literature. The disabilities of the arm, shoulder, and hand scores were moderately improved from an average of about 40 to 31, but this decrease actually did not reach statistical significance. The study was also of small power and had no comparison group, and the authors have addressed the limitations of their study appropriately. While the increase in motion was reported to be significant, this seems to represent a functionally moderate change from 79° to 88° of pronation. The VAS scores were improved from 5.3 to 3.5 with a P value of .02, but the clinical significance of this change may also be considered to be moderate with a residual VAS of 3.5, which suggests continued pain.

They also have suggested that one of the benefits of this prosthesis over some other types of DRUJ implants, such as the Scheker prosthesis, is that there are only 2 parts and, therefore, this is easier and it attains fixation by hydroxyapatite coating and bone ingrowth. While that may be the case, there is no comparison of ease of implantation, and it is conjecture at this point as to which implant may be easier to implant.

In summary, the authors demonstrate fairly good outcome of 12 of 19 implants used to treat a very difficult problem of distal radioulnar joint pain and instability. While some of these findings were statistically significant, I think some of them represent mild clinical improvement. Additionally, it must be noted that the evolution of their implant seems to have improved with the use of the C type prosthesis with a small radial pin at the base of the radial implant and increased tolerance between the distal stem and the polyethylene guide. This information will continue to help us understand how to develop a better joint prosthesis in the region of the distal radioulnar joint. These implants may provide great benefit for some patients, but the surgeon must continue to carefully select the patient and the particular prosthesis to be used when presented with these difficult problems about the distal radioulnar joint.

D. G. Dennison, MD

Suture-Button Construct for Interosseous Ligament Reconstruction in Longitudinal Radioulnar Dissociations: A Biomechanical Study

Kam CC, Jones CM, Fennema JL, et al (Univ of Miami, FL; Cleveland Clinic, OH)

J Hand Surg 35A:1626-1632, 2010

Purpose.—Longitudinal radioulnar dissociation is a triad of injuries consisting of distal radioulnar joint disruption, interosseous ligament complex (IOLC) tear, and radial head fracture. This renders the forearm longitudinally unstable, resulting in proximal migration of the radius and ulnar-sided wrist degeneration. We hypothesized that reconstruction of the central band of the IOLC in cadaver forearms using a Mini-TightRope suture-button construct would restore native forearm stability.

Methods.—We implanted 8 fresh-frozen cadaver arms with steel beads into the distal radius and ulna, mounted them on an MTS machine, and cyclically loaded them from 13 N distraction to 130 N compression. Bead motion was recorded fluoroscopically and analyzed using Image-Pro Express software. We measured distal ulnar forces using strain gauge transducers. Longitudinal radioulnar dissociation injuries were created by radial head excision and complete IOLC and triangular fibro-cartilage complex disruption. At each stage, arms were tested with and without a radial head implant. We reconstructed the central band of the IOLC using a Mini-TightRope and tightened until the distal radioulnar joint was reduced fluoroscopically. We used multiple-comparison analysis of variance with Tukey's Honestly Significant Difference test for statistical analysis.

Results.—The intact arms had an average radioulnar axial displacement of 0.7 ± 0.8 mm and distal ulnar impaction force of 16.7 ± 11.1 N (per 100 N of axial load on the forearm). After destabilization, the radioulnar displacement increased to 10.7 ± 3.9 mm (p < .001) and ulnar load increased 312%, to an average of 52.2 ± 25.7 N (p < .001). After IOLC reconstruction, average displacement decreased to 2.2 ± 0.9 mm with a distal ulnar load of 19.05 ± 13.5 N (not significantly different from intact arms).

Conclusions.—In this cadaveric study, Mini-TightRope IOLC reconstruction with or without a radial head prosthesis significantly reduced distal ulnar impaction forces to that of the native forearm, while limiting radioulnar displacement to near-anatomic levels (Figs 3 and 4).

▶ The limitations of this study are obvious. Only 8 cadaveric specimens were used, and results from biomechanical studies may be difficult to correlate with

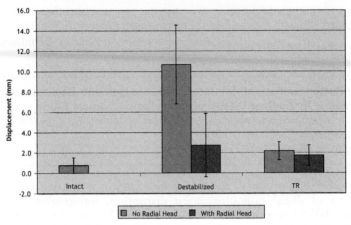

FIGURE 3.—Radioulnar displacement. TR = Mini-TightRope Reconstruction. (Reprinted from Kam CC, Jones CM, Fennema JL, et al. Suture-button construct for interosseous ligament reconstruction in longitudinal radioulnar dissociations: a biomechanical study. *J Hand Surg*. 2010;35A:1626-1632. Copyright 2010, with permission from the American Society for Surgery of the Hand.)

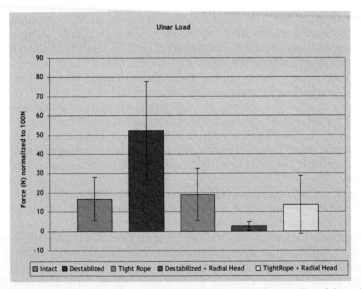

FIGURE 4.—Distal ulnar forces. (Reprinted from Kam CC, Jones CM, Fennema JL, et al. Suture-button construct for interosseous ligament reconstruction in longitudinal radioulnar dissociations: a biomechanical study. *J Hand Surg*. 2010;35A:1626-1632. Copyright 2010, with permission from the American Society for Surgery of the Hand.)

clinical outcomes. However, this study underscores the stabilizing influence of the IOLC in preventing longitudinal radioulnar dissociation. The technique of using the Mini-TightRope is also novel and can be applied with minimal soft-tissue disruption without donor site morbidity. Will the Mini-TightRope confer long-term stability to the forearm? Additional biomechanical studies examining the longevity of this construct would be beneficial before embarking on clinical trials.

E. K. Shin, MD

Application of the Brief International Classification of Functioning, Disability, and Health Core Set as a Conceptual Model in Distal Radius Fractures

Squitieri L, Reichert H, Kim HM, et al (Univ of Michigan Health System, Ann Arbor)
J Hand Surg 35A:1795-1805, 2010

Purpose.—In 2009, the World Health Organization published a conceptual outcome framework for evaluating upper extremity injury and disease, known as the Brief International Classification of Functioning, Disability, and Health (ICF) Core Set for Hand Conditions. The purpose of this study was to apply the ICF conceptual model to outcomes for distal radius fractures (DRFs) and determine the contribution of each ICF domain to patient satisfaction.

Methods.—Patient-rated and objective functional outcome data were collected at 6 weeks, 3 months, and 6 months after surgery. We measured satisfaction using a subsection of the Michigan Hand Outcomes Questionnaire (MHQ) satisfaction score. Measured study variables were linked to their corresponding ICF domain (personal factors, environmental factors, activity and participation, and body function). We then used hierarchical regression to assess the contribution of each ICF domain to variation in overall patient satisfaction at each time point.

Results.—We enrolled 53 patients with unilateral DRFs treated with the volar locking plating system. Regression analysis indicated that measured study variables explain 93% (6 weeks), 98% (3 months), and 97% (6 months) of variation in patient satisfaction. For all 3 study assessment dates, activity and participation variables (MHQ—Activities of Daily Living, MHQ—Work, and Jebsen-Taylor Score) contributed the most to variation in patient satisfaction, whereas personal and environmental factors had a considerably smaller role in predicting changes in patient satisfaction.

Conclusions.—The results demonstrated that it is possible to reliably model the relative contributions of each ICF domain to patient satisfaction over time, and the findings are consistent with previous research (ie, that most outcome variation is due to physical or functional factors). These results are strong enough to support continued use and further research using the ICF model for upper extremity outcomes.

▶ This is the first study to look at the World Health Organization (WHO) International Classification of Functioning, Disability and Health (ICF) Core Set for Hand Conditions. The ICF is "WHO's framework for measuring health and disability at both individual and population levels."[1] The attempt of the ICF is to shift "the focus from cause to impact it places all health conditions on an equal footing allowing them to be compared using a common metric—the ruler of health and disability"[1] and include the social context/impact. Given the organizations involved and the unanimous endorsement of the ICF, it appears likely that this framework will be more commonly referenced in all medical fields. The senior author of this article was the US representative to formulating the hand ICF. The authors chose 1 model of upper extremity illness (distal radius fractures treated with volar locking plates) and found that the measured study variables explained to a high degree the variations in patient satisfaction. This finding is in contrast to a prior study on distal radius fractures, which was unable to make a similar association from the general ICF and not the hand specific one.

I suspect the ICF format will be a growing part of our literature. The question remains to be answered whether it will be confined to policy and research domains of the literature or will it have an impact in the patient care domain.

There is some potential bias in that a high percentage of patients had incomplete data; at no point in the study did more than 72% of the participants have adequate data for regression analysis.

P. Blazar, MD

Reference

1. World Health Organization. International Classification of Functioning, Disability and Health (ICF). http://www.who.int/classifications/icf/en/. Accessed April 25, 2011.

Initial shortening and internal fixation in combination with a Sauvé-Kapandji procedure for severely comminuted fractures of the distal radius in elderly patients
Arora R, Gabl M, Pechlaner S, et al (Med Univ Innsbruck, Austria)
J Bone Joint Surg Br 92-B:1558-1562, 2010

We identified 11 women with a mean age of 74 years (65 to 81) who sustained comminuted distal radial and ulnar fractures and were treated by volar plating and slight shortening of the radius combined with a primary Sauvé-Kapandji procedure.

At a mean of 46 months (16 to 58), union of distal radial fractures and arthrodesis of the distal radioulnar joint was seen in all patients. The mean shortening of the radius was 12 mm (5 to 18) compared to the contralateral side. Flexion and extension of the wrist was a mean of 54° and 50°, respectively, and the mean pronation and supination of the forearm was 82° and 86°, respectively. The final mean disabilities of the arm, shoulder and hand score was 26 points. According to the Green and O'Brien rating system, eight patients had an excellent, two a good and one a fair result.

The good clinical and radiological results, and the minor complications without the need for further operations related to late ulnar-sided wrist pain, justify this procedure in the elderly patient.

▶ This study is a retrospective review of 11 patients treated primarily with volar plating for a comminuted distal radius fracture and a Sauvé-Kapandji procedure for an associated comminuted distal ulnar fracture. The authors report excellent clinical and radiographic outcomes.

The article is helpful in that it adds this combination of procedures to our armamentarium when treating difficult injuries, particularly in elderly patients. The main weakness is that it does not address the indications in a sufficient amount of detail. In particular, it is not clear whether an attempt at fixation was made initially in the operating room or whether the Sauvé-Kapandji was intended as a primary method of fixation in all cases. Furthermore, less than half of the patients had open injuries and the indications in closed fractures are not well described. Why not use plating with bone grafting in these patients? It is useful to know that patients treated in this fashion do well, but I would reserve the combination of volar plating and a Sauvé-Kapandji to open comminuted fractures or to those in whom intraoperative attempts at fixation of the ulna failed.

T. D. Rozental, MD

16 Flexor Tendon

Effects of Extensor Synovectomy and Excision of the Distal Ulna in Rheumatoid Arthritis on Long-Term Function
Jain A, Ball C, Freidin AJ, et al (Imperial College, London, UK)
J Hand Surg 35A:1442-1448, 2010

Purpose.—Objective outcomes data after excision of the distal ulna in rheumatoid arthritis are lacking. The aim of this study was to evaluate the functional results of this surgery in the long term.

Methods.—We prospectively collected data on range of motion (22 wrists), visual analog pain scores (14 wrists), and grip strength measured using a Jamar dynamometer (20 hands) in a group of 23 patients (26 wrists) preoperatively and at 3 months, 12 months, and a minimum of 5 years postoperatively (range, 5.3—10.4 y). The Jebsen-Taylor hand function test was administered to 9 patients at the same time points. A subgroup of patients also underwent extensor carpi radialis longus to extensor carpi ulnaris tendon transfer (11 wrists).

Results.—At one year, there were improvements in wrist pronation and supination, which were maintained at final follow-up. Active radial deviation decreased significantly at 3 months (p = .01) and one year (p = .02); this remained reduced at final follow-up (not significant). Wrist extension and active ulnar deviation showed slight improvements by one year, but reduced to levels below that measured preoperatively by final follow-up. Wrist flexion was significantly reduced at all time points postoperatively. Grip strength showed improvement from 10.0 kg (standard deviation [SD] 4.1 kg) preoperatively to 12.5 kg (SD 4.6 kg) 1 year after surgery and returned to preoperative levels (9.5 kg, SD 5.6 kg) by final follow-up. Wrist pain was significantly reduced from a mean score of 5 (SD 4) preoperatively to 2 (SD 2) postoperatively (p = .01). The Jebsen-Taylor hand function test showed improvements in writing and card turning.

Conclusions.—In the long term, excision of the distal ulna in rheumatoid patients results in an improvement in some aspects of hand function. There is a significant (p = .01) reduction in wrist pain but a reduction of wrist flexion.

Type of Study/Level of Evidence.—Therapeutic IV.

▶ Patients were evaluated at least 5 years after a distal ulna excision. A subset of patients were also treated with a radial extensor tendon transfer to the ulnar side of the wrist, and a subset of patients was evaluated with a Jebsen-Taylor hand function test. The results reveal overall initial improvements in pronation

119

and supination, decreases in active radial deviation and wrist flexion, and increases in active ulnar deviation and wrist extension. These results remain relatively stable at 5 years for pronation, supination, and radial deviation. Wrist flexion is decreased permanently, and wrist extension and ulnar deviation, which show initial improvement, fall back to the low preoperative measurements by 5-year follow-up.

Overall, this study provides a good glimpse of the long-term outcome after a distal ulnar excision. The general impression one gets from this article is that distal ulnar excision provides reasonable long-term outcome at 5 years. The severe degeneration of wrist motion and function that one might expect to accrue over a 5-year period does not materialize in these patients.

However, it should be noted that only two-thirds of the patients who were initially qualified to participate in this study are included. With one-third of patients from the initial cohort unavailable by final follow-up, one must at least wonder whether or not the very worst performers may be in that group. Nonetheless, this article provides an excellent assessment of what at least two-thirds of the patients are likely to accomplish with this very popular procedure.

J. C. Elfar, MD

Tissue Engineering of Flexor Tendons: The Effect of a Tissue Bioreactor on Adipoderived Stem Cell–Seeded and Fibroblast-Seeded Tendon Constructs
Angelidis IK, Thorfinn J, Connolly ID, et al (Stanford Univ Med Ctr, CA; Univ Hosp, Linköping, Sweden)
J Hand Surg 35A:1466-1472, 2010

Purpose.—Tissue-engineered flexor tendons could eventually be used for reconstruction of large tendon defects. The goal of this project was to examine the effect of a tissue bioreactor on the biomechanical properties of tendon constructs seeded with adipoderived stem cells (ASCs) and fibroblasts (Fs).

Methods.—Rabbit rear paw flexor tendons were acellularized and seeded with ASCs or Fs. A custom bioreactor applied a cyclic mechanical load of 1.25 N at 1 cycle/minute for 5 days onto the tendon constructs. Three additional groups were used as controls: fresh tendons and tendons reseeded with either ASCs or Fs that were not exposed to the bioreactor treatment and were left in stationary incubation for 5 days. We compared the ultimate tensile stress (UTS) and elastic modulus (EM) of bioreactor-treated tendons with the unloaded control tendons and fresh tendons. Comparison across groups was assessed using one-way analysis of variance with the significance level set at p<.05. Pairwise comparison between the samples was determined by using the Tukey test.

Results.—The UTS and EM values of bioreactor-treated tendons that were exposed to cyclic load were significantly higher than those of unloaded control tendons. Acellularized tendon constructs that were reseeded with ASCs and exposed to a cyclic load had a UTS of 66.76

MPa and an EM of 906.68 MPa; their unloaded equivalents had a UTS of 47.90 MPa and an EM of 715.57 MPa. Similar trends were found in the fibroblast-seeded tendon constructs that were exposed to the bioreactor treatment. The bioreactor-treated tendons approached the UTS and EM values of fresh tendons. Histologically, we found that cells reoriented themselves parallel to the direction of strain in response to cyclic strain.

Conclusions.—The application of cyclic strain on seeded tendon constructs that were treated with the bioreactor helped achieve a UTS and an EM comparable with those of fresh tendons. Bioreactor pretreatment and alternative cell lines, such as ASCs and Fs, might therefore contribute to the *in vitro* production of strong tendon material.

▶ In this study, the authors compared the effect of reseeding flexor tendon grafts with either stem cells derived from fat or fibroblasts. The grafts, after being reseeded with these cells, were cyclically loaded in a tissue bioreactor. The intended effect of the bioreactor was to provide the mechanical stimulus to these cells or to, in effect, entrain these cells into integrating into the tendon grafts.

The authors found that either cell type in conjunction with a tissue bioreactor improved the mechanical characteristics of the graft in terms of ultimate tensile strength and elastic modulus. Moreover, these conditioned grafts compare favorably with fresh grafts containing native cells.

The significance of the study is the step it takes toward the goal of providing a viable tendon substitute for reconstructive surgery. Specifically, these authors have focused on the ability to take a tendon graft that has no cells in it and then seed the graft with cells derived from fat or fibroblasts. The exact optimal preparation of these seeded grafts is the core question that the authors attempt to answer. The use of a bioreactor is novel in this regard. It provides the mechanical stimulation to allow cells that may not otherwise contribute to tendon strength to differentiate and integrate into the graft. The tendon grafts are strengthened as the result of a combination of the presence and stimulation of the cells in the bioreactor. When examined histologically, the cells are found to reorient along the axis of the tendon and are notably contributing to the overall strength of the tendon construct.

This work serves as a basis for what is very likely a viable translational approach to the need for usable grafting material for tendon reconstruction.

J. C. Elfar, MD

Flexor Tendon Pulley Reconstruction
Clark TA, Skeete K, Amadio PC (Mayo Clinic College of Medicine, Rochester, MN)
J Hand Surg 35A:1685-1689, 2010

Flexor tendon pulley reconstruction is relatively uncommon, and many technical treatment options have been described. The paucity of evidence

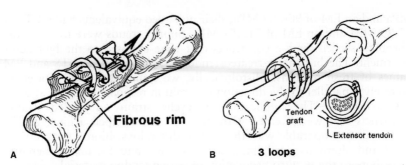

in the literature supporting one technique can make these surgical decisions and surgeries challenging. Here, we present a focused review of the triple loop pulley reconstruction technique (Fig 2).

▶ Destruction of the flexor tendon pulley causes bowstringing of the flexor tendon and loss of flexion range of the finger because of the increased distance between the flexor tendon and the center of the finger joint. The authors demonstrate 2 types of flexor tendon pulley reconstruction. One involves weaving the pulley graft through the remaining pulley rim, and the other makes an entirely new pulley loop around the phalanx (Fig 2). In the pulley loop technique, the tension on the graft tendon is important. If the pulley loop is loose, the bowstringing of the flexor tendon is not corrected and the finger loses its extension ability. If the pulley loop is too tight, it may interfere with the gliding of the flexor tendons. Adhesion of the reconstructed pulley to the flexor or extensor tendons can affect finger motion. There are several options for grafts for flexor pulley reconstruction, including the palmaris longus, plantaris, flexor digitorum superficialis tendon, and extensor retinaculum.

Injured tendons are not suitable for flexor pulley reconstruction because flexor tendon pulley reconstruction after flexor tendon repair is often associated with adhesion formation between the deep and superficial flexor tendons. I believe that injured tendons should not provide graft material for reconstruction of the flexor pulley because they may adhere to the extensor and flexor tendons. If the superficial tendon is available for a graft material for the pulley reconstruction, the part of the tendon adhering to the deep flexor tendon should be discarded and a healthy part of the tendon should be used. The tendon-weaving technique is less likely to cause adhesion to the extensor tendons because the tendon grafting is performed only on the palmar side of the finger. If the pulley rim is injured, the tendon-weaving technique is not indicated.

In the rehabilitation protocol after flexor pulley reconstruction, early motion exercises are preferable to avoid adhesion of the tendons. However, the question remains whether early motion exercise leads to loosening of the reconstructed pulley. The ideal flexor pulley reconstruction may be done in a staged flexor tendon reconstruction.[1] Passive motion exercises should start just after the first stage of the surgery to build the flexor pulley around an implanted silicone tendon. Because no tensile strength is applied to the silicone implant, it does not produce enough force to loosen the reconstructed pulley. Early mobilization has less chance of causing adhesion between the reconstructed pulley and the extensor tendon. The surgeon must consider the possibility of periosteal bone resorption of the phalanx just beneath the reconstructed pulley when the tendon loop technique is used. Bone resorption is often seen in young patients and sometimes develops into a fracture.[2]

R. Kakinoki, MD, PhD

References

1. Hunter JM. Staged flexor tendon reconstruction. *J Hand Surg Am.* 1983;8: 789-793.
2. Sanger JR, Buebendorf ND, Matloub HS, Yousif NJ. Proximal phalangeal fracture after tendon pulley reconstruction. *J Hand Surg.* 1990;15A:976-979.

The Effect of Muscle Excursion on Muscle Recovery after Tendon Repair in a Neglected Tendon Injury: A Study in Rabbit Soleus Muscles
Jeon SH, Chung MS, Baek GH, et al (Seoul Natl Univ Bundang Hosp, Gyeonggi-do, Korea)
J Orthop Res 29:74-78, 2011

We attempted to determine whether muscle excursion observed during operation can be a prognostic indicator of muscle recovery after delayed tendon repair in a rabbit soleus model. Eighteen rabbits underwent tenotomy of the soleus muscles bilaterally and were divided into three groups according to the period from tenotomy to repair. The tendons of each group were repaired 2, 4, and 6 weeks after tenotomy. The excursion of each soleus muscle was measured at the time of tenotomy (baseline), at 2, 4, 6 weeks after tenotomy, and 8 weeks after tendon repair. The amount of muscle recovery after tendon repair in terms of muscle excursion independently depended on the timing of repair and on the muscle excursion observed during repair. The regression model predicted that the muscle excursion recovered on average by 0.6% as the muscle excursion at the time of repair increased by 1% after adjusting for the timing of repair. This study suggests that measuring the muscle excursion during tendon repair may help physicians estimate the potential of muscle recovery in cases of delayed tendon repair.

▶ The authors performed tenotomy of the soleus muscle tendons and repaired thom 2, 4, or 6 weeks after tenotomy. The amount of muscle excursion was measured at the time of the repair surgery of the tendons or 8 weeks after the repair surgery. After adjusting for the timing of the repair, multiple regression analysis showed that muscle recovery time increased on average 0.6% with each 1% increase in the muscle excursion at the time of the tendon repair.

The results of this study are interesting and might be helpful for tendon surgery because they demonstrate that surgeons might be able to anticipate the final excursion of a repaired tendon during surgery. However, recovery of the excursion of the tendon after laceration may depend on various factors, including the site of the laceration and type of injured muscles. Extensor tendon laceration in zones 1 to 5 is sometimes treated successfully with a splint because the injured tendons can be stabilized by several anatomical structures, including tendon juncturae and the extensor apparatus.[1] In flexor tendon lacerations, some vincula or lumbrical muscles may prevent the transected proximal stump from retracting proximally, which may avoid myostatic contracture of the muscles. In clinical settings, we often encounter tendon interposition requiring repair of extensor tendon lacerations in zones 6 to 8 that occurred only 3 weeks previously. By contrast, the transected tendon stumps can be approximated directly in flexor tendon laceration in zones 3 to 5 that occurred 3 months previously. It may be difficult for the hand surgeon to anticipate the final excursion of a transected tendon only from the excursion of the proximal stump of the tendon at the time of tendon repair surgery.

R. Kakinoki, MD, PhD

Reference

1. Baratz ME, Schmit CC, Hughes TB. Extensor tendon injury. In. Green DP, ed, *Green hand surgery.* 5th ed. New York, NY: Churchill Livingstone; 2007:187-219.

The Effects of Exogenous Basic Fibroblast Growth Factor on Intrasynovial Flexor Tendon Healing in a Canine Model
Thomopoulos S, Kim HM, Das R, et al (Washington Univ, St Louis, MO; et al)
J Bone Joint Surg Am 92:2285-2293, 2010

Background.—Studies have demonstrated that flexor tendon repair strength fails to increase in the first three weeks following suturing of the tendon, a finding that correlates closely with the timing of many clinical failures. The application of growth factors holds promise for improving the tendon-repair response and obviating failure in the initial three weeks.

Methods.—The effects of basic fibroblast growth factor on flexor tendon healing were evaluated with use of a canine model. Operative repair followed by the sustained delivery of basic fibroblast growth factor, at two different doses, was compared with operative repair alone. Histological, biochemical, and biomechanical methods were used to evaluate the tendons twenty-one days after repair.

Results.—Vascularity, cellularity, and adhesion formation were increased in the tendons that received basic fibroblast growth factor as compared with the tendons that received operative repair alone. DNA concentration was increased in the tendons that received 1000 ng of basic fibroblast growth factor (mean and standard deviation, 5.7 ± 0.7 µg/mg) as compared with the tendons that received 500 ng of basic fibroblast growth factor (3.8 ± 0.7 μg/mg) and the matched control tendons that received operative repair alone (4.5 ± 0.9 μg/mg). Tendons that were treated with basic fibroblast growth factor had a lower ratio of type-I collagen to type-III collagen, indicating increased scar formation compared with that seen in tendons that received operative repair alone (3.0 ± 1.6 in the group that received 500-ng basic fibroblast growth factor compared with 4.3 ± 1.0 in the paired control group that received operative repair alone, and 3.4 ± 0.6 in the group that received 1000-ng basic fibroblast growth factor compared with 4.5 ± 1.9 in the paired control group that received operative repair alone). Consistent with the increases in adhesion formation that were seen in tendons treated with basic fibroblast growth factor, the range of motion was reduced in the group that received the higher dose of basic fibroblast growth factor than it was in the paired control group that received operative repair alone (16.6° ± 9.4° in the group that received 500 ng basic fibroblast growth factor, 13.4° ± 6.1° in the paired control group that received operative repair alone, and 29.2° ± 5.8° in the normal group [i.e., the group of corresponding, uninjured tendons from the contralateral forelimb]; and 15.0° ± 3.8° in the group that received 1000 ng basic fibroblast growth factor, 19.3° ± 5.5° in the paired control group that received operative repair alone, and 29.0° ± 8.8° in the normal group). There were no significant differences in tendon excursion or tensile mechanical properties between the groups that were treated with basic fibroblast growth factor and the groups that received operative repair alone.

Conclusions.—Although basic fibroblast growth factor accelerated the cell-proliferation phase of tendon healing, it also promoted neovascularization and inflammation in the earliest stages following the suturing the tendon. Despite a substantial biologic response, the administration of basic fibroblast growth factor failed to produce improvements in either the mechanical or functional properties of the repair. Rather, increased cellular activity resulted in peritendinous scar formation and diminished range of motion.

▶ The authors performed biomechanical, biological, and histological analyses of canine deep flexor tendons that were repaired without or with 2 different doses of basic fibroblast growth factor (bFGF). They used a fibrin-heparin-based delivery system that was incorporated into the transected tendon stumps. There were no clinically advantageous effects of this fibroblast growth factor (FGF) delivery system. On the contrary, the tendon excursion was reduced in the repaired tendons with a high dose of bFGF administration compared with that without FGF administration.

bFGF has several biological effects, including increased cell proliferation, collagen production, and capillary formation. Numerous studies have suggested that through these biological actions, bFGF has beneficial effects on ligament or tendon repair. The differences between the results of this study and previous studies might reflect different ways of delivering FGF to the tendon repair site. In this study, which used a unique system to deliver bFGF, bFGF bound strongly to the fibrin matrix; however, bFGF released from the system may have had a biological influence on the repaired tendon and the tissue around the tendon. bFGF remaining at the incorporated site of the tendon contributed to facilitate remodeling of the repaired tendon, although bFGF released outside the incorporated site of the tendon might also have helped the flexor tendon adhere to its surrounding tissue.

Tensile force facilitates remodeling of tendon tissue at the tendon repair site, which contributes to the maturity of the tendon tissue at the repair site. However, once adhesion between the tendon and the surrounding tissue occurs, the tensile force is not applied to the repair site of the tendon and the repair site is not repaired fully but remains immature. In a previous study by Hamada et al,[1] a suture material containing bFGF was passed across the repair site of tendons, and this material delivered FGF from inside the tendon. Three weeks after the repair, the tendons repaired by bFGF-coated sutures exhibited more ultimate force compared with those repaired by FGF-uncoated sutures. Western blot analysis showed no leakage of the exogenous FGF from the tendon to the surrounding scar tissue. The suture material functioned as a good scaffold for bFGF-delivery for tendon repair. A scaffold for the delivery of bFGF should have been used in the current experimental model. Tissue engineering techniques require cells, growth factors, and scaffolds suitable for carrying and delivering the cells and factors.[2]

R. Kakinoki, MD, PhD

References

1. Hamada Y, Katoh S, Hibino N, Kosaka H, Hamada D, Yasui N. Effects of monofilament nylon coated with basic fibroblast growth factor on endogenous intrasynovial flexor tendon healing. *J Hand Surg Am.* 2006;31:530-540.
2. Kakinoki R. Principles of tissue engineering for reconstruction of the hand. In: Chang J, Guputa G, eds. *Tissue Engineering for the Hand.* London, UK: World Scientific Publishing; 2010:21-40.

The Effect of Epitendinous Suture Technique on Gliding Resistance During Cyclic Motion After Flexor Tendon Repair: A Cadaveric Study
Moriya T, Zhao C, An K-N, et al (Mayo Clinic, Rochester, MN)
J Hand Surg 35A:552-558, 2010

Purpose.—To investigate the effects of motion following repair with a modified Kessler core suture and 5 different epitendinous suture designs on the gliding resistance, breaking strength, 2-mm gap force, and stiffness of flexor digitorum profundus tendons in a human *in vitro* model.

Methods.—The flexor digitorum profundus tendons of the index, middle, ring, and little fingers of 50 human cadavers were transected and repaired with a 2-strand modified Kessler suture and assigned to 5 groups based on type of epitendinous suture design. The 5 epitendinous designs tested were a simple, running epitendinous suture whose knot was outside the repair (simple running KO); a simple, running epitendinous suture whose knot was inside the repair (simple running KI); a cross-stitch epitendinous suture; an interlocking, horizontal mattress (IHM) epitendinous suture; and a running–locking epitendinous suture. The tendon repair strength and 2-mm gap force were measured after 1,000 cycles of tendon motion. The resistance to gap formation, a measure of repair stiffness, was obtained from the force versus gap data.

Results.—None of the repairs showed any gap formation after 1,000 cycles of tendon motion. The cross-stitch epitendinous suture, IHM epitendinous suture, and running–locking epitendinous suture all had significantly lower gliding resistance than the simple running KO epitendinous suture after 1 cycle. The simple running KI epitendinous suture had significantly lower gliding resistance than the simple running KO epitendinous suture after 100 cycles and 1,000 cycles. The differences for gap force at 2 mm and stiffness of the repaired tendon evaluation were not statistically significant. The cross-stitch epitendinous suture, IHM epitendinous suture, and running–locking epitendinous suture all had significantly higher maximal failure strength after 1,000 cycles than the simple running KI epitendinous suture.

Conclusions.—The cross-stitch, IHM, and running–locking epitendinous sutures had the best combination of higher strength and lower gliding resistance in this study. Although these findings suggest a potential for these suture types to be preferred as epitendinous sutures, these repairs should first be investigated in vivo to address their effect on tendon healing and adhesion formation.

▶ The authors demonstrate in an in vitro test model that the cross-stitch, interlocking horizontal mattress (IHM), and running-locking epitendinous sutures had the best combination of higher strength and lower gliding resistance. Previous work by Dona et al (JHS-A 2003) touted IHM as the strongest with regard to 2-mm gap and ultimate load to failure when compared with simple running, cross-stitch, and interlocking cross-stitch. The advantage of this study is that it reported the gliding resistance where the study of Dona et al only reported on strength. Although simple running sutures are commonly performed in flexor tendon surgery, a major advancement in treatment for these problems is to use a peripheral suture, which is more robust with good gliding. If one combines the findings of Dona et al with this article, IHM would be the optimal peripheral suture. Lee et al (JHS-A 2010) used the IHM in a combination zone 2 repair with a cross locked cruciate core suture that showed a very low percent increase in work of flexion (5.2%) and very high 2-mm gap force (89.8 N) and ultimate load to failure (111.5 N). A limitation of this study was that the core suture used was a modified Kessler, a relatively weak 2-strand core that may not be applicable to current repair principles.

S. K. Lee, MD

17 Elbow

Revision Arthroscopic Contracture Release in the Elbow Resulting in an Ulnar Nerve Transection: A Case Report
Gay DM, Raphael BS, Weiland AJ (Flagler Orthopedics and Sports Medicine, Palm Coast, FL; Hosp for Special Surgery, NY)
J Bone Joint Surg Am 92:1246-1249, 2010

Background.—Elbow arthroscopy is performed to remove loose bodies, treat lateral epicondylitis, for synovectomy and contracture release, and to manage osteochondritis dissecans. The rate of complications is higher with elbow arthroscopy than for similar procedures in the knee and shoulder. Neurovascular complications develop in 0% to 14% of cases, with most consisting of transient neurapraxias. Seldom does complete nerve transection occur during elbow arthroscopy. A report detailed a patient who had arthroscopic release of an elbow contracture and suffered complete transection of a previously transposed ulnar nerve.

Case Report.—Man, 45, who was left-hand dominant and worked in construction, fell, sustaining a small avulsion fracture of the coronoid process of the right ulna with no elbow dislocation. A posterior splint was applied for 4 weeks to immobilize the elbow, but the elbow's range of motion was restricted after the splint was removed. Intensive physical therapy plus a turnbuckle-type splint were used to improve flexion, but active and passive ranges of motion were still limited after 4 months. Open release of the contracture and subcutaneous ulnar nerve transposition with postoperative radiation to prevent heterotopic ossification were performed, but 4 months later the limited range of motion persisted. Neurovascular status was unharmed. Ten months after the initial injury, the patient had arthroscopic release of the residual elbow contracture. This was accomplished through the proximal anteromedial and anterolateral portals. The patient experienced numbness of the ring and small digits and weakness of the finger abduction postoperatively. Five months later, electrodiagnostic and nerve conduction velocity studies confirmed severe ulnar neuropathy at or around the right elbow.

Fifteen months after the original injury, which was 5 months after the arthroscopic release, the patient was seeking a second opinion regarding the ulnar neuropathy and residual elbow contracture. The elbow range of motion was limited to 15° of active extension and 65° of active flexion but he had full forearm rotation. He had no sensation to light touch in the distribution of the ulnar nerve and the skin over the ulnar half of the ring and small fingers was dry and cracked. Findings at that time included a positive Froment sign, weak dorsal interosseous muscles, weak finger abduction/adduction, and negative Pitres-Testut sign. There was no heterotopic ossification on radiographic evaluation. These findings suggested that some fibers of the ulnar nerve were intact or a Martin-Gruber connection was present. An open contracture release with ulnar nerve exploration and neurolysis and repair as needed was the course of action chosen.

The ulnar nerve was found to be transposed anteriorly, attaching to the medial epicondyle via scar tissue. A neuroma was located at the proximal stump. A 4.5-cm defect was present between the proximal and distal stumps of the completely transected nerve. There was no way to know if the defect occurred during portal placement or during arthroscopic capsular debridement. An open contracture release, including triceps tenolysis and posterior capsular release, was performed. A triple-cable autologous sural nerve graft was placed. The range of motion intraoperatively was markedly better, with the arm moving through a full range of motion without tension on the anteriorly transposed ulnar nerve and graft. Postoperatively the patient began intensive physical therapy and continuous passive motion. Three weeks postoperatively the patient needed manipulation of the elbow. Four months postoperatively the patient's active range of motion for the elbow was from 25° of extension to 105° of flexion. The hand had not responded with appreciable sensory or motor function, and the patient had not yet returned to his previous job.

Conclusions.—There are various portals used to perform elbow arthroscopy, depending on the pathologic condition being treated. Risks are associated with each of these sites. Before the arthroscopy was performed in this patient, an ulnar nerve transposition was done, placing the ulnar nerve directly in the path of the proximal anteromedial portal. To lower the risk of nerve injury, it is important to proceed through arthroscopic release cautiously in patients who have had an open contracture release.

▶ Elbow arthroscopy for contracture release has become a more popular treatment option for addressing the stiff elbow following trauma. This is a technically demanding operation in the setting of posttraumatic contracture because the elbow has markedly decreased volume and compliance. The neurovascular structures therefore have decreased displacement when the joint is insufflated. This case report highlights the possibility of iatrogenic nerve injury during elbow arthroscopy. The authors of this article remind the reader of technical considerations when performing this operation. The surgeon should consider his or her own technical abilities and experience when performing elbow arthroscopy, especially in posttraumatic contractures when the normal anatomy may be altered. The ulnar nerve should be identified prior to placement of the medial portals. This may be done by direct palpation or open surgical dissection. If the ulnar nerve has been previously transposed, it has been suggested by other authors that elbow arthroscopy should be avoided. On another note, it has also been suggested that an arthroscopic procedure should not be attempted if there has been a previous operation on the lateral side of the elbow because of possible adherence of the radial nerve to the anterior aspect of the capsule.

E. Cheung, MD

Osteochondritis Dissecans of the Capitellum
Baker CL III, Romeo AA, Baker CL Jr (Hughston Clinic, Columbus, GA; Rush Univ Med Ctr, Chicago, IL)
Am J Sports Med 38:1917-1928, 2010

Osteochondritis dissecans of the capitellum is a well-recognized cause of elbow pain and disability in the adolescent athlete. This condition typically affects young athletes, such as throwers and gymnasts, involved in high-demand, repetitive overhead, or weightbearing activities. The true cause, natural history, and optimal treatment of osteochondritis dissecans of the capitellum remain unknown. Suspicion of this condition warrants investigation with proper radiographs and magnetic resonance imaging. Prompt recognition of this disorder and institution of nonoperative treatment for early, stable lesions can result in healing with later resumption of sporting activities. Patients with unstable lesions or those failing nonoperative therapy require operative intervention with treatment based on lesion size and extent. Historically, surgical treatment included arthrotomy with loose body removal and curettage of the residual osteochondral defect base. The introduction of elbow arthroscopy in the treatment of osteochondritis dissecans of the capitellum permits a thorough lesion assessment and evaluation of the entire elbow joint with the ability to treat the lesion and coexistent pathology in a minimally invasive fashion. Unfortunately, the prognosis for advanced lesions remains more guarded, but short-term results after newer reconstruction techniques are promising (Fig 6).

▶ The authors present a review of osteochondritis dissecans (OCD) lesions, including proposed causes, clinical presentation, and treatment options, along with historical accounts.

OCD lesions typically affect high-demand overhead athletes or those involved in weight-bearing activities. Other causes of elbow pain should be ruled out, including Panner disease. No single cause had been attributed to

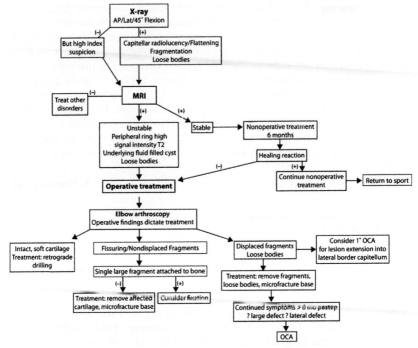

FIGURE 6.—Treatment algorithm showing the author's preferred approach for evaluation and treatment of osteochondritis dissecans of the capitellum. OCA, osteochondral autograft. (Reprinted from Baker CL III, Romeo AA, Baker CL Jr. Osteochondritis dissecans of the capitellum. *Am J Sports Med.* 2010;38:1917-1928, with permission from The Author(s).)

OCD lesions, but repetitive microtrauma and vascular insult appear to be the most influential factors.

Patients present with elbow pain, localized at the radiocapitellar joint, which may include mechanical symptoms. Radiographic studies are warranted, including full-extension anteroposterior and lateral radiographs, with the addition of 45° flexion anteroposteriorly.

MRI (MR arthrogram) should be utilized to define the size, extent, and stability of the OCD lesion. Unstable OCD lesions demonstrate a peripheral ring or underlying fluid-filled cyst on T2-weighted images.

Nonoperative treatment is indicated for stable lesions with an open physis, including a 6-month rest period with nonsteroidal anti-inflammatory drugs and gentle stretching exercises. Serial radiographs with repeat MRI at 6 months are recommended to assess lesion healing and stability.

Operative treatment (open and arthroscopic) includes drilling, removal of unstable lesions or fixations, reconstruction using cartilage grafts, and closing wedge osteotomy of the lateral condyle. Poor prognostic factors include large lesions that extend into the lateral border of the capitellum, allowing engagement of the radial head; these lesions should be reconstructed rather than removing the large fragment. The authors also review surgical technique of arthroscopic treatment of OCD lesions.

This is an excellent review article of the treatment and outcomes of OCD lesions, including a treatment algorithm for stable and unstable lesions.

J. Jacobson, MD

Osteochondritis Dissecans of the Capitellum: Minimum 1-Year Follow-Up After Arthroscopic Debridement
Schoch B, Wolf BR (Univ of Iowa Hosps and Clinics, Iowa City)
Arthroscopy 26:1469-1473, 2010

Purpose.—The purpose of our study is to show that arthroscopic debridement is an appropriate intervention for midterm to long-term subjective symptom relief of osteochondritis dissecans (OCD) of the elbow.

Methods.—A retrospective case series of 13 patients undergoing arthroscopic treatment of OCD of the elbow over a 10-year period was studied. Patients were assessed with a mean follow-up of 3.6 years (range, 12 months to 8 years). The disability/symptom section of the Disabilities of the Arm, Shoulder and Hand (DASH) was used to measure patient-reported outcome. Additional questions were used to assess other injuries to the elbow and return to sports activities.

Results.—Of 13 patients, 8 reported participating in repetitive valgus stress sports associated with overhead throwing. Two participated in gymnastics. Ten patients provided follow-up data greater than 1 year after surgical intervention. The mean follow-up DASH score for surgically treated patients was 8.6 (range, 0.0 to 22.41). Four patients reported a complete return to their sports activities, and six reported complete cessation of at least 1 sport. By use of intraoperative reports, the OCD lesions were graded according to the Classification System for OCD Lesions established by the American Sports Medicine Institute. No difference in mean DASH score between grades was found.

Conclusions.—In our small group of patients, arthroscopic debridement of OCD of the capitellum resulted in a functional elbow with subjective symptom relief for the majority of patients, as evidenced by DASH scores. However, despite a functional outcome, many patients reported ceasing at least some sporting activities because of their elbow.

Level of Evidence.—Level IV, therapeutic case series.

▶ This article adds to the support in the literature for the practice of simple debridement of capitellar osteochondritis dissecans. There are more than a few series in the literature of articles detailing more intricate treatment protocols involving stabilization of the lesion in attempts to heal the original lesions. Although these studies hold promise, this study reminds us that debridement continues to be a steady and dependable way to improve symptoms and function in these patients.

M. I. Loebenberg, MD

18 Elbow: Arthroplasty

Revision interposition arthroplasty of the elbow
Larson AN, Adams RA, Morrey BF (Mayo Clinic, Rochester, MN)
J Bone Joint Surg [Br] 92-B:1273-1277, 2010

Between 1996 and 2008, nine patients with severe post-traumatic arthritis underwent revision of a failed interposition arthroplasty of the elbow with a further interposition procedure using an allograft of tendo Achillis at a mean of 5.6 years (0.7 to 13.1) after the initial procedure. There were eight men and one woman with a mean age of 47 years (36 to 56).

The mean follow-up was 4.7 years (2 to 8). The mean Mayo Elbow Performance score improved from 49 (15 to 65) pre-operatively to 73 (55 to 95) (p = 0.04). The mean Disability of the Arm, Shoulder and Hand score was 26 (7 to 42). One patient was unavailable for clinical follow-up and one underwent total elbow replacement three months post-operatively. Of the remaining patients, one had an excellent, two had good, three fair and one a poor result. Subjectively, five of the nine patients were satisfied. Four continued manual labour.

Revision interposition arthroplasty is an option for young, active patients with severe post-traumatic arthritis who require both mobility and durability of the elbow.

▶ The authors present a retrospective review of 9 patients who underwent revision interposition arthroplasty following prior interposition arthroplasty. The study adds to the limited literature on this subject. The typical patient was young and had a satisfactory initial result from a primary interposition arthroplasty but had developed further symptoms. Mean time between primary and revision interposition arthroplasty was 5.6 years. Based on intraoperative findings, tendo Achillis was a more durable allograft than fascia lata. Of the 4 patients with a previous tendo Achillis interposition, 1 had graft and fibrocartilage remaining in the joint and 3 had remnants of the graft anteriorly and posteriorly on the humerus with a bare articulation. In the 5 patients with a previous fascia lata graft, 2 had only fibrous tissue in the joint and 3 had no evidence of the previous graft. Following revision arthroplasty, 4 patients were still employed in heavy labor, 1 continued with sedentary work, and the others remained retired or disabled. Revision interposition arthroplasty may be considered as one salvage option for patients with posttraumatic arthritis who wish to continue with active lifestyles. Revision to total elbow arthroplasty is another option, but lifting restrictions associated with an elbow prosthesis are unsuitable to the active patient or manual laborer, and the revision rate for total elbow arthroplasty in this population is very high. Other alternatives include resection arthroplasty and arthrodesis, both of which are poorly tolerated because of compromised function.

E. Cheung, MD

The Kudo 5 total elbow replacement in the treatment of the rheumatoid elbow: results at a minimum of ten years
Qureshi F, Draviaraj KP, Stanley D (Northern General Hosp, Sheffield, UK)
J Bone Joint Surg [Br] 92-B:1416-1421, 2010

Between September 1993 and September 1996, we performed 34 Kudo 5 total elbow replacements in 31 rheumatoid patients. All 22 surviving patients were reviewed at a mean of 11.9 years (10 to 14). Their mean age was 56 years (37 to 78) at the time of operation. All had Larsen grade IV or V rheumatoid changes on X-ray. Nine (three bilateral replacements and six unilateral) had died from unrelated causes. One who had died before ten years underwent revision for dislocation.

Of the 22 total elbow replacements reviewed six had required revision, four for aseptic loosening (one humeral and three ulnar) and two for infection. Post-operatively, one patient had neuropraxia of the ulnar nerve and one of the radial nerve. Two patients had valgus tilting of the ulnar component.

With revision as the endpoint, the mean survival time for the prosthesis was 11.3 years (95% confidence interval (10 to 13) and the estimated survival of the prosthesis at 12 years according to Kaplan-Meier survival analysis was 74% (95% confidence interval 0.53 to 0.91).

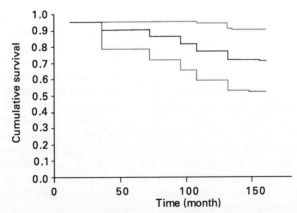

FIGURE 1.—Kaplan-Meier survival analysis using revision as the endpoint. (Reprinted from Qureshi F, Draviaraj KP, Stanley D. The Kudo 5 total elbow replacement in the treatment of the rheumatoid elbow: results at a minimum of ten years. *J Bone Joint Surg [Br]*. 2010;92-B:1416-1421, with permission and copyright © of the British Editorial Society of Bone and Joint Surgery.)

TABLE 1.—Details of the 22 Surviving Patients and their Results

Case	Gender	Age (yrs)	Follow-up (mths)	Side	Range of Flexion/ Extension (°)	Pain	Mayo Score	Revision	Time to Failure (mths)
1	F	41	161	R	26 to 150	None	95	-	
2	F	41	132	L	-		-	Loose ulna	132
3	F	53	156	R	-		-	Loose humerus	96
4	F	46	149	R	30 to 140	None	90		
5	F	43	156	R	30 to 140	None	100		
6	F	67	145	L	10 to 140	Mild	80		
7	F	37	146	R	30 to 120	None	80		
8	F	66	152	L	20 to 140	None	95		
9	F	65	150	L	20 to 140	Moderate	70		
10	F	72	148	L	30 to 120	None	80		
11	F	51	152	R	-		-	Loose ulna	72
12	F	72	146	L	30 to 140	Mild	70		
13	F	64	146	L	30 to 130	Moderate	60		
14	F	63	154	L	-		-	Loose ulna	36
15	F	58	141	R	45 to 110	Mild	70		
16	F	68	142	L	20 to 120	None	95		
17	F	54	133	R	20 to 120	None	80		
18	F	53	135	R	30 to 120	None	80		
19	M	78	139	L	20 to 140	Mild	80		
20	F	44	142	R	-		-	Infected	12
21	F	61	127	L	-		-	Infected	108
22	M	41	120	R	20 to 140	None	85		

Of the 16 surviving implants, ten were free from pain, four had mild pain and two moderate. The mean arc of flexion/extension of the elbow was 106° (65° to 130°) with pronation/supination of 90° (30° to 150°) with the joint at 90° of flexion. The mean Mayo elbow performance score was 82 (60 to 100) with five excellent, ten good and one fair result.

Good long-term results can be expected using the Kudo 5 total elbow replacement in patients with rheumatoid disease, with a low incidence of loosening of the components (Fig 1, Table 1).

▶ The authors provide a review of the survival and outcomes of an unlinked elbow prosthesis at an average of nearly 12 years postoperatively (Table I). The population exclusively comprised rheumatoid patients. In contrast to earlier designs, failure by aseptic loosening was seen in 3 of 4 cases because of ulnar-sided loosening rather than humeral loosening. The authors suggest this may be to improve designs that transmit forces from a well-fixed humeral component to the ulnar component. The authors note good results at more than 10 years of follow-up with survival of 74% at 12 years (Fig 1).

J. E. Adams, MD

Use of metal proximal radial endoprostheses for treatment of non-traumatic disorders: a case series

Gokaraju K, Miles J, Parratt MTR, et al (Royal Natl Orthopaedic Hosp (RNOH), Stanmore, UK)
J Bone Joint Surg [Br] 92-B:1685-1689, 2010

We have reviewed five adult patients treated with endoprosthetic reconstruction of the proximal radius following resection of non-traumatic lesions. The patients had a mean age of 33.4 years (20 to 60) at the time of surgery and the mean follow-up was 7.6 years (0.8 to 16).

Following surgery, all elbows were clinically stable and there was 100% survivorship of the prosthesis. Evaluation of function was assessed clinically and by the Mayo Elbow Performance Score, achieving a mean of 86% (70 to 100).

Results at medium-term follow-up are encouraging with regards to elbow stability, implant survivorship and functional outcome.

▶ This is a report of a small series of 5 patients who underwent reconstruction of large, nontraumatic, proximal radial defects using a custom endoprosthesis. The diagnoses included metastatic renal cell carcinoma, recurrent benign fibrous histiocytoma, Ewing sarcoma, chondroblastoma, and radioulnar synostosis from previous infection. The patients were followed for a mean of 7.6 years. The authors reported that all elbows were clinically stable and still in service at follow-up. In general, the postoperative function was good, and the pain scores were low. The authors conclude that the medium-term results of this form of treatment were encouraging.

Resection of large proximal radius defects is indeed a difficult reconstructive dilemma. Options for treatment include allograft reconstruction, nonvascularized autograft reconstruction, vascularized autograft reconstruction, endoprosthetic reconstruction, or simply leaving the proximal radius unreconstructed. Although this study highlights a method of reconstruction that may be successful in the medium term, it is difficult to draw firm conclusions from this series of patients, given the heterogeneity of resultant defects and variability in the techniques used. For instance, the defects ranged from 4.8 cm to 11 cm. Furthermore, the endoprostheses used among this group of patients were both cemented and uncemented, and some were hydroxylapatite coated and some were not. One prosthesis used an extracortical plate. The authors' concluding statement that these endoprosthetic devices restore "normal biomechanical forces through the elbow and forearm" is not supported by any data and should not be considered valid.

The authors are to be commended for their successful work with these extremely difficult proximal radial defects. What we can take away from this study is that endoprosthetic reconstruction of large, nontraumatic, proximal, radial defects is a treatment alternative requiring implant customization tailored to the size and nature of the defect. It is reasonable to expect good medium-term function in some patients.

P. Murray, MD

19 Elbow: Trauma

Preoperative Computer-Assisted Design Templating of Complex Articular Olecranon Osteotomy: Case Report
Garg R, Hammoud S, Lipman J, et al (Hosp for Special Surgery, NY; Weill Med College of Cornell Univ, NY)
J Hand Surg 35A:1990-1994, 2010

Preoperative 3-dimensional modeling methods are commonly used in orthopedic surgery but there have been limited reports of their use for planning upper extremity surgery. In this report, we describe a case of a malunited olecranon fracture and its management using custom preoperative computed tomographic templating and mechanical modeling. One year after surgery, the patient demonstrated nearly full painless restoration of function and motion.

▶ This study is a case report of malunion after tension band wiring of a highly comminuted olecranon fracture that led to a discrepancy between the radius of curvature of the semilunar notch and the trochlea with a resultant block to motion. The authors have used a 3-dimensional (3D) CT scan, did solid modeling of the uninjured elbow with a 3D printer, and based their corrective osteotomy on the normal contralateral elbow. This is a novel technique with applications in planning the correction of articular complex malunions. There is emerging literature of preoperative planning with the help of solid models available and may prove useful in selected cases.

A. Cil, MD

Quantitative Measurements of the Coronoid in Healthy Adult patients
Guitton TG, Van Der Werf HJ, Ring D (Massachusetts General Hosp, Boston, MA)
J Hand Surg 36A:232-237, 2011

Purpose.—We investigated the hypothesis that a quantitative 3-dimensional computed tomography (CT) modeling technique that can measure size, shape, and proximal articular surface area can be used to develop formulas that could predict the volume and proximal surface area of the intact coronoid based on anatomical and demographic data available in patients with fracture of the coronoid process.

Methods.—We used a consecutive series of 50 CT scans with a slice thickness of 1.25 mm or less obtained in patients with fracture of the distal humerus, but no injury to the coronoid, to create 3-dimensional models. The volume and articular surface area of the coronoid were measured, and predictive formulas were based on anatomical measurements. We calculated gender using multiple linear regression.

Results.—There were significant correlations between total coronoid volume and coronoid articular surface area for coronoid width, radial neck diameter, radial head diameter, height, weight, and gender. Multiple linear regression modeling with the factors radial head diameter, radial neck diameter, coronoid width, height, weight, and gender resulted in formulas that could account for 71.8% of the variation in coronoid volume and 66.2% of the variation in coronoid articular surface area. The average relative percent difference was 1.32% for the coronoid volume and 0.68% for the coronoid articular surface area.

Conclusions.—The volume and articular surface area of the coronoid can be estimated based on anatomical measurements and gender. This may lead to better estimates of lost fragments when modeling the fractured coronoid and CT scan of the opposite limb is not available.

▶ Coronoid fracture classifications dictate fixation indications of these fractures based on the percentage of the coronoid involved. The authors have used quantitative 3-dimensional CT scans of intact coronoids of 50 patients to develop a linear regression model capable of estimating the volume and proximal articular surface area of the coronoid based on coronoid width, radial head diameter, radial neck diameter, height, weight, and gender. The outlined technique seems to be labor intensive but can help better define fracture patterns and fracture morphology that can improve the management of coronoid fractures. This study did not account for articular cartilage, as it cannot be identified on CT scans. It has recently been shown that the coronoid cartilage height at the tip of the bony coronoid was 2.96 mm, and the thickness at the tip was 2.63 mm.[1] The cartilage thickness not only allows for proper classification but also possibly results in fixation of the coronoid fractures, which was thought would do fine without fixation.

A. Cil, MD

Reference

1. Rafehi S, King G, Athwal G. An anatomic study of coronoid cartilage thickness with special reference to fractures. *FASEB J.* 2010;24:635.

Pediatric Elbow Dislocation Associated with Proximal Radioulnar Translocation: A Report of Three Cases and a Review of the Literature
Combourieu B, Thevenin-Lemoine C, Abelin-Genevois K, et al (Armand Trousseau Hosp, Paris, France)
J Bone Joint Surg Am 92:1780-1785, 2010

Background.—Elbow dislocation in children accounts for just 3% of elbow injuries. Only 12 cases of proximal radioulnar translocation have been reported in children. It is often misdiagnosed initially, leading to delayed treatment and a poor functional result. Three cases were reported.

Case Reports.—*Case 1*: Girl, 6, had fallen on her right elbow and complained of a painful, swollen right elbow. No neurologic or vascular problems were found, but anteroposterior and lateral radiographs revealed proximal radioulnar dislocation of the right elbow. Closed reduction was performed with the patient placed under general anesthesia, then the arm was immobilized in a posterior splint with the forearm in neutral position and the elbow flexed at 90° for 2 months. Transient ulnar nerve palsy occurred but resolved within 6 months. Three-month assessment showed normal radiographic appearance and 20% loss of pronation. Complete range of elbow and forearm motion was regained at 1 year.

Case 2: Boy, 12, suffered elbow trauma but was not seen for 2 months. Posterior dislocation was diagnosed and reduced with the patient under general anesthesia, but the reduction was not recognized as being incomplete. Two months later the child had a stiff elbow and radiographic evidence of anterior calcification. On clinical evaluation a flexion contracture of 90° and maximal flexion of 135° were seen. There was no pronation and supination and the forearm was blocked at 60° of pronation. The patient had partial ulnar nerve palsy, paresthesia of the fourth and fifth fingers, and slight muscular weakness. Proximal radioulnar dislocation was diagnosed radiographically, followed by open reduction. Intraarticular adhesions and scarring were found between the radius and ulna, requiring dissection before reduction of the radial head and olecranon could be performed. Radial head reduction was completed using a lateral approach. The annular ligament was reconstructed using local fibrous tissue. Rehabilitation with flexion-and-extension postural splints and early mobilization increased the patient's range of motion from 0° of extension to 150° of flexion and from 70° of pronation to 145° of supination. Ulnar nerve dysfunction resolved within 1 year. The patient had normal articular congruency with slight growth disturbance of the radial head.

Case 3: Boy, 9, fell on his left elbow and came for treatment of a painful, deformed elbow in 30° of flexion with the forearm in neutral position. Incomplete motor and sensory ulnar nerve paralysis was found. Radiographs demonstrated a proximal radioulnar dislocation, which was managed using closed reduction via longitudinal traction with manual reduction of the radial head. Normal articular congruency was found postoperatively. A long arm cast was used to immobilize the cast in 90° of flexion for 3 weeks. Ulnar nerve paralysis had resolved within 3 months, and the boy had full range of motion after 5 months. However, radiographs revealed a growth disturbance of the radial head and anterior calcifications at final evaluation.

Conclusions.—Minimal deformity accompanies proximal radioulnar translocations, so its diagnosis is often delayed. Restricted supination on physical examination may be the most important clue to its presence. Associated injuries include radial head fractures, radial neck fractures, coronoid process fractures, and ulnar nerve palsy. When the diagnosis is missed, delay in treatment can produce decreased elbow motion and other complications. Although a satisfactory outcome is normally achieved after closed reduction, growth disturbances of the radial head may impair long-term functional results.

▶ In this article, 3 elbow dislocations with proximal radioulnar joint dislocation in children are presented. The authors recommend closed reduction in acute cases. If a concentric reduction cannot be achieved by closed means, open reduction is recommended. Based on their limited experience, they recommend a release of the anterior fibrous scar and interosseous scarring without a formal release of the interosseous ligament. Because of the severe ligamentous injury, ligament repair or reconstruction may be necessary to achieve a stable concentric reduction.

D. A. Zlotolow, MD

Long-Term Results of Radial Head Resection Following Isolated Radial Head Fractures in Patients Younger Than Forty Years Old

Antuña SA, Sánchez-Márquez JM, Barco R (Hospital Universitario La Paz, Madrid, Spain)
J Bone Joint Surg Am 92:558-566, 2010

Background.—In the past, radial head resection was the surgical treatment of choice for radial head fractures that could not be internally fixed. More recently, radial head implant arthroplasty has gained popularity for the treatment of isolated radial head fractures. The purpose of the present study was to review the long-term results of radial head resection after radial head fractures not associated with elbow instability in patients younger than forty years of age.

Methods.—Twenty-six patients younger than forty years of age who had sustained an isolated fracture of the radial head (including six patients who had sustained a Mason type-II fracture and twenty who had sustained a Mason type-III fracture) that had been treated with primary radial head resection were reviewed retrospectively at a minimum of fifteen years (mean, twenty-five years). Outcomes were evaluated according to the Mayo Elbow Performance Score and the Disabilities of the Arm, Shoulder and Hand score. Radiographic assessment of osteoarthritic changes and the carrying angle was also performed.

Results.—Twenty-one patients (81%) had no elbow pain, three had mild pain, and two had moderate pain. The mean arc of motion was from 9° to 139° of flexion. All but one patient had a functional arc of motion. The mean pronation was 84°, and the mean supination was 85°. Nineteen elbows had normal strength in comparison with the unaffected side. The mean Mayo Elbow Performance Score was 95 points; the score was classified as good or excellent for twenty-four elbows (92%) and as fair for two. The mean Disabilities of the Arm, Shoulder and Hand score was 6 points. Three patients complained of wrist pain, which was mild in two patients and moderate in one. In four patients, some degree of elbow instability could be detected on physical examination. The mean carrying angle of the involved elbow was significantly greater than that of the uninjured elbow (21° compared with 10°). Radiographic changes of arthritis were considered mild in seventeen elbows and moderate in nine. We could not detect significant differences in functional outcome on the basis of the degree of radiographic change.

Conclusions.—Radial head resection in young patients with isolated fractures without instability yields long-term satisfactory results in >90% of cases. Osteoarthritic changes are uniformly present but typically are not associated with functional impairment.

▶ There is controversy regarding the long-term outcome of radial head resection for the treatment of radial head fractures. Prior studies have included patients of mixed ages and some of whom had associated elbow or forearm instability. The strengths of this study include the uniform patient population younger than 40 years who had an isolated radial head fracture. This study supports the findings of previous authors who have noted that osteoarthritis is almost uniformly present after radial head resection. However, there was no correlation between the degree of degenerative changes and functional impairment. The patients in this study had an average radial shortening of 3.1 mm on the involved side. Three patients had > 5 mm of shortening, all with radiographic evidence of distal radioulnar arthritis and wrist pain, and one demonstrated instability on clinical examination. Of note, there were no postoperative complications and no patient underwent additional surgery of the elbow or wrist. Thus, this was found to be a remarkably well-tolerated treatment option for the vast majority of patients, with a high rate of patient satisfaction. The authors discuss the fact that others have suggested that internal fixation or arthroplasty, rather than excision, should be considered for the healthy active patient in the presence of a stable elbow or forearm articulation. Reasons to consider this approach include the reported association of radial head resection with delayed complications such as pain, instability, proximal radial translation, decreased strength, osteoarthritis, or cubitus valgus. The authors also note that it is quite possible that some associated ligamentous or articular injuries were missed, and according to van Riet and Morrey, 50% to 75% of patients with types II and III fractures have concomitant pathology.

E. Cheung, MD

Partial Articular Fracture of the Radial Head

Athwal GS, King GJW (Univ of Western Ontario, London, Ontario, Canada)
J Hand Surg Am 35:1679-1680, 2010

Background.—The management of displaced isolated partial articular fractures of the radial head remains controversial. A case was presented and the evidence supporting nonsurgical or surgical approaches was reviewed.

> *Case Report.*—Man, 40, fractured the right radial head after falling onto an outstretched hand. He can flex the elbow from 25° to 130° and has 80° of supination and 80° of pronation with no tenderness at the medial elbow, forearm, or distal radioulnar joint. Radiographs and computed tomograms show a simple partial articular anterolateral radial head fracture involving 40% of the radial head articular surface. There is a 2-mm incongruity.

Evidence.—A nonsurgical approach yielded satisfactory outcomes in 88% of 49 patients with displaced partial articular fractures of the radial head in a study with a 14- to 25-year follow-up. Eighty-two percent of the patients had no subjective complaints, 8 had occasional elbow pain, and 1 had daily pain. The average arc of elbow flexion and extension was slightly less on the injured side than contralaterally, but forearm rotation was comparable. Degenerative changes were significantly more prevalent on the injured side but showed no correlation with pain or motion. Similar findings were noted in 76% of 34 patients with displaced partial articular fracture of the radial head after a mean of 10 years. Comparing nonsurgical management with open reduction and internal fixation in 26 patients with type 2 fractures, 9 of the 10 surgery patients and 7 of the 16 nonsurgical patients had a good or excellent outcome.

Eight patients with Mason type 2 fractures were managed surgically and had mean Mayo elbow scores of 97 out of 100 points a mean of 30 months later. All 8 had good or excellent outcomes. Eleven patients assessed a mean of 9 years postoperatively had good or excellent outcomes. A review of 30 patients an average of 58 months after surgery on Broberg and Morrey modified Mason type 2 fractures revealed 4 of 15 patients with comminuted fractures had an unsatisfactory outcome. However, all 15 of the patients with single fragment fractures had a satisfactory outcome. A mean of 22 years after 16 patients had surgery for an isolated displaced radial head fracture, the mean arc of ulnohumeral motion was significantly less in the injured arm than in the contralateral arm. The mean arc of forearm rotation had a similar limitation in the injured arm. Complications in this series included a deep infection, a superficial infection, a transient posterior interosseous nerve palsy, and the need to remove hardware early because of excessively long screws placed in the proximal radioulnar joint, restricting forearm rotation.

Conclusions.—Displaced fractures are not common and may include associated but undiagnosed ligament injuries. None of the available evidence was gained from randomized prospective or case-control studies that compared nonsurgical and surgical approaches. Further evidence is needed to clearly characterize fracture displacement and develop reliable and validated ways to measure it. For the patient in question, the best available evidence should be summarized and presented to him, along with the information that intraarticular osteotomy, radial head excision, and prosthetic replacement can still be done if nonsurgical treatment does not resolve the problem.

▶ The authors present a concise summary of the literature on the surgical and nonsurgical treatment of Mason type 2 radial head fractures, given the clinical scenario of a 40-year-old male with an isolated radial head fracture with 2-mm intra-articular step-off. The authors conclude that existing evidence consists of retrospective case series and comparative cohorts, with variation in fracture characterization, classification, treatment, follow-up time, and evaluation. There are no randomized prospective or case-control studies comparing surgical with nonsurgical management for this fracture pattern. Long-term retrospective outcome studies have documented generally excellent results for both operative and nonsurgical treatment. Therefore, the patient should be counseled on both treatment options and then allowed to decide. If the patient is undecided, then the authors generally recommend conservative treatment.

E. Cheung, MD

Anatomical plate configuration affects mechanical performance in distal humerus fractures

Penzkofer R, Hungerer S, Wipf F, et al (Trauma Ctr Murnau, Germany; Stryker Trauma AG, Switzerland; et al)
Clin Biomech 25:972-978, 2010

Background.—Because of strong loads acting in the elbow joint, intra-articular fractures with a methaphyseal comminuted fracture site at the distal humerus demand a lot from the osteosynthetic care. Ambiguities arise concerning to the anatomic position of the implants and the resulting mechanic performance. The aim of this biomechanical study was to compare the performance of different anatomical plate configurations for fixation of comminuted distal humerus fractures within one system.

Methods.—In an artificial bone model two perpendicular and one parallel plating configuration of a dedicated elbow plating system were compared with respect to system rigidity (flexion and extension) and dynamic median fatigue limit (extension). The flexion tests were conducted under 75° and the extension tests under 5°. Furthermore, the relative displacements were recorded. As a fracture model an AO C 2.3-fracture on an artificial bone (4th Gen. Sawbone) was simulated via double osteotomy in sagittal and transversal plane.

Findings.—Large differences in mechanical performance were observed between flexion and extension loading modes. In extension the parallel configuration with lateral and medial plates achieved the highest bending stiffness and median fatigue limit. In flexion the highest bending stiffness was reached by the construct with a medial and a postero-lateral plate. Failure of the implant system predominantly occurred at the screw—bone interface or by fatigue of the plate around the screw holes.

Interpretation.—All three plate configurations provided sufficient mechanical stability to allow early postoperative rehabilitation with a reduced loading protocol. Although the individual fracture pattern determines the choice of plate configuration, the parallel configuration with lateral and medial plates revealed biomechanical advantages in extension only.

▶ The authors present a biomechanical study comparing parallel and perpendicular plating techniques for comminuted distal humerus fractures. The biomechanical model includes artificial humeri (sawbones), an unstable AO C2.3 fracture with metaphyseal comminution, and fixation with parallel or perpendicular plating (using a single plating system, VariAx Elbow, Stryker).

The fixation techniques included one with a posteromedial and lateral plate, one with posterolateral and medial plate (PLM), and medial-lateral parallel plating.

Results included higher stiffness in extension for all configurations when compared with flexion. The least gap displacement in flexion was observed in the PLM perpendicular plating, yet this configuration had the greatest gap displacement in extension. The authors concluded that the most stable configuration is parallel plating for forces in extension.

The study does not alter the current knowledge regarding fixation techniques for distal humerus fractures. The model leaves a gap where metaphyseal comminution occurs, which does allow for testing of the model, but does not mimic the clinical situation in which comminution is compressed or the humerus is shortened to gain stability in the construct. The plate system used allows for variable locked fixation utilizing 2 types of titanium, which did show failure at the screw head and plate interface in each construct.

J. Jacobson, MD

New Intramedullary Locking Nail for Olecranon Fracture Fixation—An In Vitro Biomechanical Comparison With Tension Band Wiring
Nowak TE, Burkhart KJ, Mueller LP, et al (Johannes Gutenberg Univ Mainz, Germany)
J Trauma 69:E56-E61, 2010

Background.—The aim of this study was to determine the difference in displacement of a newly designed intramedullary olecranon fracture fixation device compared with multifilament tension band wiring after 4 cycles and 300 cycles of dynamic continuous loading.

Methods.—In eight pairs of fresh-frozen cadaver ulnae, oblique olecranon fractures were created and stabilized using either newly designed intramedullary olecranon nail or multifilament tension band wiring. The specimens were then subjected to continuous dynamic loading (from 25 N to 200 N) using matched pairs of cadaveric upper extremities. The Wilcoxon test was used to determine statistical differences of the displacement in the fracture gap.

Results.—After 4 cycles and 300 cycles, the displacement in the fracture model was significantly higher in the tension band wiring group than in the intramedullary nailing group.

Conclusions.—The newly designed interlocking nailing system showed higher stability in comparison with multifilament tension band wiring after continuous dynamic loading.

▶ The authors present a biomechanical study comparing a new intramedullary locked olecranon nail with tension band wiring with Kirschner wires. The elbow model with oblique fracture was taken through an arc of motion of 0° to 90°, with a maximum force of 200 N applied to the triceps tendon.

Locked intramedullary nail had significantly less fragment displacement when compared with tension band wiring at 0° extension, 45°, and 90° flexion. The maximum displacement for the tension band was 2.2 mm at full extension compared with the intramedullary nail with 0.3-mm displacement.

This biomechanical study shows mechanical advantages of locked intramedullary nail to tension band wiring for oblique simple olecranon fractures. The clinical applicability for other fracture types and cost are unknown. The clinical significance of 2.2-mm displacement during fracture healing is likely minimal. The locked nail may minimize prominent hardware as seen with tension band wiring.

J. Jacobson, MD

Radiation Therapy for Heterotopic Ossification Prophylaxis Acutely After Elbow Trauma: A Prospective Randomized Study

Hamid N, Ashraf N, Bosse MJ, et al (Carolinas Med Ctr, Charlotte, NC; et al)
J Bone Joint Surg Am 92:2032-2038, 2010

Background.—Heterotopic ossification around the elbow can result in pain, loss of motion, and impaired function. We hypothesized that a single dose of radiation therapy could be administered safely and acutely after elbow trauma, could decrease the number of elbows that would require surgical excision of heterotopic ossification, and might improve clinical results.

Methods.—A prospective randomized study was conducted at three medical centers. Patients with an intra-articular distal humeral fracture or a fracture-dislocation of the elbow with proximal radial and/or ulnar fractures were enrolled. Patients were randomized to receive either single-fraction radiation therapy of 700 cGy immediately postoperatively (within seventy-two hours) or nothing (the control group). Clinical and radiographic assessment was performed at six weeks, three months, and six months postoperatively. All adverse events and complications were documented prospectively

Results.—This study was terminated prior to completion because of an unacceptably high number of adverse events reported in the treatment group. Data were available on forty-five of the forty-eight patients enrolled in this study. When the rate of complications was investigated, a significant difference was detected in the frequency of nonunion between the groups. Of the nine patients who had a nonunion, eight were in the treatment group. The nonunion rate was 38% (eight) of twenty-one patients in the treatment group, which was significantly different from the rate of 4% (one) of twenty-four patients in the control group (p = 0.007). There were no significant differences between the groups with regard to the prevalence of heterotopic ossification, postoperative range of motion, or Mayo Elbow Performance Score noted at the time of study termination.

Conclusions.—This study demonstrated that postoperative single-fraction radiation therapy, when used acutely after elbow trauma for prophylaxis against heterotopic ossification, may play a role in increasing the rate of nonunion at the site of the fracture or an olecranon osteotomy. The clinical efficacy of radiation therapy could not be determined on the basis of the sample size. Further research is needed to determine the role of limited-field radiation for prophylaxis against heterotopic ossification after elbow trauma.

▶ This study illustrates how valuable a further review of accepted practice can be. Despite several studies in the literature demonstrating safety and efficacy, this is a larger study than previous reports and has been well structured to limit the weaknesses in the existent literature, which may have resulted in assumptions of efficacy that this report now refutes. This study makes clear that the standard radiation therapy of 700 cGy in the elbow results in unacceptably high rates of nonunion. Although this dose was extrapolated from studies around the hip joint, which demonstrated better inhibition effects when compared with lower doses, it appears now to be too high for regular use in the elbow. The 700 cGy appears to have been chosen as the highest dose that could be given at one time without significant complications and is a much higher dose than the fractionated treatments usually used in other inhibition efforts, as in the treatment of metastatic lesions. This study announces that further studies to examine alternative fractionation protocols are necessary.

M. I. Loebenberg, MD

Reconstruction of Massive Bone Losses of the Elbow with Vascularized Bone Transfers

Cavadas PC, Landin L, Thione A, et al (Clínica Cavadas, Valencia, Spain)
Plast Reconstr Surg 126:964-972, 2010

Background.—Massive bone loss of the elbow in young patients is a complex injury. A series of five cases of massive loss of the elbow joint reconstructed with single or double vascularized bone transfers is reported.

Methods.—Five patients with nonacute massive bone loss of the distal humerus (two cases) or distal humerus and proximal ulna (three cases) were reconstructed with a single (two cases) or double (three cases) microvascular vascularized bone transfer from the iliac crest, the fibula, or the scapula. Collateral ligament reconstruction was performed in a second stage. Follow-up was 1 to 3 years.

Results.—All free flaps survived. There was one septic complication not affecting flap survival. The number of surgical procedures was 3.2 (range, two to five). Active range of motion was 86 degrees (range, 70 to 100 degrees), without significant pain and acceptable lateral stability. Treatment time was 7 to 13 months.

Conclusions.—Vascularized bone transfer can restore the articular gross anatomy in cases of massive destruction of the elbow. Midterm functional results have been favorable in a short series of young patients.

▶ Fortunately, the cases reported in this article are rare. Unfortunately, when they do present, they quickly generate a feeling of deep hopelessness in the treating physicians, because of both the catastrophic damage and the limitations of our own techniques to adequately restore function. In this article, very talented and dedicated surgeons illustrate their own intense efforts to provide some sort of solution to this problem. They present impressive results that have restored some range of motion and significantly improved stability in these elbows. Although it certainly requires multispecialty skills, the reconstructions are imaginative and appear to be admirable innovations. The short-term nature of the follow-up leaves open the question of the durability of this architecture and whether the stability of the joint can be maintained over time. Nonetheless, this article does provide some apparently viable options for these often forsaken cases.

M. I. Loebenberg, MD

Vascularized medial femoral condyle corticoperiosteal flaps for the treatment of recalcitrant humeral nonunions
Kakar S, Duymaz A, Steinmann S, et al (Mayo Clinic, Rochester, MN)
Microsurgery 31:85-92, 2011

Background.—Several methods have been used in the management of humeral nonunions. With the advent of modern microsurgical techniques, vascularized bone grafting is becoming increasingly used to improve local biology. We report our experience in the use of a vascularized corticoperiosteal bone flap from the medial femoral supracondylar region in the treatment of recalcitrant humeral nonunions.

Methods.—A retrospective review was performed of all patients treated with this technique over a 4-year period within our institution. Patient demographics, nonunion characteristics, complications, and long-term outcomes were analyzed.

Results.—Six patients underwent vascularized periosteal graft reconstruction. Prior to this, all had failed an average of three procedures with the length of nonunion ranging from 6 to 68 months. All six nonunions healed by an average of 6.8 months (range 2–12 months). Two patients required additional secondary procedures. Functional outcome improved in all patients as adjudged by disabilities of the arm, shoulder, and hand, Mayo elbow performance, and Constant Murley scores.

Conclusions.—The vascularized medial femoral condyle corticoperiosteal flap provides an additional treatment option for the management of humeral nonunions.

▶ This is a retrospective review of 6 patients treated at a single institution for a humeral nonunion with a vascularized medial femoral condyle corticoperiosteal free tissue transfer. All nonunions healed radiographically at an average of 6.8 months. The bone defect ranged from 8 to 22 mm. The average follow-up was 35 months. The Mayo Clinic Performance Index for the elbow was excellent in all 5 patients, while excellent shoulder function was observed in 3 patients and good and fair shoulder function was present in the other 2 patients.

The authors provide a well-illustrated description of this procedure. Moreover, this procedure is extremely versatile for the short atrophic defect. Often, surgeons are faced with an atrophic humeral nonunion, whereby minimal or no bone defect exists. Free fibular transfer is neither practical nor necessary for the reconstruction of small atrophic humeral defects, but a vascularized transfer of bone is still attractive. The vascularized medial femoral condyle corticoperiosteal free tissue transfer provides a modest portion of vascularized periosteum and bone, which can be contoured around the nonunited humeral shaft.

The challenge with the flap is the diameter of the pedicle: the descending genic-ulate artery. Alternatively, the superomedial geniculate artery, a medial branch of the popliteal artery, can be used. The authors contend that avoiding harvest of the free vascularized fibular transfer prevents notable donor site morbidity. This has not, in my experience, been a deterrent to the use of the free fibular transfer, when appropriate. High donor site morbidity following harvest of the free fibular flap is not generally expected. Complication rates as high as 50% may be seen in series of patients requiring free fibular transfers, but this is generally because of the large bony defects and complicated circumstances seen in patients needing free fibulas and should not be necessarily inferred as a shortcoming of the procedure. Rather, the vascularized medial femoral condyle corticoperiosteal free flap should be considered as another potential successful alternative for the reconstruction of atrophic humeral nonunions having limited or no bony defects.

P. Murray, MD

Dual Plating for Fractures of the Distal Third of the Humeral Shaft
Prasarn ML, Ahn J, Paul O, et al (Orthopaedic Trauma Service at the Hosp for Special Surgery, NY; et al)
J Orthop Trauma 25:57-63, 2011

In this study, we present a novel method for performing dual plating of extra-articular fractures of the distal third of the humerus. Since 2006, we have treated 15 such fractures with dual plates from a single posterior midline incision. In the first part of the study, we provide the surgical protocol we have used in addressing these fractures. In the second part, the charts of these patients were reviewed retrospectively to examine their clinical and radiographic Outcomes. Using this technique, we have achieved an excellent union rate without significant complications while allowing early and aggressive range of motion.

▶ This article discusses the treatment in 15 patients with distal humeral shaft fractures with a dual plating technique. The authors have shown that this tech-nique can be performed safely, with good results.

Several questions remain unanswered after reading this article. Firstly, is operative treatment of these fractures necessary? Only arbitrary criteria exist to determine if surgery is indicated. There is no clear consensus in the literature on whether conservative treatment with functional bracing[1] or operative treat-ment[2] will yield the best clinical results. Some degree of malalignment is common following conservative treatment, but this does not necessarily lead to a functional deficit.[1,2] Radial nerve palsy is a feared complication from open reduction and plate fixation of humerus fractures.[2] If plate fixation is chosen, one should be aware of this potentially devastating complication.

The second, and most pertinent, question that remains unanswered after reading this article is if it is really necessary to use a dual plating technique. The authors of this article have certainly shown that dual plating can lead to excellent results, without a clear additional risk of complications. Rubel et al showed a biomechanical advantage, with dual plating offering stronger fixation over a single posterior plate.[3] However, Levy et al[4] showed results comparable to the article discussed with a single posterolateral plate.

Finally, the authors used demineralized bone graft in most patients. The data do not seem to show an added value of its use, but the numbers are too small to draw any valid conclusions.

In conclusion, the authors have shown a seemingly safe and efficient dual plating technique to fix distal humeral diaphyseal fractures. The first, most lateral plate is used to obtain and maintain anatomic reduction and adds to the stability of the final construct. The second plate offers the larger part of the stability. This article did not prove that 2 plates are necessary for every fracture, and further study is needed to answer this question. The authors have, however, provided an extra option that can be very useful in the treatment of more unstable distal humeral diaphysis fractures.

R. P. van Riet, MD, PhD

References

1. Sarmiento A, Horowitch A, Aboulafia A, Vangsness CT Jr. Functional bracing for comminuted extra-articular fractures of the distal third of the humerus. *J Bone Joint Surg Br.* 1990;72:283-287.
2. Jawa A, McCarty P, Doornberg J, Harris M, Ring D. Extra articular distal-third diaphyseal fractures of the humerus. A comparison of functional bracing and plate fixation. *J Bone Joint Surg Am.* 2006;88:2343-2347.
3. Rubel IF, Kloen P, Campbell D, et al. Open reduction and internal fixation of humeral nonunions: a biomechanical and clinical study. *J Bone Joint Surg Am.* 2002;84-A:1315-1322.
4. Levy JC, Kalandiak SP, Hutson JJ, Zych G. An alternative method of osteosynthesis for distal humeral shaft fractures. *J Orthop Trauma.* 2005;19:43-47.

Biomechanical comparison of interfragmentary compression in transverse fractures of the olecranon
Wilson J, Bajwa A, Kamath V, et al (James Cook Univ Hosp, Middlesbrough, UK)
J Bone Joint Surg [Br] 93-B:245-250, 2011

Compression and absolute stability are important in the management of intra-articular fractures. We compared tension band wiring with plate fixation for the treatment of fractures of the olecranon by measuring compression within the fracture. Identical transverse fractures were created in models of the ulna. Tension band wires were applied to ten fractures and ten were fixed with Acumed plates. Compression was measured using a Tekscan force transducer within the fracture gap. Dynamic testing was carried out by reproducing cyclical contraction of the triceps of 20 N and of the brachialis of 10 N. Both methods were tested on each sample. Paired t-tests compared overall compression and compression at the articular side of the fracture.

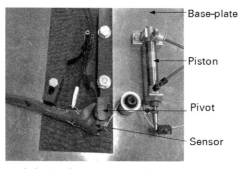

Base–plate

Piston

Pivot

Sensor

FIGURE 1.—Photograph showing the components of the dynamic testing jig with the model ulna and sensor mounted, following tension band wiring fixation. (Reproduced with permission and copyright © of the British Editorial Society of Bone and Joint Surgery, Wilson J, Bajwa A, Kamath V, et al. Biomechanical comparison of interfragmentary compression in transverse fractures of the olecranon. *J Bone Joint Surg [Br]*. 2011;93-B:245-250.)

The mean compression for plating was 819 N (sd 602, 95% confidence interval (CI)) and for tension band wiring was 77 N (sd 19, 95% CI) (p = 0.039). The mean compression on the articular side of the fracture for plating was 343 N (sd 276, 95% CI) and for tension band wiring was 1 N (sd 2, 95% CI) (p = 0.038).

During simulated movements, the mean compression was reduced in both groups, with tension band wiring at -14 N (sd 7) and for plating -173 N (sd 32). No increase in compression on the articular side was detected in the tension band wiring group.

Pre-contoured plates provide significantly greater compression than tension bands in the treatment of transverse fractures of the olecranon, both over the whole fracture and specifically at the articular side of the fracture. In tension band wiring the overall compression was reduced and articular compression remained negligible during simulated contraction of the triceps, challenging the tension band principle (Fig 1).

▶ Tension band wiring has been the gold standard[1] for treating transverse olecranon fractures for a long time. It is cheap, easy, and generally believed to have a low risk of severe complications. Clinical results of tension band wiring are comparable to those of other types of fixation. However, fracture displacement occurs more frequently with tension band wiring than with plate fixation,[2] and protruding hardware, necessitating hardware removal, is common.[3]

Several technical variations of tension band wiring have been described in an effort to improve stability of the construct and to decrease hardware-related problems. The literature concerning these variations has, however, not conclusively proven one technique to be superior over another. Unfortunately, the authors of this study did not clearly specify which configuration was used, but from Fig 1 it seems that bicortical pins were used, with a figure-of-eight configuration of the tension band wire.

This study confirms previous findings from Hutchinson et al, showing that the posterior tension band does not provide compression at the articular surface at the level of the fracture.[4] Perhaps more importantly, this study shows that locking plate fixation does provide compression at both the posterior and the articular side.

One of the questions that remains after reading this interesting article is the necessity of locking plates and screws in fixing olecranon fractures. Locking plates are usually thicker, and a low-profile fixation would certainly be preferable because of the subcutaneous position of the plate. Fixation of olecranon fractures with one-third tubular plates has been shown to be significantly stronger than fixation with tension band wires.[5] Fixation with one-third tubular plates also leads to superior clinical results when compared with tension band wiring.[2] Biomechanically, it has not been shown that locking plates offer an advantage over lower-profile nonlocking plates.[6,7]

Another question that should be studied is the role of relatively newer options, such as low-profile tension band screws and cables and specifically designed olecranon nails. Olecranon nails have also been shown to provide a stronger fixation than tension band wiring,[8,9] and good clinical results were found in up to 93%.[10]

In conclusion, despite the excellent track record of tension band wiring, this and other studies have shown that there is room for improvement. Direct comparison between different techniques of fixation is needed to determine if tension band wiring should indeed be the gold standard. The available literature suggests that plate fixation is stronger and leads to comparable results with a decreased chance of complications.

R. P. van Riet, MD, PhD

References

1. Chalidis BE, Sachinis NC, Samoladas EP, Dimitriou CG, Pournaras JD. Is tension band wiring the "gold standard" for the treatment of olecranon fractures? A long term functional outcome study. *J Orthop Surg Res.* 2008;22:3-9.
2. Hume MC, Wiss DA. Olecranon fractures. A clinical and radiographic comparison of tension band wiring and plate fixation. *Clin Orthop Relat Res.* 1992;285: 229-235.
3. Villanueva P, Osorio F, Commessatti M, Sanchez-Sotelo J. Tension-band wiring for olecranon fractures: analysis of risk factors for failure. *J Shoulder Elbow Surg.* 2006;15:351-356.
4. Hutchinson DT, Horwitz DS, Ha G, Thomas CW, Bachus KN. Cyclic loading of olecranon fracture fixation constructs. *J Bone Joint Surg Am.* 2003;85-A: 831-837.
5. Horner SR, Sadasivan KK, Lipka JM, Saha S. Analysis of mechanical factors affecting fixation of olecranon fractures. *Orthopedics.* 1989;12:1469-1472.
6. Edwards SG, Martin BD, Fu RH, et al. Comparison of olecranon plate fixation in osteoporotic bone: do current technologies make a difference? *J Orthop Trauma.* 2011;25:306-311.
7. Buijze GA, Blankevoort L, Tuijthof GJ, Sierevelt IN, Kloen P. Biomechanical evaluation of fixation of comminuted olecranon fractures: one-third tubular versus locking compression plate. *Arch Orthop Trauma Surg.* 2010;130:459-464.
8. Molloy S, Jasper LE, Elliott DS, Brumback RJ, Belkoff SM. Biomechanical evaluation of intramedullary nail versus tension band fixation for transverse olecranon fractures. *J Orthop Trauma.* 2004;18:170-174.

9. Nowak TE, Mueller LP, Burkhart KJ, Sternstein W, Reuter M, Rommens PM. Dynamic biomechanical analysis of different olecranon fracture fixation devices—tension band wiring versus two intramedullary nail systems: an in-vitro cadaveric study. *Clin Biomech (Bristol, Avon).* 2007;22:658-664.

10. Gehr J, Friedl W. Intramedullary locking compression nail for the treatment of an olecranon fracture. *Oper Orthop Traumatol.* 2006;18:199-213.

Combination of Arthrolysis by Lateral and Medial Approaches and Hinged External Fixation in the Treatment of Stiff Elbow

Liu S, Fan C-Y, Ruan H-J, et al (Shanghai Jiaotong Univ School of Medicine, People's Republic of China)
J Trauma 70:373-376, 2011

Background.—Various methods are available to treat the stiff elbow. However, there is no consensus on which one is most useful. This study involves the effects of combination of arthrolysis by lateral and medial approaches and hinged external fixation in the treatment of stiff elbow.

Patients.—We treated 12 patients with stiff elbows using a combination of arthrolysis by lateral and medial approaches and hinged external fixation. The arthrolysis was applied to the elbow for complete soft-tissue release, and the hinged external fixation mainly for rehabilitation and stability of the elbow after arthrolysis. With the help of the hinged external fixation, nonsurgical treatment including exercises was effectively performed to maintain the stability and the results of arthrolysis. Before surgery, the mean extension was −35 degrees and the mean flexion 70 degrees. One patient had a loss of 70 degrees in pronation.

Results.—Satisfactory follow-up was given to 11 patients with the mean length of 15 month. The mean postoperative extension was −8 degrees whereas flexion 122 degrees. Two of 11 patients had a transient ulnar paresthesia and returned to normal after 8-month follow-up. The loss of pronation in one patient reduced to 30 degrees afterward. There were no complicating infections. All patients reported satisfactory effect.

Conclusion.—The combination of arthrolysis by lateral and medial approaches and hinged external fixation in the treatment of stiff elbow is safe and effective.

▶ This is an interesting study looking at medial and lateral release with an external fixation. The authors did not perform a posterolateral release; they performed only anterolateral, anteromedial, and posteromedial releases. Hinged external fixators were then placed for range of motion. The added time and cost of the hinged fixator is of question because there was no control group to compare against. The authors certainly achieved a great result, but one wonders if exercises and a simple hinged splint would have achieved the same result. There were no significant complications, with no complicating infections. If an extensive release is done and instability occurs, a hinged fixator can maintain postoperative stability, but it would be interesting to see how a similar group of patients would have performed without a fixator.

S. P. Steinman, MD

Failed Distal Biceps Tendon Repair Using a Single-Incision EndoButton Technique and Its Successful Treatment: Case Report
Desai SS, Larkin BJ, Najibi S (Newport Orthopedics Inst, Newport Beach, CA; Henry Ford Health Systems, Detroit, MI; St John's Health Ctr, Santa Monica, CA)
J Hand Surg 35A:1986-1989, 2010

Surgical repair has become a mainstay in the treatment of ruptures of the distal biceps tendon and multiple surgical techniques have been described advocating anatomic or near-anatomic repair. Fixation with an EndoButton technique has been shown to have superior fixation strength and durable clinical outcomes. Here, we describe a case of failed EndoButton fixation of the distal biceps tendon, and its successful treatment.

▶ This case report is useful in that rupture of a distal biceps tendon after Endo-Button repair has not yet been reported. Single-incision approach to distal biceps tendon repairs has gained popularity over the last decade in an effort to minimize the risk of heterotopic ossification with the 2-incision approach. The theoretic disadvantages of single-incision approach, such as radial nerve injury and higher rupture rates, have not been borne out by the literature or in my practice. The improvement in soft tissue to bone fixation techniques has made rerupture very uncommon. One of the reasons I use suture anchor rather than EndoButton fixation for distal biceps tendon repairs is my desire to limit cortical compromise with drill holes in the radial tuberosity region. Anchor pullout failure (which I have not yet seen in this application) is a simple fix, but the authors are fortunate that the patient did not fracture through the drill holes, as this would be a challenge to correct.

T. R. McAdams, MD

Screw fixation of radial head fractures: Compression screw versus lag screw—A biomechanical comparison
Burkhart KJ, Nowak TE, Appelmann P, et al (Johannes Gutenberg-Univ, Langenbeckstraße, Mainz, Germany)
Injury 41:1015-1019, 2010

Introduction.—Secondary loss of reduction and pseudarthrosis due to unstable fixation methods remain challenging problems of surgical stabilisation of radial head fractures. The purpose of our study was to determine whether the 3.0 mm Headless Compression Screw (HCS) provides superior stability to the standard 2.0 mm cortical screw (COS).

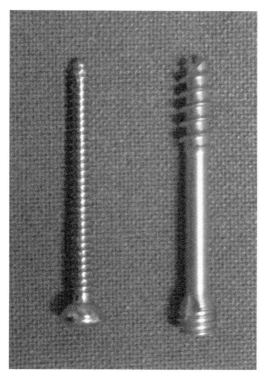

FIGURE 1.—The studied implants—the 2.0 mm cortical screw on the left and the 3.0 mm headless compression screw on the right. (Reprinted from the Injury, International Journal of the Care of the Injured, Burkhart KJ, Nowak TE, Appelmann P, et al. Screw fixation of radial head fractures: compression screw versus lag screw—a biomechanical comparison. *Injury.* 2010;41:1015-1019. Copyright 2010, with permission from Elsevier.)

Materials and Methods.—Eight pairs of fresh frozen human cadaveric proximal radii were used for this paired comparison. A standardised Mason II-Fracture was created with a fragment size of 1/3 of the radial head's articular surface that was then stabilised either with two 3.0 mm HCS (Synthes) or two 2.0 mm COS (Synthes) according to a randomisation protocol. The specimens were then loaded axially and transversely with 100 N each for 4 cycles. Cyclic loading with 1000 cycles as well as failure load tests were performed. The Wilcoxon test was used to assess statistically significant differences between the two groups.

Results.—No statistical differences could be detected between the two fixation methods. Under axial loads the COS showed a displacement of 0.32 mm vs. 0.49 mm for the HCS. Under transverse loads the displacement was 0.25 mm for the COS vs. 0.58 mm for the HCS group. After 1000 cycles of axial loading there were still no significant differences. The failure load for the COS group was 291 N and 282 N for the HCS group.

Conclusion.—No significant differences concerning the stability achieved by 3.0 mm HCS and the 2.0 mm COS could be detected in the experimental setup presented (Fig 1).

▶ The authors have shown that, in their cadaveric model, there is no difference in compression ability between headless compression screws and cortical screws (COS) (Fig 1). However, I strongly feel the headless screws provide a greater advantage over the COS lag technique in the application of fixation of radial head fracture. The prominence of the screw head in the COS may be problematic even when placed in the safe zone. If one tries to countersink the screw head, additional trauma may be imparted to a sometimes very small fragment. The increased cost of the headless screws is justified, in my opinion. Elbow stiffness and mechanical pain are all too common after these seemingly benign Mason II fractures, and every effort should be made to allow early motion after stable fixation with the least amount of risk for impingement or scar formation around a prominent screw head. One must remember that the most important factor in operative repair of displaced Mason II fractures of the radial head, above and beyond the type of screw used, is anatomic reduction of the intra-articular chondral surface. I find the radiocapitellar joint quite unforgiving in this regard.

T. R. McAdams, MD

20 Brachial Plexus

Axillary Nerve Reconstruction in 176 Posttraumatic Plexopathy Patients
Terzis JK, Barmpitsioti A (Eastern Virginia Med School, Norfolk)
Plast Reconstr Surg 125:233-247, 2010

Background.—In posttraumatic brachial plexus palsy, shoulder stabilization is of utmost importance before reanimation of the distal upper extremity. The aim of this study was to present the authors' experience with axillary nerve reconstruction in 148 patients with posttraumatic plexopathy. Functional outcomes were assessed and correlated with the following factors: severity score, denervation time, and donor nerve used.

Methods.—The medical records of 176 patients who underwent axillary nerve reconstruction performed by a single surgeon between 1978 and 2006 were reviewed. The results were analyzed in 148 patients who had adequate follow-up (>24 months). Nerve reconstruction was performed using 94 intraplexus donor nerves and 55 extraplexus donor nerves; axillary-to-axillary repair was performed in 13 patients, and 15 patients had microneurolysis. One hundred forty patients had interposition nerve grafts. A total of 135 patients had concomitant neurotization of the suprascapular nerve.

Results.—Results were good or excellent in 45.95 percent of patients. The intraplexus donors yielded significantly better shoulder function than the extraplexus donors. The length of the nerve graft had a direct influence on deltoid recovery. Patients with a severity score higher than 10 attained significantly better results than patients with multiple root avulsions. Surgery earlier than 4 months yielded significantly better functional outcomes than delayed operation of more than 8 months.

Conclusions.—Early primary axillary nerve reconstruction offers rewarding glenohumeral joint stability and an acceptable range of shoulder function. Concomitant neurotization of the suprascapular nerve yielded improved outcomes in shoulder abduction and external rotation.

▶ This is a well-written article on the outcome of axillary nerve reconstruction in a large number of patients that was performed by one surgeon. This article will be of great help to the brachial plexus surgeons. Though some of the findings in this article have been reported previously, this is one of the largest series of patients with outcomes focused on restoration of shoulder function with a selection of factors that correlated positively or negatively to the outcome. The authors correlated the outcome of nerve reconstruction to the severity score of injury, denervation time, and donor nerve used. They found that surgery performed earlier than 4 months compared with surgery performed after 8 months (early primary axillary nerve reconstruction and intraplexus donor transfers compared with extraplexus donors) yielded significantly better shoulder function. A longer graft influenced the outcome negatively, but patients with higher severity scores attained significantly better results than patients with multiple root avulsions. When suprascapular nerve neurotization was performed, a significant improvement in shoulder abduction and external rotation was observed.

B. Elhassan, MD

Complications of Intercostal Nerve Transfer for Brachial Plexus Reconstruction

Kovachevich R, Kircher MF, Wood CM, et al (Mayo Clinic College of Medicine, Rochester, MN; Mayo Clinic, Rochester, MN)
J Hand Surg 35A:1995-2000, 2010

Purpose.—Although numerous publications discuss outcomes of intercostal nerve transfer for brachial plexus injury, few publications have addressed factors associated with intercostal nerve viability or the impact perioperative nerve transfer complications have on postoperative nerve function. The purposes of this study were to report the results of perioperative intercostal nerve transfer complications and to determine whether chest wall trauma is associated with damaged or nonviable intercostal nerves.

Methods.—All patients who underwent intercostal nerve transfer as part of a brachial plexus reconstruction procedure as a result of injury were identified. A total of 459 nerves in 153 patients were transferred between 1989 and 2007. Most nerves were transferred for use in biceps innervation, free-functioning gracilis muscle innervation, or a combination of the two. Patient demographics, trauma mechanism, associated injuries, intraoperative nerve viability, and perioperative complications were reviewed.

Results.—Complications occurred in 23 of 153 patients. The most common complication was pleural tear during nerve elevation, occurring in 14 of 153 patients. Superficial wound infection occurred in 3 patients, whereas symptomatic pleural effusion, acute respiratory distress syndrome, and seroma formation each occurred in 2 patients. The rate of complications increased with the number of intercostal nerves transferred. Nerves were harvested from previously fractured rib levels in 50 patients. Rib fractures were not associated with an increased risk of overall complications but were associated with an increased risk of lack of nerve viability. In patients with rib fractures, intraoperative nerve stimulation revealed 148 of 161 nerves to be functional; these were subsequently transferred. In patients with preoperative ipsilateral phrenic nerve palsy, the risk of increased complications was marginally significant.

Conclusions.—Brachial plexus reconstruction using intercostal nerves can be challenging, especially if there is antecedent chest wall trauma.

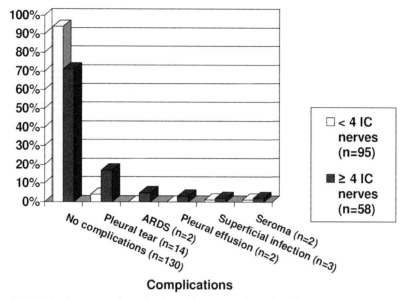

Complications

FIGURE 1.—Occurrence of complications with respect to the number of ICNs harvested. (Reprinted from Kovachevich R, Kircher MF, Wood CM, et al. Complications of intercostal nerve transfer for brachial plexus reconstruction. *J Hand Surg.* 2010;35A:1995-2000. Copyright 2010, with permission from the American Society for Surgery of the Hand.)

Complications were associated with increasing numbers of intercostal nerves transferred. Ipsilateral rib fracture was adversely associated with intercostal nerve viability; it was not significantly associated with complication risk and should not be considered a contraindication to transfer. Preoperative phrenic nerve palsy was marginally associated with the likelihood of complications but not postoperative respiratory dysfunction when associated with intercostal nerve transfer.

Type of Study/Level of Evidence.—Therapeutic IV (Fig 1).

▶ The authors have retrospectively reviewed complications associated with intercostal nerve grafts for reconstruction of patients with brachial plexus palsy. Their experience challenges several previously stated caveats regarding the use of intercostal nerves, including the preoperative presence of ipsilateral phrenic nerve palsy or rib fractures as contraindications. While the authors found that there was a higher incidence of respiratory distress when the phrenic nerve was paralyzed, this increase was not statistically significant. They point out the benefit of intraoperative electrical stimulation of the intercostal nerve to be certain that the nerve has not been damaged as a consequence of rib fractures. This is an important point because these patients have frequently suffered polytrauma, and when seen by us months later for consideration for brachial plexus repair, they may not relate that they had rib fractures or we may not ask this question to the patient. Not mentioned in the abstract was a discussion of how the authors managed pleural tears, the most frequent complication, occurring in 10% of their patients (Fig 1). They elected to insert a chest tube for some days. Since typically only the parietal pleura suffers a rent and not the visceral pleura, there is no real risk for a continuing leak of air. There is no need to remove the rib, and there is a good repairable muscle layer. For these small tears, most surgeons today would insert a small catheter through the rent, close the muscle layers over the interspace, and withdraw the catheter as the anesthesiologist fully expanded the lung. It is rather futile to try to suture a parietal pleural tear. This only serves to enlarge the tear. Over a 20-year experience, no patient of mine has developed a postoperative pneumothorax. The authors do acknowledge that the management of pleural tears is controversial, but I think the controversy relates to large defects rather than the small rents that can complicate intercostal nerve transfers.

V. R. Hentz, MD

Reconstruction of Complete Palsies of the Adult Brachial Plexus by Root Grafting Using Long Grafts and Nerve Transfers to Target Nerves
Bertelli JA, Ghizoni MF (Governador Celso Ramos Hosp, Florianópolis, Brazil; Univ of Southern Santa Catarina (Unisul), Tubarão, Brazil)
J Hand Surg 35A:1640-1646, 2010

Purpose.—We report on the results we obtained with reconstruction for total paralysis of the brachial plexus using long nerve grafts that connect nonavulsed roots to the musculocutaneous and radial nerve. Nerve transfers were performed to restore function of the suprascapular nerve, triceps long head, and pectoralis major muscle.

Methods.—We studied 22 young adults with complete brachial plexus palsy who had surgical repair an average of 5 months after trauma. Nerve grafts connected the C5 root to the musculocutaneous nerve. The C6 root was connected by grafts to the radial nerve. When the C6 root was avulsed, the levator scapulae motor branch was connected by grafts to the triceps long head motor branch. In 13 patients, the platysma motor branch was transferred to the medial pectoralis nerve through a long nerve graft. The suprascapular nerve was repaired through transfer of the accessory nerve. Outcomes were assessed an average of 27 months after surgery, focusing on recovery of muscle strength, categorized using the Medical Research Council scale.

Results.—All but one patient recovered some shoulder abduction, with a mean range of recovered shoulder abduction of 57°. Pectoralis major reinnervation was observed in 9 of the 13. Twenty patients recovered full elbow flexion and achieved at least grade M3 strength. Among the 10 patients in whom the C6 root was grafted to the radial nerve, 4 patients recovered active elbow extension with biceps co-contraction. All patients in whom the levator scapulae nerve was connected to the triceps long head recovered active elbow extension, albeit weak. Double lesions of the musculocutaneous nerve were identified in 4 patients.

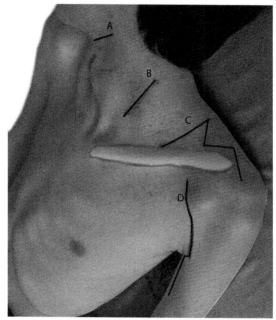

FIGURE 1.—Schematic representation of the skin incisions used to dissect **A** the platysma motor branch, **B** the upper roots of the brachial plexus and the levator scapulae motor branch, **C** the accessory and suprascapular nerves, and **D** the musculocutaneous nerve, radial nerve, and triceps long head motor branch. (Reprinted from Bertelli JA, Ghizoni MF. Reconstruction of complete palsies of the adult brachial plexus by root grafting using long grafts and nerve transfers to target nerves. *J Hand Surg.* 2010;35A:1640-1646. Copyright 2010, with permission from the American Society for Surgery of the Hand.)

Conclusions.—Accessory to suprascapular nerve transfer, levator scapulae nerve transfer to the triceps long head and C5 root grafting to the musculocutaneous nerve is now our preferred method of reconstruction in total palsies of the brachial plexus.

Type of Study/Level of Evidence.—Therapeutic IV (Fig 1).

▶ This article supports the change in the paradigm for treatment of many varieties of brachial plexus injuries in adults. The shift has been away from reconnecting ruptured roots to divisions and/or cords via multiple cable grafts and toward more targeted innervation of specific motor branches, even if this requires very long nerve grafts. Bertelli and Ghizoni have used extraplexal sources of motor axons, such as the nerve to the platysma or to the levator scapulae to try to provide better shoulder and elbow control. The placement of their incisions (Fig 1) is novel. The results of these transfers are less successful than those for restoration of elbow flexion. They have been particularly successful in restoring shoulder abduction (mean abduction was 57°) only by spinal accessory nerve transfer to the suprascapular nerve in these patients who lack glenohumeral stabilizers. I agree with the authors that it remains important to explore the plexus rather than forgoing ruptured roots as a source of motor axons and depending entirely on extraplexal nerve transfers, particularly in patients with global palsies.

V. R. Hentz, MD

21 Elbow: Cubital Tunnel Syndrome and Ulnar Nerve

Endoscopic Cubital Tunnel Release
Cobb TK (Orthopaedic Specialists, Davenport, IA)
J Hand Surg 35A:1690-1697, 2010

A minimally invasive endoscopic approach has been successfully applied to surgical treatment of cubital tunnel syndrome. This procedure allows for smaller incisions with faster recovery time. This article details relevant surgical anatomy, indications, contraindications, surgical technique, complications, and postoperative management.

▶ This review of the surgical technique of endoscopic cubital tunnel release is careful in its elaboration of the dangers and complications of this procedure. Like most minimally invasive procedures, the early literature, presented by the most experienced and talented surgeons, demonstrates similar or better outcomes with less morbidity. In general, I am hesitant to be critical of these new techniques because, in most cases, they tend to become more standard and at least influence the techniques of the more standard approaches. Nonetheless, I am not sure that this has been the experience with minimally invasive nerve surgery, where complications can often be catastrophic in nature. Few patients with elbow injuries are as unhappy as those with sensory neuromas or large nerve injuries. Although this technique can clearly diminish the morbidity of the procedure, I have several remaining questions about the procedure. It seems to me that the subcutaneous dissection in the endoscopic technique is similar to that in open releases, and thus only the skin incision is saved. I am not sure if any release can occur deep to the fascial release of the flexor carpi ulnaris, an area commonly explored. I think that assiduous hemostasis at the end of the procedure is a critical factor in limiting postoperative morbidity, and I am not sure that I fully understand how this is accomplished with limited visualization of the operative field. I think the author's note of caution and his advice that cadaver experience is mandatory reflect my concerns about the danger of this technique in a novice's hands.

M. I. Loebenberg, MD

24 Elbow: Cubital Tunnel Syndrome and Ulnar Nerve

Endoscopic Cubital Tunnel Release

M.J. Loebenberg, MD

22 Shoulder: Anatomy and Instability

Outcome of the Open Bankart Procedure for Shoulder Instability and Development of Osteoarthritis: A 5- to 20-Year Follow-up Study
Ogawa K, Yoshida A, Matsumoto H, et al (Keio Univ, Tokyo, Japan)
Am J Sports Med 38:1549-1557, 2010

Background.—The etiologic factors, time of development, and extent of the progression of postoperative osteoarthritis (OA) in traumatic shoulder instability remain controversial.

Hypothesis.—Most OA seen postoperatively occurs before surgery and progresses very slowly.

Study Design.—Cohort study; Level of evidence, 3.

Methods.—Review of 167 joints of 163 patients undergoing the open Bankart procedure, who had no history of shoulder surgery and were younger than 45 years at follow-up, was done at a mean follow-up of 8.7 years (range, 5-20 years). The shoulders were directly examined and radiographed. A statistical analysis was performed to examine the correlation between OA development/progression and patients' demographic characteristics and various factors, and to evaluate the correlation between these factors.

Results.—Recurrence of instability occurred in 8 of 167 joints (4.8%). Preoperative computed tomography (CT) showed OA in 44 shoulders (26.3%), among which 12 shoulders (7.2%) showed OA on the preoperative radiographs. Consequently, CT-proven OA in the remaining 32 shoulders was incipient OA that was not revealed radiographically. Radiographs taken at follow-up revealed OA in 30 shoulders (18.0%), of which 24 (80%) had had OA proven by preoperative imaging. Preoperative CT-proven OA in 20 shoulders never became visible on postoperative radiographs. The severity of OA slightly increased in 14 joints (32%) during the postoperative period. The number of preoperative subluxations and the total number of preoperative dislocations/subluxations were significantly greater, and the percentages of male patients and glenoid bone defect greater than 20% of the anteroposterior diameter were higher for the 30 shoulders with postoperative OA.

Conclusion.—Most postoperatively detected OA developed before surgery. The preoperative factors are profoundly involved in the development of OA. The role of surgery in favoring the OA development appears to be inconclusive. The development and progression of OA cannot be prevented by surgical intervention, but the progression of postoperative OA is extremely slow.

▶ This article retrospectively examines the long-term outcome of open Bankart repair for shoulder instability in 167 shoulders. Long-term follow-up and examination was performed at a mean of 8.7 years (range, 5-20 years). This article is a follow-up to one published in 2006 and hypothesizes that most osteoarthritis seen in follow-up occurs prior to surgical treatment.

All patients had preoperative radiographs and CT of which 7% and 26% showed mild arthritic changes, respectively. This finding confirms that most preoperative arthritic changes are not easily visualized on routine radiographs. At final follow-up, 30 of the 167 shoulders demonstrated arthritic changes of which 24 had arthritic changes evident on radiographs preoperatively. Arthritis severity had increased in 14 of these shoulders. The presence of postoperative osteoarthritis was predicted by an increasing number of dislocations or subluxations, being male, and glenoid defect greater than 20% of the glenoid.

This is an interesting article that suggests that posttraumatic arthritis is present in many shoulders that later develop postoperative radiographically evident arthritic changes. In this study, the mean time to surgery was 4 years (range, 1-15 years), and mean number of total dislocation/subluxation events prior to surgery was 19.1 (range, 2-156).

The delay in operative treatment from the point of the initial injury to the time of surgery was lengthy in many patients. This article should stimulate further research into the role of early versus delayed operative intervention to prevent the development of arthritic changes in the treatment of shoulder instability.

A. M. Smith, MD

Pathoanatomy of First-Time, Traumatic, Anterior Glenohumeral Subluxation Events

Owens BD, Nelson BJ, Duffey ML, et al (Keller Army Hosp, West Point, NY; Univ of Minnesota, Minneapolis; Pennsylvania State Univ, PA; et al)

J Bone Joint Surg Am 92:1605-1611, 2010

Background.—Relative to dislocations, glenohumeral subluxation events have received little attention in the literature, despite a high incidence in young athletes. The pathoanatomy of first-time, traumatic, anterior subluxation events has not been defined, to our knowledge.

Methods.—As part of a prospective evaluation of all cases of shoulder instability sustained during one academic year in a closed cohort of military academy cadets, a total of thirty-eight first-time, traumatic, anterior glenohumeral subluxation events were documented. Clinical subluxation events were defined as incomplete instability events that did not require a manual reduction maneuver. Twenty-seven of those events were evaluated with plain radiographs and magnetic resonance imaging within two weeks after the injury and constitute the cohort studied. Magnetic resonance imaging studies were independently evaluated by a musculoskeletal radiologist blinded to the clinical history. Arthroscopic findings were available for the fourteen patients who underwent arthroscopic surgery.

Results.—Of the twenty-seven patients who sustained a first-time, traumatic, anterior subluxation, twenty-two were male and five were female, and their mean age was twenty years. Plain radiographs revealed three osseous Bankart lesions and two Hill-Sachs lesions. Magnetic resonance imaging revealed a Bankart lesion in twenty-six of the twenty-seven patients and a Hill-Sachs lesion in twenty-five of the twenty-seven patients. Of the fourteen patients who underwent surgery, thirteen had a Bankart lesion noted during the procedure. Of the thirteen patients who chose nonoperative management, four experienced recurrent instability. Two of the thirteen patients left the academy for nonmedical reasons and were lost to follow-up. The remaining seven patients continued on active-duty service and had not sought care for a recurrent instability event at the time of writing.

Conclusions.—First-time, traumatic, anterior subluxation events result in a high rate of labral and Hill-Sachs lesions. These findings suggest that clinical subluxation events encompass a broad spectrum of incomplete events, including complete separations of the articular surfaces with spontaneous reduction. A high index of suspicion for this injury in young athletes is warranted, and magnetic resonance imaging may reveal a high rate of pathologic changes, suggesting that a complete, transient luxation of the glenohumeral joint has occurred.

▶ The authors review the pathoanatomy of glenohumeral subluxation in 27 military academy cadets. Shoulder subluxation was defined as "incomplete instability events that did not require a manual reduction maneuver." Patients were followed clinically and with radiographs and MRI.

MRI demonstrated a Bankart lesion in 26 of 27 patients and a Hill-Sachs lesion in 25 of 27 patients. Thirteen patients chose nonoperative management of which 2 had recurrent instability. Fourteen patients were treated with operative arthroscopy.

The authors concluded that first time clinically significant subluxation events result in a high rate of labral and Hill-Sachs lesions. The authors further suggest that the high rate of pathoanatomy changes suggest a complete transient dissociation of the humeral head relative to the glenoid fossa and propose that these events be called transient luxation.

This is an interesting article that documents significant pathology in patients with a shoulder instability event that did not require a manual reduction maneuver. I would concur with the authors that a high index of suspicion is necessary to make a conclusive diagnosis. Further research is needed to guide the treatment of these patients.

A. M. Smith, MD

Position and Duration of Immobilization After Primary Anterior Shoulder Dislocation: A Systematic Review and Meta-Analysis of the Literature
Paterson WH, Throckmorton TW, Koester M, et al (Campbell Clinic-Univ of Tennessee Dept of Orthopaedics, Memphis; Slocum Ctr for Orthopedics & Sports Medicine, Eugene, OR; et al)
J Bone Joint Surg Am 92:2924-2933, 2010

Background.—Immobilization after closed reduction has long been the standard treatment for primary anterior dislocation of the shoulder. To determine the optimum duration and position of immobilization to prevent recurrent dislocation, a systematic review of the relevant literature was conducted.

Methods.—Of 2083 published studies that were identified by means of a literature review, nine Level-I and Level-II studies were systematically reviewed. The outcome of interest was recurrent dislocation. Additional calculations were performed by pooling data to identify the ideal length and position (external or internal rotation) of immobilization.

Results.—Six studies (including five Level-I studies and one Level-II study) evaluated the use of immobilization in internal rotation for varying lengths of time. Pooled data analysis of patients younger than thirty years old demonstrated that the rate of recurrent instability was 41% (forty of ninety-seven) in patients who had been immobilized for one week or less and 37% (thirty-four of ninety-three) in patients who had been immobilized for three weeks or longer (p = 0.52). An age of less than thirty years at the time of the index dislocation was significantly predictive of recurrence in most studies. Three studies (including one Level-I and two Level-II studies) compared recurrence rates with immobilization in external and internal rotation. Analysis of the pooled data demonstrated that the rate of recurrence was 40% (twenty-five of sixty-three) for patients managed with conventional sling immobilization in internal rotation and 25% (twenty-two of eighty-eight) for those managed with bracing in external rotation (p = 0.07).

Conclusions.—Analysis of the best available evidence indicates there is no benefit of conventional sling immobilization for longer than one week for the treatment of primary anterior shoulder dislocation in younger patients. An age of less than thirty years at the time of injury is significantly predictive of recurrence. Bracing in external rotation may provide a clinically important benefit over traditional sling immobilization, but the difference in recurrence rates did not achieve significance with the numbers available.

▶ Anterior shoulder instability continues to be an area of significant interest because of its common prevalence and high recurrence rate, especially in younger active patients. Traditionally, first-time anterior dislocations of the shoulder have been treated with a period of immobilization following closed reduction, although the optimal duration and position of such immobilization have recently been called into question. To attempt to answer these important questions, the authors performed a systematic review and meta-analysis of the literature, limited to prospective level I and level II studies dealing with shoulder immobilization in first-time anterior shoulder dislocations.

Of an initial 2083 studies retrieved, 9 articles were identified for detailed review, with the primary outcome end point of interest being recurrent dislocation. Pooled data were examined to strengthen the statistical power of these conclusions, whereby an age of lesser than or greater than 30 years was used as a cutoff for stratification. Six of these studies looked at the use of a sling in internal rotation for varying lengths of time. Pooled data in patients younger than 30 years demonstrated a recurrence rate of 41% in those patients immobilized for 1 week or less versus 37% in those immobilized for 3 weeks or longer ($P = .52$). Three studies examined the effect of immobilization in external rotation versus internal rotation, in which pooled data again demonstrated a recurrence rate of 40% for internal rotation versus 25% for those braced in external rotation ($P = .07$). Age less than 30 years at the time of index dislocation was significantly predictive of recurrence in most studies.

The authors concluded that there is no demonstrable benefit to sling immobilization for more than 1 week in younger patients and have confirmed that younger age was indeed predictive of recurrent dislocation, as has been previously well documented. Although the rates of recurrent instability in patients immobilized in internal versus external rotation did not show a statistically significant benefit, they did observe a 15% lower risk of recurrence in those patients immobilized in external rotation. They concluded, however, that based on the best currently available evidence, they could not recommend external rotation immobilization for first-time anterior dislocations.

Several limitations are apparent in the present study. Pooled data were limited to only 2 studies in each case, patient populations were not completely homogeneous, and patients were treated with different postinjury rehabilitation protocols, all of which may have ultimately influenced the rate of recurrence. The major limitation of this analysis, however, is that the pooled data evaluated were from a best case scenario and only included patients who were completely compliant with the external rotation immobilization protocol. The greatest difficulty we have experienced in our own patient population with attempted treatment in this manner is a lack of strict compliance with an external rotation protocol, calling into question the external validity of these conclusions. However, given the high rate of recurrence, particularly in younger patients, any reduction of recurrence risk may be of clinical importance. Despite these limitations, this remains an area that deserves further scrutiny and attention to determine if there is indeed a subset of the population that may benefit from these interventions.

J. T. Bravman, MD

L. S. Oh, MD

Recurrent Shoulder Instability: Current Concepts for Evaluation and Management of Glenoid Bone Loss

Provencher MT, Bhatia S, Ghodadra NS, et al (Naval Med Ctr San Diego, CA; Rush Univ Med Ctr, Chicago, IL)
J Bone Joint Surg Am 92:133-151, 2010

Background.—The most common cause of recurrent instability of the glenohumeral joint is a Bankart tear, which is a soft tissue injury of the glenoid labrum attachment. Often osseous injury of the glenoid and humeral head is also found. The integrity of the osseous architecture of the glenoid is a vital component in the success of surgical repair. Glenoid bone deficiency with recurrent shoulder instability is a recognized cause of failed shoulder stabilization surgery. All patients with recurrent shoulder instability should be assessed for the presence of osseous injuries to the glenoid. This includes obtaining a complete history, performing a thorough physical examination, and diagnosing and quantifying any anterior glenoid deficiency. Appropriate preoperative imaging is essential for detecting and quantifying osseous abnormalities in patients with recurrent shoulder stability. The surgical approach can then be determined. The principles guiding surgical management include the extent of osseous deficiencies, consideration of the combined glenoid and humeral bone defects, the surgeon's personal experience with specific reconstructive techniques, and patient-specific factors such as work and athletic demands. Techniques for soft-tissue stabilization, type and orientation of the glenoid bone graft, and treatment of accompanying pathologic conditions must be considered to obtain a well-functioning shoulder joint after repair.

Diagnosis.—Patients must provide a thorough orthopedic history. Glenoid bone loss should be suspected when the patient suffered a high-energy injury, especially if the arm was abducted 70° or more and extended 30° or more when initially dislocated. Shoulder instability that occurs within the range of 20° to 60° of abduction is also indicative of glenoid bone loss. Patients may report that it is gradually easier to subluxate the glenohumeral joint and report a long history of shoulder instability or coping with instability. Other shoulder disorders must also be considered.

The physical examination should compare the affected shoulder with the contralateral shoulder to confirm instability and identify other shoulder disorders. The shoulder is visually inspected to identify deformity, rotator cuff atrophy, or scapular dyskinesia. A careful neurovascular evaluation of the entire upper extremity, testing of active and passive shoulder motion, and assessment of rotator cuff strengths are part of this complete physical examination. Special maneuvers such as the Jobe relocation test, sulcus sign, Gagey hyperabduction sign, and apprehension sign can be useful. The shoulder apprehension is done in various degrees of shoulder abduction and external rotation. Normally patients with glenoid bone loss have a positive apprehension test in 90° of shoulder abduction and 90° of external rotation, but patients with apprehension findings in 30° to 90° of shoulder abduction and in lesser external rotation may also have bone loss. Other assessments include anterior translation of the humeral head over the glenoid rim, which, when strongly positive, may indicate glenoid bone loss is likely and should be investigated with advanced imaging studies.

In addition to basic radiographic views of the shoulder, specialized glenoid views in which the radiographic beam is angled oblique to the glenoid face may find osseous glenoid rim lesions. The West Point view, Didiée view, and the special oblique (Garth) view are the most useful radiographic views. Two-dimensional computed tomography (CT) and magnetic resonance imaging (MRI) may be helpful in detecting glenoid bone loss and newly formed glenoid rim fragments but can be inadequate for quantifying bone loss. A three-dimensional CT scan is the gold standard for glenoid imaging because it permits digital subtraction of the humeral head from images of the glenohumeral complex. It provides the most information about the extent and magnitude of glenoid bone loss and about the type of glenoid bone injury or loss.

Glenoid bone loss has been classified radiographically as type I, a displaced avulsion fracture with an attached capsule; type II, a medially displaced fragment malunited to the glenoid rim; and type III, an erosion of the glenoid rim. In type III lesions the bone loss can be less (type IIIA) or greater (type IIIB) than 25%. Three-dimensional CT scans can better define the amount of loss. Arthroscopic quantification of glenoid bone loss use the glenoid bare spot method, found to be the most accurate way to quantify Bankart lesions that occur parallel to the long axis of the glenoid. Rim defects occurring at a 45° angle to the long axis of the glenoid can be overestimated using this method, but occur infrequently. To circumvent problems associated with the glenoid bare spot method, the secant chord theory-n-based method was developed. Studies show that a relatively small amount of bone loss can be clinically relevant. Considering the glenoid in 5% increments, each 5% increment comprises about 1.5 to 2.0 mm of bone.

Treatment.—The most important factors determining treatment selection are degree of glenoid bone injury or loss, patient expectations, and the anticipated postoperative activity level. Nonsurgical treatment is appropriate for patients with less than 20% glenoid bone loss who have low activity demands, are sedentary, or are older; those who are high surgical risks; and those with a history of voluntary glenohumeral dislocation. When nonoperative approaches fail or the patient is highly active and has glenoid osseous deficiency, surgical repair is usually needed. When considering future surgical treatment in cases where a previous surgical repair failed to address shoulder instability and there is recurrent instability, glenoid bone loss must be ruled out.

Arthroscopic repair is often sufficient for patients with 0% to 20% (even up to 25%) glenoid bone loss. Patients with 15% o 25% glenoid bone loss may also benefit from arthroscopic techniques but require a cautious approach because of the possibility of instability-related failure. Sound osseous fragment fixation is imperative. Open capsulolabral repair is the gold standard in these cases. Bone augmentation techniques may be needed if the osseous Bankart fragment has partially or fully resorbed. Patient expectations and desires are an important component in managing glenoid bone loss.

Patients with more than 20% to 25% bone loss require open bone augmentation procedures such as the Latarjet, iliac crest bone-grafting, or allograft technique to reconstitute the glenoid osseous arc. Excellent results in terms of shoulder stability and function have been obtained with transfer of the coracoid. Other bone graft options, such as autogenous iliac crest graft and various frozen and fresh osteochondral allografts, have also been described. Future developments include allografts such as the distal tibial allograft technique and arthroscopic glenoid bone grafting.

Concomitant Pathologic Conditions.—Patients must be thoroughly evaluated for the presence of concomitant shoulder disorders before any surgery is begun. MRI or magnetic resonance arthrography (MRA) can identify injuries such as glenoid labrum articular disruptions (GLAD lesions), anterior labral periosteal sleeve avulsions (ALPSA lesions), and humeral avulsions of the glenohumeral ligaments (HAGL lesions).

Conclusions.—The diagnosis and management of glenoid bone loss in patients with recurrent shoulder instability are evolving. Glenoid bone loss is likely to be present in patients with a history of instability, multiple dislocations, progressively easier dislocation, and humeral head engagement symptoms. Radiographic studies can confirm and evaluate glenoid bone loss, with three-dimensional reformatted CT being the most accurate approach. Several procedures are available, depending on the extent of bone loss, surgeon preferences, and patient activity level, among other factors.

▶ To evaluate glenoid bone loss in the context of recurrent shoulder instability, specialized glenoid views are useful: West Point view, Didiée view, and apical oblique (Garth) view. A 3-dimensional CT is considered the gold standard for glenoid imaging. Usually, the inferior aspect of the glenoid is modelized as a true circle on an en face view with the center at the glenoid bare spot. The amount of glenoid bone loss can be calculated by a digital surface area calculation that determines the amount of glenoid bone loss on the basis of the amount of glenoid surface area that is involved. Another technique is to calculate the distance from the bare spot to the anterior edge of the lesion and to divide this distance by the radius of the circle (d/R). The length of the osseous lesion has also been described as an important marker of glenohumeral stability. If the length (x) is greater than half of the widest anteroposterior diameter (R), the resistance to recurrent shoulder dislocation is ≤70% of that of an intact glenohumeral joint. Finally, the distance from the bare spot to the anterior rim (A) and from the bare spot to the posterior rim (B) can be measured; percent bone loss is calculated as ($[B - A]/2B$) × 100%. Same measures can be performed arthroscopically, but the glenoid bare spot is not identifiable in all shoulders. A 25% glenoid bone injury or loss comprises about 6 to 8 mm of the glenoid.

This underscores the finding that only a relatively small amount of bone loss is required for clinical relevance.

In patients with 0% to 20% of glenoid bone loss, it may be possible to treat the instability successfully with arthroscopic repair. Patients with between 15% and 25% glenoid bone loss may still be treated with arthroscopic techniques, but instability-rated failure has been associated with this amount of glenoid bone loss. If the osseous Bankart fragment has resorbed, bone augmentation techniques may be needed. In patients with greater than 20% to 25% bone loss, open bone augmentation procedure should be considered. The different techniques have been discussed.

P. Mansat, MD, PhD

Reduction of Acute Anterior Dislocations: A Prospective Randomized Study Comparing a New Technique with the Hippocratic and Kocher Methods
Sayegh FE, Kenanidis EI, Papavasiliou KA, et al ("Papageorgiou" General Hosp, Nea Efkarpia, Thessaloniki, Greece)
J Bone Joint Surg Am 91:2775-2782, 2009

Background.—There are several methods to reduce anterior shoulder dislocations, but few studies have compared the efficacy, safety, and reliability of the different techniques. As a result, deciding which technique to use is seldom based on objective criteria. The aim of the present study was to introduce a new method to reduce an anterior shoulder dislocation, which we have termed "FARES" (Fast, Reliable, and Safe), and to compare it with the Hippocratic and Kocher methods in terms of efficacy, safety, and the intensity of pain felt by the patient during reduction.

Methods.—Between September 2006 and June 2008, a total of 173 patients with an acute anterior shoulder dislocation (with or without a fracture of the greater tuberosity) were enrolled in the study. One hundred and fifty-four patients, who met all inclusion criteria, were randomly assigned to one of the three study groups (FARES, Hippocratic, and Kocher) and underwent reduction of the dislocation by first or second-year orthopaedic surgery residents. A visual analog scale was used to determine the intensity of the pain felt by the patient during reduction.

Results.—Demographically, the groups were comparable in terms of age, male:female ratio, the mechanism of dislocation, and the mean time between the injury and the first attempt at reduction. Reduction was achieved with the FARES method in 88.7% of the patients, with the Hippocratic method in 72.5%, and with the Kocher method in 68%. This difference was significant, in favor of the FARES method (p = 0.033). The mean duration of the reduction maneuver was significantly shorter for the FARES method (2.36 ± 1.24 minutes for the FARES method, 5.55 ± 1.58 minutes for the Hippocratic method, and 4.32 ± 2.12 minutes for the Kocher method; p < 0.001), and the mean visual analog pain score was significantly lower for the FARES method

(1.57 ± 1.43 for the FARES method, 4.88 ± 2.17 for the Hippocratic method, and 5.44 ± 1.92 for the Kocher method; p < 0.001). No complications were noted in any group.

Conclusions.—The FARES method is a significantly more effective, faster, and less painful method of reduction of an anterior shoulder dislocation in comparison with the Hippocratic and Kocher methods. It is easily performed by only one physician, it is applicable to anterior shoulder dislocations as well as simple fracture-dislocations, and its use is associated with no more morbidity than that associated with the other two methods.

► In this level I study the authors wanted to evaluate their personal method of reduction of traumatic anterior shoulder dislocation with or without greater tuberosity fracture (fast, reliable, and safe [FARES] method). One hundred fifty-four patients were included in the study. Patients were randomized in 3 groups according to the method of reduction: the FARES technique, the Hippocratic technique, and the Kocher technique. Objectives of the study were to evaluate the efficiency of the different technique of reduction and the level of pain induced by these methods without the use of analgesic or sedation.

In the FARES method, the shoulder dislocation is reduced; the physician holds the patient's hand while the arm is at the side, the elbow is extended, and the forearm is in neutral rotation; the physician gently applies longitudinal traction and slowly moves the arm into abduction; past 90° of abduction, the arm is gently externally rotated while abduction and the vertical oscillation to relax the muscles were continued. Reduction is usually achieved at around 120° of abduction; once reduction was achieved, the arm was gently internally rotated to bring the forearm to lie across the chest. No sedation or analgesics are used.

In the Hippocratic method, an assistant exerted countertraction by holding a sheet wrapped around the patient's chest and under the patient's axilla.

The Kocher method is performed with the elbow flexed and the arm pressed against the side of the body; the forearm is slowly rotated outward until resistance is felt, and then it was lifted forward in the sagittal plane as far as possible; reduction is achieved by internally rotating the arm.

The FARES method was used for 53 patients, the Hippocratic method for 51 patients, and the Kocher method for 50 patients. The FARES method was more efficient in reducing the shoulder dislocation compared with the 2 other methods (P = .033), faster (P < .001), and less painful (P < .001).

This study shows that the FARES method is a valuable technique to reduce traumatic anterior shoulder dislocation, accessible to first- or second-year orthopedic surgery residents. However, we do not know the intra-articular morbidity of these 3 methods of joint reduction without anesthesia, which could impair the prognosis of these dislocations.

P. Mansat, MD, PhD

23 Shoulder: Arthroplasty

A multicentre study of the long-term results of using a flat-back polyethylene glenoid component in shoulder replacement for primary osteoarthritis
Young A, Walch G, Boileau P, et al (European Multicentre Study, Nice, France)
J Bone Joint Surg [Br] 93-B:210-216, 2011

We report the long-term clinical and radiological outcomes of the Aequalis total shoulder replacement with a cemented all-polyethylene flat-back keeled glenoid component implanted for primary osteoarthritis between 1991 and 2003 in nine European centres. A total of 226 shoulders in 210 patients were retrospectively reviewed at a mean of 122.7 months (61 to 219) or at revision. Clinical outcome was assessed using the Constant score, patient satisfaction score and range of movement. Kaplan-Meier survivorship analysis was performed with glenoid revision for loosening and radiological glenoid loosening (SD) as endpoints. The Constant score was found to improve from a mean of 26.8 (SD 10.3) preoperatively to 57.6 (SD 20.0) post-operatively (p < 0.001). Active forward flexion improved from a mean of 85.3° (SD 27.4) pre-operatively to 125° (SD 37.3) post-operatively (p < 0.001). External rotation improved from a mean of 7° (SD 6.5) pre-operatively to 30.3° (SD 21.8°) post-operatively (p < 0.001). Survivorship with revision of the glenoid component as the endpoint was 99.1% at five years, 94.5% at ten years and 79.4% at 15 years. Survivorship with radiological loosening as the endpoint was 99.1% at five years, 80.3% at ten years and 33.6% at 15 years.

Younger patient age and the curettage technique for glenoid preparation correlated with loosening. The rate of glenoid revision and radiological loosening increased with duration of follow-up, but not until a follow-up of five years. Therefore, we recommend that future studies reporting radiological outcomes of new glenoid designs should report follow-up of at least five to ten years.

▶ This study is a retrospective case series with level IV evidence of patients who underwent total shoulder arthroplasty (TSA) with an all-polyethylene flat-back glenoid component between 1991 and 2003. Some of the authors had previously reported results of TSA with the same glenoid component, but with shorter follow-up, in 2003. In that earlier study, with a mean follow-up of 44 months, an 11.5% rate of radiologic loosening and a 1.3% rate of revision were reported. In this study, with a mean follow-up of 122.7 months, a 45.6% rate of radiologic loosening and a 9.1% rate of revision were reported. All patients received a third-generation humeral component with a cemented keeled flat-back glenoid component implanted either by bone-sacrificing curettage (62.4%) or bone-sparing compaction of the glenoid bone. Outcomes included Constant score, subjective shoulder value, and radiographic evaluation for radiolucency. The mean Constant score improved from 26.8 to 57.6. The survivorship of the glenoid component was 99.1% at 5 years, 94.5% at 10 years, and 79.4% at 15 years. A significant increase in the rate of revision for glenoid loosening occurred between 5 and 10 years. Glenoid revision was significantly associated with a younger age at the time of surgery (60.4 vs 66.9 years). Radiolucency surrounding the glenoid component was associated with cementing technique, as the compaction technique showed a decreased occurrence of definite radiologic loosening (31% vs 54.9%). Similarly, the presence of loosening was associated with a significant decrease in clinical outcome scores.

Strengths of this study include long-term follow-up (10-15 years), multicenter involvement, a validated shoulder and elbow outcome score (Constant score), and a large homogenous patient population (263 shoulders with primary osteoarthritis). Limitations include variations in surgical technique and data collection between centers, the inclusion of 38 patients with either partial or full thickness supraspinatus rotator cuff tears, and selection bias because of its retrospective design. This study is further evidence against the use of a flat-back glenoid component design, which has an unacceptably high rate of revision due to loosening. The authors correctly conclude that loosening of the glenoid continues to be the main problem affecting the longevity of TSA.

J. M. Wiater, MD

Thermal Effects of Glenoid Reaming During Shoulder Arthroplasty in Vivo
Olson S, Clinton JM, Working Z, et al (Univ of Washington Med Ctr, Seattle)
J Bone Joint Surg Am 93:11-19, 2011

Background.—Glenoid component loosening is a common cause of failure of total shoulder arthroplasty. It has been proposed that the heat generated during glenoid preparation may reach temperatures capable of producing osteonecrosis at the bone-implant interface. We hypothesized that temperatures sufficient to induce thermal necrosis can be produced with routine drilling and reaming during glenoid preparation for shoulder arthroplasty in vivo. Furthermore, we hypothesized that irrigation of the glenoid during reaming can reduce this temperature increase.

Methods.—Real-time, high-definition, infrared thermal video imaging was used to determine the temperatures produced by drilling and reaming during glenoid preparation in ten consecutive patients undergoing total shoulder arthroplasty. The maximum temperature and the duration of temperatures greater than the established thresholds for thermal necrosis were documented. The first five arthroplasties were performed without irrigation and were compared with the second five arthroplasties, in which continuous bulb irrigation was used during drilling and reaming. A one-dimensional finite element model was developed to estimate the depth of penetration of critical temperatures into the bone of the glenoid on the basis of recorded surface temperatures.

Results.—Our first hypothesis was supported by the recording of maximum surface temperatures above the 56°C threshold during reaming in four of the five arthroplasties done without irrigation and during drilling in two of the five arthroplasties without irrigation. The estimated depth of penetration of the critical temperature (56°C) to produce instantaneous osteonecrosis was beyond 1 mm (range, 1.97 to 5.12 mm) in four of these patients during reaming and one of these patients during drilling, and two had estimated temperatures above 56°C at 3 mm. Our second hypothesis was supported by the observation that, in the group receiving irrigation, the temperature exceeded the critical threshold in only one specimen during reaming and in two during drilling. The estimated depth of penetration for the critical temperature (56°C) did not reach a depth of 1 mm in any of these patients (range, 0.07 to 0.19 mm).

Conclusions.—Temperatures sufficient to induce thermal necrosis of glenoid bone can be generated by glenoid preparation in shoulder arthroplasty in vivo. Frequent irrigation may be effective in preventing temperatures from reaching the threshold for bone necrosis during glenoid preparation.

▶ The authors of this article present a study in support of a simple solution to a technical concern in glenohumeral arthroplasty. Although the authors do not suggest that glenoid loosening or lucent radiographic lines are because of thermal osteonecrosis related to reaming, the solution they suggest is so easy that it should adapted by all, even if its clinical value remains hypothetical. I think this article could have added to its value with a clearer explanation of their reaming technique. Further studies might be helpful to see whether interval reaming generates less heat than continuous reaming, whether reaming pressure affects temperatures, and to what degree bone quality plays in the increased temperatures associated with reaming.

In addition, when a glenoid is implanted, the increased bone temperatures seen in reaming are invariably followed by the much higher and longer increased temperatures associated with the polymerization of cement. Does this mean that the reaming temperatures are not clinically significant, or is it a double hit that should be avoided? Either way, this simple technique should be quickly adopted by all.

M. I. Loebenberg, MD

24 Shoulder: Arthroscopy

Magnetic resonance arthrography of the shoulder: accuracy of gadolinium versus saline for rotator cuff and labral pathology
Helms CA, McGonegle SJ, Vinson EN, et al (Duke Univ Med Ctr, Durham, NC)
Skeletal Radiol 40:197-203, 2011

Objective.—The purpose of this study was to evaluate the necessity of intra-articular gadolinium versus saline alone in magnetic resonance arthrography (MRA) of the shoulder.

Materials and Methods.—Our database was reviewed for 100 consecutive shoulder MRA examinations performed between January 2007 and December 2007. Patient information was blinded and images were retrospectively reviewed by at least two radiologists with dedicated musculoskeletal training. T2-weighted (T2W) images were initially analyzed in isolation to simulate MRA with saline alone. After a delay, the full study was analyzed including T1-weighted (T1W) and T2W images. If there was a significant discordance between the two analyses with regard to rotator cuff or labral pathology, the study was again reviewed by all evaluators in consensus to determine if the T1W images offered additional diagnostic information and increased diagnostic confidence.

Results.—Of the 100 MRA examinations, there were 15 discordant cases. Two cases were discordant with regard to rotator cuff pathology and 13 were discordant on the basis of labral pathology. When the discordant cases were reviewed in consensus, the T2W images appeared to display rotator cuff and labral pathology as definitively as the T1W images. Interobserver and intraobserver variability was favored to have played a role in causing the discordances.

Conclusions.—MRA of the shoulder performed with joint distention provided by saline alone appears to offer equivalent diagnostic information to MRA performed with gadolinium enhancement. This protocol modification improves efficiency by eliminating several image series and provides a small cost savings by eliminating gadolinium.

▶ Probably the most valuable information from this article is the methodology; the authors used a clever design using isolated T2-weighted (T2W) image analysis after infusion of gadolinium to simulate saline-only magnetic resonance arthrography (MRA). This way they evaluated the T2W images first (simulating saline MRA) and then, the full study with T1-weighted (T1W) and T2W images. They then compared both readings in order to identify discrepancies. This approach allowed elimination of interpatient variability, avoided the infusion of different fluids (saline and gadolinium) on different patient groups, and allowed an easy identification of an adequate sample (a consecutive series of 100 MRA).

The authors found 15 discrepancies and concluded that such discrepancies were attributable to interobserver variations since, when viewed together, no difference could be seen between the T1W and the T2W images. They concluded that the improved accuracy of MRA compared with conventional MRI was primarily because of adequate joint distention and the improved intra-articular contrast resolution offered by intra-articular fluid, not necessarily intra-articular gadolinium. T1W images offered no additional information and could therefore be eliminated from studies, shortening the image time. Gadolinium could be also eliminated from the studies and replaced by saline.

The study could not verify the findings with surgical information, was retrospective in nature, and did not take into account the possible additional information that T1W MRA could give to other specialists (as surgeons in preoperative planning). Real saline was not used; saline has been found to provide lower quality images by some authors,[1] so the conclusions of this article should be taken cautiously. Lesions other than rotator cuff and labral pathology were not tested (ie, bony deficiencies associated with instability, usually studied with other image tests that could be with a complete MRA image set). Whereas MRA has superior sensitivity on the diagnosis of specific rotator cuff and labral injuries,[2] image interpretation is influenced by the experience of the reader.[3] Discrepancies found on the article could be because of image interpretation variations as the authors concluded by consensus, but this consensus could be somewhat biased by the more experienced radiologists during the consensus session.

A. M. Foruria, MD, PhD

References

1. Zanetti M, Hodler J. Contrast media in MR arthrography of the glenohumeral joint: intra-articular gadopentetate vs saline: preliminary results. *Eur Radiol.* 1997;7:498-502.
2. Magee T. 3-T MRI of the shoulder: is MR arthrography necessary? *AJR Am J Roentgenol.* 2009;192:86-92.
3. Theodoropoulos JS, Andreisek G, Harvey EJ, Wolin P. Magnetic resonance imaging and magnetic resonance arthrography of the shoulder: dependence on the level of training of the performing radiologist for diagnostic accuracy. *Skeletal Radiol.* 2010;39:661-667.

Percutaneous SLAP Lesion Repair Technique Is an Effective Alternative to Portal of Wilmington

Galano GJ, Ahmad CS, Bigliani L, et al (Columbia Univ, NY)

Orthopedics 33:803, 2010

Athletes with superior labral tear from anterior to posterior (SLAP) lesions place large demands on their rotator cuff and often have partial articular-sided rotator cuff tears as part of an internal impingement process. A percutaneous technique that facilitates SLAP repair may decrease the rotator cuff morbidity associated with establishment of the standard Wilmington portal. The current study reports the clinical outcome of patients with SLAP lesions treated with a percutaneous repair technique. Twenty-two patients with SLAP lesions underwent percutaneous repair. Mean patient age was 26.9 years. Standard posterior viewing and anterior working portals were used. Anchor placement and suture passing were performed with a 3-mm percutaneous and transtendinous approach to the superior labrum. Knot tying was performed via the standard anterior working portal. Clinical outcomes were assessed with validated shoulder evaluation instruments. Mean follow-up was 31.1 months (± 6.6 months). Improvement of shoulder evaluation scores from pre- to postoperative were as follows: American Shoulder and Elbow Surgeons score improved from 49.5 to 83.6, visual analog scale improved from 5.4 to 1.5, and Simple Shoulder Score improved from 6.4 to 11.0. All were significant improvements ($P<.05$). There was no significant difference in functional scores between Type II lesions versus combined lesions, or between patients with or without a concurrent low-grade rotator cuff tear. Ninety percent of athletes were able to return to sport at pre-injury level of function. Percutaneously-assisted arthroscopic SLAP lesion repair may minimize surgical morbidity to the rotator cuff and provides excellent results.

▶ Superior labral tear from anterior to posterior (SLAP) lesions and their treatment have been a topic of recent increased attention in shoulder arthroscopy. The current best recommendation for treatment of unstable type II SLAP tears is surgical fixation; however, there exists considerable debate regarding what indeed constitutes a true SLAP tear, what type of surgical intervention is most appropriate, and how these decisions should be altered based on age and/or concomitant pathology. When the decision for surgical fixation of a SLAP lesion has been made, it has been well described and accepted that a superior transrotator cuff portal (either situated more posterior, coined the Port of Wilmington, or more anterior, coined the accessory transrotator cuff portal) aids in technical execution of this procedure. Attention has been recently drawn to potential direct adverse effects of creating a transrotator cuff portal through which a cannula is inserted. A solution to avoid such complications has been proposed by way of a percutaneous technique for anchor insertion and suture passage without the use of a cannula during transrotator cuff instrumentation.

This article reports the clinical outcomes of a cohort of patients treated with this technique, where the authors hypothesized that results would be as good or better than those demonstrated with a more traditional transrotator cuff portal with respect to validated shoulder measures and return to sport. Twenty-two patients were included for analysis with a mean age of 27 years and average follow-up of 31 months. They reported statistically significant improvements in all outcome measures (American Shoulder and Elbow Surgeons, visual analog scale, and Simple Shoulder Test), with 90% of patients able to return to their prior level of sport. There was no deterioration of results or significant difference in outcomes based on the configuration of the SLAP tear or in those patients (6 of 22) with a concomitantly debrided partial-thickness undersurface rotator cuff tear.

Although this technique has been reported previously, this is the first study that has reported validated outcome measures with significant follow-up using the technique. For this, the authors should be applauded. However, there are several limitations of this study, which the authors are extremely forthright in discussing. This is a small cohort of patients without homogeneous pathology that were followed for a relatively short period. Additionally, no direct comparison was made to a control group, nor to a historical control group to compare the actual values of the validated measures collected regarding outcomes. Lastly, no postoperative imaging or second look was performed. Thus, it remains unknown whether the rotator cuff defect created, although certainly smaller than that created with a traditional portal, has been reported with the more traditional Port of Wilmington technique. A prospective randomized study will ultimately be required to address whether there is indeed superiority of this percutaneous technique over a traditional Port of Wilmington technique. However, the article clearly demonstrates that this is a valuable technique capable of producing significant improvement in outcome measures and sheds light on an issue that deserves increased attention and awareness as we move forward in treating this complex pathology.

J. T. Bravman, MD

L. S. Oh, MD

Retrospective Analysis of Arthroscopic Management of Glenohumeral Degenerative Disease
Van Thiel GS, Sheehan S, Frank RM, et al (Rush Univ Med Ctr, Chicago, IL)
Arthroscopy 26:1451-1455, 2010

Purpose.—The purpose of this study was to examine the results of arthroscopic debridement for isolated degenerative joint disease of the shoulder.

Methods.—We retrospectively identified 81 patients who had arthroscopic debridement to treat glenohumeral arthritis. Of these patients, 71 (88%) were available for follow-up. The preoperative Simple Shoulder

Test score, American Shoulder and Elbow Surgeons score, Short Form 12 score, visual analog scale score for pain, and range of motion were recorded. These were compared against postoperative scores by use of the statistical paired t test. In addition, patients completed postoperative University of California, Los Angeles; Constant; and Single Assessment Numeric Evaluation scores. Forty-six preoperative radiographs were blindly evaluated and classified. Finally, the need for subsequent shoulder arthroplasty was recorded.

Results.—The mean follow-up for the 55 patients who did not progress to arthroplasty was 27 months. The mean preoperative and postoperative American Shoulder and Elbow Surgeons, Simple Shoulder Test, and pain visual analog scale scores all significantly improved ($P < .05$). Furthermore, range of motion significantly improved ($P < .05$) in flexion, abduction, and external rotation. Additional postoperative scores were as follows: University of California, Los Angeles, 28.3; Single Assessment Numeric Evaluation, 71.1; Constant score for affected shoulder, 72.0; and Constant score for unaffected shoulder, 78.5. Of the patients, 16 (22%) underwent arthroplasty at a mean of 10.1 months after debridement. Radiographic review showed that 13 shoulders with a mean joint space of 1.5 mm and grade 2.4 arthrosis went on to have shoulder arthroplasty. In contrast, 33 shoulders with a mean joint space of 2.6 mm and grade 1.9 arthrosis did not go on to have shoulder arthroplasty.

Conclusions.—Patients with residual joint space and an absence of large osteophytes can avoid arthroplasty and have increased function with decreased pain after arthroscopic debridement for degenerative joint disease. Significant risk factors for failure include the presence of grade 4 bipolar disease, joint space of less than 2 mm, and large osteophytes.

Level of Evidence.—Level IV, case series.

▶ In this retrospective level IV study, the authors tried to demonstrate the value of arthroscopic debridement of the shoulder to slow down the evolution of isolated degenerative joint disease of the glenohumeral joint and improve patient shoulder function. Eighty-one patients were identified, but only 71 were available for follow-up, 47 men and 24 women with an average age of 47 years (18-77 years). Of these 71 patients, only 46 preoperative radiographs were available for evaluation of the amount of joint space narrowing and to classify the disease according to the classification by Samilson and Prieto. Inclusion criteria consisted of patients who had a pre- and postoperative diagnosis of glenohumeral degenerative joint disease. Exclusion criteria included a postoperative diagnosis of adhesive capsulitis, concomitant labral or rotator cuff repair, and previous shoulder surgery within the last year. The surgical technique of arthroscopic debridement was not described, but associated procedures were cited: 44 capsular releases, 14 biceps tenodeses/tenotomies, 11 microfractures, 12 loose body/osteophytes removals, and 28 subacromial decompressions. Of the 71 patients, 16 (22%) had undergone shoulder replacement at a mean of 10 months (2.5-27 months) after the arthroscopic surgery, whereas 55 had not. Of the 55 patients, 37 had preoperative range of motion recorded and had a significant increase in range of motion at 27 months of average follow-up. The mean Constant score ratio of the 55 affected shoulder to the unaffected shoulder was 0.9. Main prognosis factors of the efficiency of the arthroscopic debridement were importance of joint space and importance of articular cartilage damage. It is difficult to conclude anything at the end of this study, but we can assume that arthroscopic debridement can give satisfactory short-term results in patients with glenohumeral arthritis with joint space of more than 2-mm and less than grade 4 bipolar disease according to the classification by Samilson and Prieto.

P. Mansat, MD, PhD

Arthroscopic Stabilization for First-Time Versus Recurrent Shoulder Instability
Grumet RC, Bach BR Jr, Provencher MT (Rush Univ Med Ctr, Chicago, IL; Naval Med Ctr, San Diego, CA)
Arthroscopy 26:239-248, 2010

Purpose.—The purpose of this study was to systematically review the evidence on the outcomes of arthroscopic repair for anterior shoulder instability in first-time dislocators when compared with patients with recurrent instability.

Methods.—We designed a systematic review with a specific methodology to investigate the outcomes of surgery for those with only a first-time dislocation versus those who underwent surgery after multiple instability events. We performed a literature search from January 1966 to December 2008 using Medline, CINAHL (Cumulative Index to Nursing and Allied Health Literature), and the Cochrane Central Register of Controlled Trials. Key words included the following: first time, primary shoulder, or recurrent shoulder instability, shoulder dislocation, Bankart repair, arthroscopic Bankart repair, and labral repair. The inclusion criteria were cohort studies (Level I to II) that evaluated the outcomes of patients undergoing arthroscopic stabilization after the first dislocation or multiple recurrent episodes. Studies that lacked a comparison group or were retrospective (Level III studies or higher) were excluded.

Results.—There were 15 studies that met the inclusion criteria and were included in the final analysis: 5 in the first-time dislocation group and 10 in the recurrent instability group. Study design, patient demographics, mean number of dislocations, surgical technique, and rehabilitation protocol, as well as subjective and objective outcome measures, were recorded.

Conclusions.—There were no differences in recurrence or complication rate among patients undergoing surgery after the primary dislocation when compared with those undergoing surgery after multiple recurrent episodes. Clinical outcome measures significantly improved within all independent studies from preoperatively to postoperatively. However, because of variation in the outcome measurement tools used, no direct comparison between the study groups could be performed. Additional randomized controlled studies are needed to compare the functional outcome, quality of life, and ability to return to preinjury activity level among patients undergoing early versus delayed repair for anterior shoulder instability.

▶ It has been suggested that early surgical management of first-time shoulder dislocation improves outcome when compared with that of recurrent instability because of the anterior soft-tissue attenuation and bone loss that can occur with recurrent instability episodes. The authors present a systematic review of levels I and II studies in an effort to compare the outcomes of arthroscopic stabilization of first-time anterior shoulder dislocation versus stabilization of recurrent shoulder instability. Their literature search revealed 5 studies meeting the inclusion criteria for the first-time dislocation group and 10 studies in the recurrent instability group. The study design, patient demographics, number of dislocations, surgical technique, rehabilitation protocol, and outcome measures were noted for each study. The authors conclude based on their literature review that no difference in reported postsurgical recurrence rate exists between patients undergoing arthroscopic management of first-time dislocations and those treated for recurrent instability.

The authors present a valuable review of the literature concerning arthroscopic stabilization of anterior shoulder instability. When reviewing the authors' conclusions, however, it is important to recognize several of the article's limitations. The studies included in the review use varying methods of fixation, including older transglenoid suture and bioabsorbable tack techniques. The authors address this disparity by drawing their conclusions on a comparison of recurrence rates between studies using similar techniques. Only one of the studies in the first-time dislocation group, however, used modern suture anchor fixation. The authors also point out that the variation in outcome measures applied across the study groups makes direct comparison difficult. A prospective study using a modern suture anchor technique directly comparing the outcome of arthroscopic management of first-time versus recurrent shoulder dislocation would be valuable.

T. J. Fox, MD
L. S. Oh, MD

25 Shoulder: Biomechanics and Examination

Subscapularis Function Following the Latarjet Coracoid Transfer for Recurrent Anterior Shoulder Instability
Elkousy H, Gartsman GM, Labriola J, et al (Fondren Orthopedic Group, Houston, TX)
Orthopedics 33:802, 2010

The Latarjet procedure may be performed with both subscapularis split ting and subscapularis transecting approaches. The subscapularis splitting approach may better preserve subscapularis function and anatomy. The goal of this study was to determine the functional status of the subscapularis after the Latarjet procedure with a subscapularis splitting approach using the quantified belly press test.

Thirty patients with traumatic anterior shoulder instability were prospectively enrolled in the study. All patients underwent a Latarjet procedure through a subscapularis splitting approach. Both operative and nonoperative extremities were tested preoperatively with a belly press test using an Isobex muscle strength analyzer (Medical Device Solutions AG, Oberburg, Switzerland). Fifteen patients returned for postoperative Isobex belly press testing at a minimum of 6 months. Average patient age was 23.3 years, and average followup interval was 13 months. We detected no significant differences in pre- vs postoperative subscapularis strength in the surgical shoulder (decreased by 0.3 kg [95% CI, −1.0 to 1.7 kg; P=.630]). There was no difference in control vs surgical arm at preoperative (control +0.3 kg stronger; 95% CI, −0.8 to 0.1 kg; P=.124) vs postoperative (control +0.3 kg stronger; 95% CI, −1.1 to 0.5 kg; P=.444) measurements. Neither sex (P=.593) nor surgery in the dominant arm (P=.459) had an effect on recovery of subscapularis strength. Finally, the surgical arm at follow-up was not significantly different from reported height- and weight-based normative values for either men (P=.481) or women (P=.298).

This study suggests that subscapularis strength is not significantly altered by the Latarjet procedure with a subscapularis splitting approach.

▶ The authors attempted to quantify subscapularis strength preoperatively and postoperatively after a subscapularis splitting approach for a Latarjet reconstruction using an isometric belly press test with a computerized strength analyzer. As expected, the authors found no difference between preoperative and postoperative measurements, nor between the operated and nonoperated extremities. Only half of the patients enrolled returned for follow-up, although it is reasonable to assume that their results would have been similar. The study would have been much better if the authors had compared this group of patients with one that had had a subscapularis transection approach.

S. P. Steinman, MD

Quantifying scapula orientation and its influence on maximal hand force capability and shoulder muscle activity
Picco BR, Fischer SL, Dickerson CR (Univ of Waterloo, Ontario, Canada)
Clin Biomech 25:29-36, 2010

Background.—Non-neutral scapular orientations are often implicated as potential causes of shoulder pathologies. However, their specific influence on shoulder functional capabilities is largely unknown. This study objectively measured scapular orientation and quantified its influence on shoulder muscle activity levels and hand force capabilities during vertical and horizontal manual exertions.

Methods.—Ten healthy male university students performed 24 exertions in combinations of scapular orientation (protracted, neutral and retracted), exertion direction (up, down, medial, lateral) and intensity (maximal or 40 N). Scapular orientation was quantified using an acromion marker cluster method. An orientation by intensity repeated measures ANOVA identified differences in quantified scapular orientation. A two-way multivariate ANOVA identified the influence of scapular orientation and hand force direction on muscle activity and hand force capability.

Findings.—Participants assumed consistent retracted, neutral, and protracted scapular orientations during exertions, and these three orientations were different from each other ($F(2, 99)=158.57$; P-value: 0.0001). Scapular orientation and exertion direction influenced muscle recruitment almost universally (P-value: 0.05). Scapular orientation did not influence hand force capability ($F(2, 99)=1.34$; P-value: 0.05), but a hand force direction effect on force existed ($F(3, 99)=144.19$; P-value: 0.0001).

Interpretation.—These findings support recommendations of health practitioners who advocate neutral scapular orientations to reduce injury risk, as a neutral orientation achieved a balanced overall muscle use pattern between retraction and protraction. Also, lowered muscle activity and higher maximal forces suggest that downward exertion forces may be preferable when possible.

▶ The authors should be commended on an interesting study of the effect of scapula position on strength. Scapulothoracic dyskinesia continues to be a challenge for physicians who treat shoulder injuries, and this article demonstrates how a nonneutral position of the scapula adversely affects strength of the shoulder. However, scapulothoracic mechanics are much more complicated than the simple (but reproducible) setup used by the authors. In addition, many scapulothoracic problems arise after fatigue failure and not after single maximal load application. It would be interesting to see how strength deteriorates after repetitive loads or after prolonged scapular malposition with taping in retraction or protraction. Regardless, the concept of a neutral scapula position is appropriate. I have used the S3 brace to stabilize the scapula with some success. Different types of kinesiotaping can also be helpful to better position and stabilize the scapula. Further biomechanical studies like this one may help us to better understand the effects of scapular malposition on strength and more specifically, aid in our ability to treat this difficult entity.

T. R. McAdams, MD

and higher maximal forces suggest that downward eccentric forces may be
preferable when possible.

T. P. McClatchie, MD

26 Shoulder: Rotator Cuff

Revision Arthroscopic Rotator Cuff Repair: Repair Integrity and Clinical Outcome

Keener JD, Wei AS, Kim HM, et al (Washington Univ, St Louis, MO)
J Bone Joint Surg Am 92:590-598, 2010

Background.—Literature regarding the outcomes of revision rotator cuff repair is limited. The purposes of the present study were to report the tendon repair integrity and clinical outcomes for a cohort of patients following revision arthroscopic rotator cuff repair and to examine factors related to tendon healing and the influence of healing on clinical outcomes.

Methods.—Twenty-one of twenty-nine consecutive revision arthroscopic rotator cuff repairs with a minimum of two years of postoperative follow-up were retrospectively reviewed. Outcomes were evaluated on the basis of a visual analog pain scale, the range of motion of the shoulder, the Simple Shoulder Test, the American Shoulder and Elbow Surgeons score, and the Constant score. Ultrasonography was used to examine repair integrity at a minimum of one year following surgery. Ten shoulders underwent arthroscopic repair of a recurrent single-tendon posterior rotator cuff tear, whereas eleven shoulders had repair of both the supraspinatus and infraspinatus.

Results.—The mean age of the twenty-one subjects was 55.6 years; thirteen subjects were male and eight were female. Complete preoperative and postoperative clinical data were available for nineteen subjects after an average duration of follow-up of thirty-three months. Significant improvements were seen in terms of postoperative pain ($p < 0.05$), the Simple Shoulder Test score ($p < 0.05$), the American Shoulder and Elbow Surgeons function ($p < 0.05$) and total scores ($p < 0.05$), active forward elevation ($p < 0.05$), and active external rotation ($p < 0.05$). Postoperative ultrasound data were available for all twenty-one shoulders after a mean duration of follow-up of twenty-five months. Ten (48%) of the twenty-one shoulders had an intact repair. Seven (70%) of the ten single-tendon repairs were intact, compared with three (27%) of the eleven supraspinatus/infraspinatus repairs ($p = 0.05$). Patient age ($p < 0.05$) and the number of torn tendons ($p = 0.05$) had significant effects on postoperative tendon repair integrity. Shoulders with an intact repair had better postoperative Constant scores (p < 0.05) and scapular plane elevation strength (p < 0.05) in comparison with those with a recurrent tear.

Conclusions.—Revision arthroscopic rotator cuff repair results in reliable pain relief and improvement in shoulder function in selected cases. Approximately half of the revision repairs can be expected to be intact at a minimum of one year following surgery. Patient age and the number of torn tendons are related to postoperative tendon integrity. The postoperative integrity of the rotator cuff can have a significant influence on shoulder abduction strength and the Constant score.

▶ In this retrospective case series, authors have evaluated the tendon repair integrity and clinical outcome of 21 revision complete arthroscopic rotator cuff repairs with double-row repair in 18 of them. All shoulders were immobilized for 6 weeks. Significant improvements were noted in terms of the visual analog scale pain score, the Simple Shoulder Test score, the American Shoulder and Elbow Surgeons function, and total scores. At a minimum of 1 year after the revision surgery, 48% of the patients were found to have intact repairs, with 70% of single tendon repairs intact versus 27% of the multiple tendon repairs being intact with ultrasound. Because of the insufficient power to detect a significant difference between intact repair and recurrent tears, functional results were not found to be different between intact repair and recurrent tear groups except for the scapular plane elevation strength and final Constant scores. Overall, revision arthroscopic rotator cuff repair was found to provide substantial improvement in terms of both shoulder pain and function. As expected, the 2 factors that correlated with repair integrity were the age of the subject and the number of torn tendons, validating the outcomes from primary arthroscopic rotator cuff repair studies. Of note, the recurrent tears in this patient group was not a failure, and they were well tolerated by patients despite the fact that they were surgical candidates after their initial rotator cuff repair failure, which remains unexplained.

A. Cil, MD

Suprascapular Neuropathy
Boykin RE, Friedman DJ, Higgins LD, et al (Massachusetts General Hosp, Boston; New York Univ School of Medicine; Brigham and Women's Hosp, Boston, MA)
J Bone Joint Surg Am 92:2348-2364, 2010

Suprascapular neuropathy has often been overlooked as a source of shoulder pain.

The condition may be more common than once thought as it is being diagnosed more frequently.

Etiologies for suprascapular neuropathy may include repetitive overhead activities, traction from a rotator cuff tear, and compression from a space-occupying lesion at the suprascapular or spinoglenoid notch.

Magnetic resonance imaging is useful for visualizing space-occupying lesions, other pathological entities of the shoulder, and fatty infiltration of the rotator cuff.

Electromyography and nerve conduction velocity studies remain the standard for diagnosis of suprascapular neuropathy; however, data on interobserver reliability are limited.

Initial treatment of isolated suprascapular neuropathy is typically non-operative, consisting of physical therapy, nonsteroidal anti-inflammatory drugs, and activity modification; however, open or arthroscopic operative intervention is warranted when there is extrinsic nerve compression or progressive pain and/or weakness.

More clinical data are needed to determine if treatment of the primary offending etiology in cases of traction from a rotator cuff tear or compression from a cyst secondary to a labral tear is sufficient or whether concomitant decompression of the nerve is warranted for management of the neuropathy.

▶ In this current concepts article, authors have done an excellent review of a hot topic in shoulder surgery. Suprascapular neuropathy has gained recent interest because of increased awareness of the problem by MRI findings and application of electromyogram and nerve conduction studies. Overall, etiology involves either compression or traction to the nerve. Recent anatomic dissections have delineated the role of massive rotator cuff tears by causing traction on the nerve. Moreover, once thought to be a predominantly motor nerve, recent evidence suggests that there are sensory branches to the glenohumeral and acromioclavicular joints, as well as to the skin. Initial nonoperative treatment can be tried in patients without a discrete structural lesion with good success. Failures of nonoperative treatment and space-occupying lesions in the suprascapular or spinoglenoid notch are better candidates for operative intervention. Historically, operative intervention has been open decompression; however, emerging literature suggests arthroscopy as an effective means to decompress the nerve. It is still not clear from the available literature whether concomitant decompression of the nerve is warranted in conditions where the primary structural lesion (paralabral cyst, massive rotator cuff tear, etc) can effectively be treated.

A. Cil, MD

Novel Nanostructured Scaffolds as Therapeutic Replacement Options for Rotator Cuff Disease
Taylor ED, Nair LS, Nukavarapu SP, et al (Univ of Virginia, Charlottesville; Univ of Connecticut Health Ctr, Farmington)
J Bone Joint Surg Am 92:170 179, 2010

Background.—Rotator cuff injuries are common causes of upper extremity disability and can produce considerable pain and dysfunction. Surgical repair for rotator cuff injuries can be accomplished via open, mini-open, or arthroscopic techniques. Open techniques require a larger dissection and longer operating time. Arthroscopic repairs are associated with a limited working area, longer learning curve, and higher percentage of recurrent lesions compared to the open or mini-open repairs. Surgical repairs using autografts, cadaveric allografts, or patch grafts made of biological and synthetic materials have been developed but donor site morbidity, limited availability of autografts, and risk of disease transmission have limited their usefulness. A novel therapeutic strategy to support and accelerate the healing of a torn rotator cuff was developed via a tissue-engineering approach using a nanostructured resorbable polymeric scaffold. The scaffold was fabricated, biological characterization was achieved in vitro, an original rodent model was developed, and biomechanical characterization was done in vivo.

Methods.—A biodegradable polymeric solution was used to create resorbable polymer scaffolds from poly(85 lactic acid-*co*-15 glycolic acid) (PLAGA) using electrospinning. The PLAGA solution was prepared in a 3:1 solvent mixture of tetrahydrofuran and dimethylformamide and charged to 30 kV. Ultra-thin fibers with diameters of 400 to 800 nm collected randomly on a grounded collecting plate. Patellar tendon cells were cultured, trypsinized after 80% confluency, and seeded on the newly developed nanofiber matrices. These were then irradiated with ultraviolet light for 15 minutes on a side to reduce bacterial contamination. A scanning electron microscope (SEM) was used to assess the development of a cellular network and determine adhesion properties. Cell-seeded matrix scaffolds were washed with phosphate-buffered saline solution and fixed in 3% glutaraldehyde solution, washed and air dried, then coated with gold. The SEM was again employed to qualify cellular material that developed and remained adhered to the scaffold after washings. MTS assays were done to quantify the proliferation of cells. The number of live cells was also noted. The Young modulus of the matrices was determined using a biomechanical testing machine. Samples were incubated in cell culture media, and biomechanical properties were then determined. Suture strength was also assessed to determine the mode of failure and maximum force that could be withstood at the graft-suture interface.

Forty-eight Sprague-Dawley rats underwent operative procedures and repairs. In some, the supraspinatus was reapproximated primarily; in others, a 3 × 3-mm scaffold sample was sutured over the primary repair. Rodents were allowed to move freely in their cages, then were killed and biomechanical values were assessed.

Results.—The SEM assessments revealed increases in the presence of a cellular network on the matrices that had been prepared in vitro. Between 7 and 28 days after fabrication, MTS proliferation assays showed that there was a significant increase in the measured absorbance from the scaffold, indicating cellular activity and proliferation. There were qualitative indications of the presence of increased numbers of viable cells with time. Measurements after 7, 14, and 28 days showed increased mechanical properties of the cell-seeded scaffolds. These scaffolds also had higher

Young modulus than cell-free scaffolds. There was a trend toward a decline in the amount of load required to cause construct failure over time, but the values were not significant.

The in vivo tests showed that there were no wound complications or premature deaths among the rats. All subjects regained full use of the upper extremity and could reach overhead to feed. The repair junctions of both those animals having primary supraspinatus repair alone and those having augmented repairs showed similar biomechanical results after 4 weeks. Between weeks 4 and 8 a significant increase in the Young modulus was noted for the augmented repairs.

Conclusions.—A bioabsorbable nanostructured scaffold was developed that could serve as an augmentation device for regenerating torn rotator cuffs. Tissue-engineering accelerates the repair and regeneration of damaged tissue using these bioresorbable scaffolds, which can be augmented with cells and bioactive factors. Ideally they will mimic the properties of the damaged tissue and perform as a temporary augmentation device.

▶ This article presents the results of a pilot study investigating the use of a nanostructured, resorbable scaffold for rotator cuff repair in a rodent model. The authors first fabricated a nanofiber polymeric scaffold via a process called electrospinning from poly(85 lactic acid-co-15 glycolic acid) and verified the ability of the material to develop a cellular matrix. The Young modulus was then calculated with and without cells. The authors developed a rodent rotator cuff model to test the scaffold in vivo.

The authors found that over time, a cellular network developed on the matrices of the scaffold. A higher Young modulus was noted in matrices seeded with cells when compared with cell-free scaffolds. In vivo testing in the rodent model was performed comparing primary direct repair of the rotator cuff with direct repair with augmentation with the scaffold. At 4 weeks, both groups demonstrated similar biomechanical findings. However, from 4 to 8 weeks, there was an increase in the Young modulus of the group undergoing rotator cuff augmentation of the repair with the nanostructured scaffold.

This is an interesting study that should stimulate further research into the use of nanostructured scaffolds for use in rotator cuff repair.

A. M. Smith, MD

Treatment of Biceps Tendon Lesions in the Setting of Rotator Cuff Tears: Prospective Cohort Study of Tenotomy Versus Tenodesis

Koh KH, Ahn JH, Kim SM, et al (Sungkyunkwan Univ School of Medicine, Kangnam-Gu, Seoul, Korea)
Am J Sports Med 38:1584-1600, 2010

Background.—During rotator cuff repair, biceps tendon lesions are frequently encountered. However, there is still controversy about optimal treatment for these lesions.

Purpose.—To compare the results of tenotomy and suture anchor tenodesis prospectively.

Study Design.—Cohort study; Level of evidence, 2.

Methods.—From January 2006 to June 2007, 90 patients (age, >55 years) with a rotator cuff tear and biceps tendon lesion (tear more than 30%, subluxation or dislocation, or degenerative superior labrum anterior to posterior lesion type II) were evaluated prospectively. The first 45 patients treated consecutively underwent biceps tenodesis, and the next 45 underwent biceps tenotomy. Postoperatively, patient evaluations were conducted with a focus on (1) "Popeye" deformity, (2) arm cramping pain, and (3) elbow flexion powers (measured with a hand dynamometer). Overall shoulder function was assessed with the American Shoulder and Elbow Surgeons (ASES) score and the Constant score.

Results.—At final follow-up, 43 in the tenodesis and 41 in the tenotomy groups were available for evaluation. There was no difference between groups in demographic data such as age, sex, dominant arm, and the time from symptom to surgery and in preoperative ASES score, Constant score, and rotator cuff tear size. A Popeye deformity occurred in 4 (9%) in the tenodesis group and in 11 (27%) in the tenotomy group ($P = .0360$). Mild cramping pain was observed in 2 in the tenodesis group and 4 in the tenotomy group ($P = .4274$). Mean elbow flexor power ratio (vs the contralateral side) showed no difference between the 2 groups, with mean values of 0.92 ± 0.15 (tenodesis) and 0.94 ± 0.19 (tenotomy) ($P = .7475$). The ASES and Constant scores were improved from 38.9 ± 14.2 and 52.1 ± 21.3 to 84.7 ± 13.6 and 82.9 ± 13.5 in the tenodesis group ($P < .0001$) and from 35.2 ± 10.5 and 48.1 ± 21.3 to 79.6 ± 15.8 and 78.3 ± 14.1 in the tenotomy group ($P < .0001$), respectively.

Conclusion.—Suture anchor tenodesis of the long head of the biceps tendon appears to lead to less Popeye deformity than tenotomy. No other clinical variables showed a difference between the 2 modalities.

▶ This is a very well-done study out of Seoul, Korea, looking at biceps tenotomy versus tenodesis. This is a prospective cohort study with level II evidence. Over a 2-year period, the authors looked at the treatment of biceps tendon lesions in the setting of rotator cuff tears in the over 55 patient population. They had 43 patients in the tenodesis group and 41 in the tenotomy group. The only significant difference was a lower rate of Popeye deformity in the tenodesis group when compared with the tenotomy group. Specifically, the tenodesis had a 9% rate of Popeye deformity compared with 27% rate in the tenotomy group. No other statistically significant differences could be found after looking at pain, strength, the American Shoulder and Elbow Surgeons score, and Constant score. I think this is an excellent article that finally puts to rest the issue of tenodesis versus tenotomy. It would suggest that in the younger patient population, a tenodesis is probably warranted more for cosmetic purposes. However, in the older population with potentially poorer quality long head of biceps tendon, it is very reasonable to perform a tenotomy without the need of considering a tenodesis. This article provides justification for either technique in the setting of treating biceps lesions with rotator cuff tears.

Again, it was a very well-done study and very well-written article. The question for the orthopedic surgeon is whether it is worth the extra 10 minutes of time to perform the biceps tenodesis when from a functional and pain standpoint, it probably does not make any difference over just performing a biceps tenotomy.

S. F. M. Duncan, MD, MPH, MBA

Arthroscopic Rotator Cuff Repair With Metal and Biodegradable Suture Anchors: A Prospective Randomized Study
Milano G, Grasso A, Salvatore M, et al (Catholic Univ, Rome, Italy; Villa Valeria Clinic, Rome, Italy)
Arthroscopy 26:S112-S119, 2010

Purpose.—The purpose of this study was to compare the clinical outcome of arthroscopic rotator cuff repair with metal and biodegradable suture anchors.

Methods.—Arthroscopic rotator cuff repair was performed in 110 patients with a full-thickness rotator cuff tear. They were divided into 2 groups of 55 patients each, according to suture anchors used: metal anchors in group 1 and biodegradable anchors in group 2. Results were evaluated by use of the Disabilities of the Arm, Shoulder and Hand (DASH) and Work-DASH self-administered questionnaires, as well as the Constant score normalized for age and sex. On analyzing the results at 2 years' follow-up, we considered the following independent variables: baseline scores; age; sex; arm dominance; location, shape, and retraction of cuff tear; fatty degeneration; treatment of biceps tendon; rotator cuff repair technique (anchors or anchors and side to side); and number of anchors. Univariate and multivariate statistical analyses were performed to determine which variables were independently associated with the outcome. Significance was set at $P < .05$.

Results.—Of the patients, 9 (8.2%) were lost to follow-up. Comparison between groups did not show significant differences for each variable considered. Overall, according to the results, the mean DASH scores were 17.6 ± 17.2 points in group 1 and 22.8 ± 19.9 points in group 2; the mean Work-DASH scores were 24.9 ± 28.1 points and 22.5 ± 24.1 points, respectively; and the mean Constant scores were 104 ± 20.5 points and 98.6 ± 14.3 points, respectively. Differences between groups 1 and 2 were not significant. Univariate and multivariate analysis showed that only baseline score, age, tear location, and fatty degeneration significantly and independently influenced the outcome.

Conclusions.—At a short-term follow-up, differences between arthroscopic repair of full-thickness rotator cuff tears with metal and biodegradable suture anchors were not significant.

Level of Evidence.—Level I, high-quality randomized controlled trial with no statistically significant differences but narrow confidence intervals.

▶ This prospective randomized controlled trial attempts to answer the question if biodegradable suture anchors are as effective as metal suture anchors. The authors included 110 arthroscopic rotator cuff repairs with randomization into either metal suture anchors (5.5-mm metal corkscrew, Arthrex Inc.; group 1) or biodegradable suture anchors (5.5-mm Bio-Corkscrew, Arthrex Inc.; group 2). Outcomes were assessed using the Disabilities of the Arm, Shoulder and Hand (DASH), Work DASH, and Constant scores. No data on range of motion, strength, or radiographic outcomes were reported.

Results were available for 101 patients at a mean follow-up of 24 months. There were no differences between the 2 study groups with regard to age, size of the tear, tear pattern, type of repair, fatty degeneration, or number of anchors used. There was no difference in any of the outcome measures between the 2 study groups. The DASH score was slightly lower (17.6 vs 22.8) in the metal suture anchor group and approached statistical significance. However, a 5-point difference on the DASH is unlikely to be clinically significant. The authors also reviewed the effects of multiple factors on the outcome scores and found significant association of sex, age, tear location, tear shape, type of repair, and number of anchors.

This study did not demonstrate any clinical difference between the use of biodegradable and metal suture anchors. The study falls short of a complete analysis, as there is no radiographic analysis, and as they identified in the introduction, one of the biggest concerns regarding the use of biodegradable anchors is the development of osteolysis around the anchor, resulting in loosing. There are many studies demonstrating equivalent performance of biodegradable implants in cadavers at time 0; however, the question remains regarding the potential survival of the biomechanics properties in the in vivo setting. The Bio-Corkscrew anchors used in this study have largely been replaced by PEEK or Biocomposite anchors to help decrease the risk of osteolysis while retaining the benefit of an implant that does not interfere with future MRI studies. This article neither confirms nor refutes the use of biodegradable implants in rotator cuff repair and, therefore, has little impact on clinical practice.

T. Duquin, MD

Comparative Analysis of Single-Row Versus Double-Row Repair of Rotator Cuff Tears
Pennington WT, Gibbons DJ, Bartz BA, et al (Midwest Orthopedic Specialty Hosp, Franklin; et al)
Arthroscopy 26:1419-1426, 2010

Purpose.—Our goal in this analysis was to compare clinical outcomes and radiographic healing rates of double-row (DR) transosseous-equivalent versus single-row (SR) Mason-Allen configuration (MAC) arthroscopic repair techniques.

Methods.—A prospective, nonrandomized assessment of 132 arthroscopic rotator cuff repair patients included 78 SR repair patients and 54 with DR repair. Tears measured between 1.5 and 4.5 cm. Patients were evaluated with a visual analog scale; University of California, Los Angeles score; American Shoulder and Elbow Surgeons score; active range of motion; and dynamometric strength. Scores and measurements were obtained preoperatively and at 3, 6, 12, and 24 months postoperatively. The SR repairs were performed with the arthroscopic MAC. For DR repairs, two 5.5-mm fully threaded Bio-Corkscrew anchors (Arthrex, Naples, FL), single loaded with FiberWire (Arthrex), were used for the medial row. The lateral row was secured with PushLock bioabsorbable anchors (Arthrex). Forty-four patients in the SR group and 37 patients in the DR group returned for magnetic resonance imaging (MRI) evaluation of repair integrity between 12 and 28 months postoperatively.

Results.—DR repairs resulted in higher outcome scores, though not significantly. Patient satisfaction rates were 95% in the SR group and 92% in the DR group. MRI showed a statistically significantly improved healing rate with SR repair compared with DR repair in our entire patient population ($P \leq .017$). A more homogeneous subset of patients with tears between 2.5 and 3.5 cm showed a significantly improved healing rate for the DR repair ($P \leq .03$).

Conclusions.—Our short-term results suggest that SR MAC repair provides comparable clinical results to DR repair. Although our MRI data suggest improved healing rates in our SR repairs in the entire patient population, when similar-sized tears were compared, the DR repair group showed improved radiographic healing.

Level of Evidence.—Level III, retrospective comparative study.

▶ This retrospective review attempts to answer the long-debated question if double-row (DR) rotator cuff repair is superior to single-row (SR) repair. A total of 132 arthroscopic rotator cuff repairs were included in the study (54 DR repairs with suture-bridge technique and 78 SR repairs with modified Mason-Allen suture technique). Outcome was assessed with range of motion, strength, the American Shoulder and Elbow Surgeon shoulder index, the University of California, Los Angeles shoulder scale, and the visual analog scale scores. MRI was performed on 56% of the SR repairs and 66% of the DR repairs at a mean of 21 months (12-28 months).

Results showed no difference in range of motion, strength, or outcome scores at 1-year follow-up. The only statistically significant difference was in the strength of the supraspinatus at 2 years, which was greater in the DR repair group (16 lb vs 13 lb). There were no other differences in motion, strength, or outcome scores between the groups. MRI results showed a higher healing rate in the SR group when all tears were included (80% vs 68%). However, there was a bias toward larger tears in the DR group because there was no randomization and the surgeon selected which type of repair to perform based on the intraoperative findings. When tears 2.5 to 3.5 mm were compared, the DR group had a higher healing rate than the SR group (76% vs 72%). There was no analysis performed for tears < 2.5 mm or > 3.5 mm.

The debate regarding DR and SR repairs continues, and this study does little to support either side of the issue. The biomechanical properties of DR repairs have been shown to be superior to those of SR with regard to strength and restoration of the tendon footprint. However, there have been no clinical studies that have shown superiority of DR repairs on clinical outcome measures. Healing rates have previously been shown to be superior with DR repairs when controlling for tear size, which is supported by this study. The improved strength of the supraspinatus at 2 years in this study may indicate the influence tendon healing will have on the long-term clinical results. This study provides limited clinical support to the use of DR repairs, and the limited benefit may not justify the increased cost of implants and time associated with DR repairs.

T. Duquin, MD

Latissimus Dorsi Tendon Transfer for Irreparable Rotator Cuff Tears: A Modified Technique to Improve Tendon Transfer Integrity: Surgical Technique
Tauber M, Moursy M, Forstner R, et al (Paracelsus Med Univ, Salzburg, Austria)
J Bone Joint Surg Am 92:226-239, 2010

Background.—Latissimus dorsi tendon transfer is a well-established method for the treatment of massive irreparable posterosuperior defects of the rotator cuff. Subsequent rupture of the transferred tendon may contribute to the rate of failure of the index procedure. We hypothesized that modification of our technique of tendon harvesting would lead to greater fixation stability and a reduced failure rate.

Methods.—Forty-two patients (mean age, fifty-eight years) with a massive irreparable posterosuperior tear of the rotator cuff were managed with a latissimus dorsi tendon transfer. Sharp separation of the latissimus tendon from the humerus was performed in twenty-two patients (Group A), whereas the tendon harvest was carried out with a modified technique that involved removal of some bone along with the tendon at the humeral insertion in a subsequent group of twenty patients (Group B). The mean duration of follow-up was forty-seven months. Outcome measures included the Constant and American Shoulder and Elbow Surgeons (ASES) scores and a patient subjective satisfaction scale. Standard radiographs were made to determine the stage of osteoarthritis and proximal migration of the humeral head, and magnetic resonance imaging was performed to assess the integrity of the transferred muscle.

Results.—In Group A, the mean Constant score improved from 43.4 preoperatively to 64.8 points at the time of follow-up and the mean ASES score improved from 49.3 to 69.6 points (p < 0.05). In Group B, the mean Constant score increased from 40.2 to 74.2 points and the mean ASES score, from 47.2 to 77.1 points (p < 0.05). The Constant pain score improved from 5.6 to 11.9 points in Group A and from 5.2 to 13.8 points in Group B. The results in Group B were significantly superior to those in Group A (p < 0.05). Magnetic resonance imaging revealed complete rupture at the tendon insertion with tendon retraction in four patients in Group A and none in Group B. The final outcome was rated as poor in 27% of the patients in Group A and in 10% in Group B.

Conclusions.—Latissimus dorsi tendon transfer achieves satisfactory clinical results in most patients who have a massive irreparable posterosuperior tear of the rotator cuff. Harvesting the tendon along with a small piece of bone enables direct bone-to-bone transosseous fixation, resulting in better tendon integrity and clinical results.

▶ This technique of latissimus dorsi transfer for irreparable rotator cuff tears is a follow-up of a previous study that was published in *The Journal of Bone and Joint Surgery* in 2009. The authors developed a technique of harvesting the latissimus tendon with a fragment of bone and found improved healing and clinical results when compared with the traditional tenotomy. In the original study, there were 42 patients (22 tenotomies/20 bone fragments) with a mean follow-up of 47 months. Both groups had increased American Shoulder and Elbow Surgeons and Constant scores, but the bone fragment group had significantly higher scores on all outcome measures, with MRI scans showing rupture of the tendon in 18% of the tenotomy group and none in the bone fragment group. The authors recommend the use of the bone fragment technique for latissimus tendon transfer.

The technique is described well in the article, and the theory makes sense for a tendon transfer that involves reattachment to bone. Similar to the argument for lesser tuberosity osteotomy in total shoulder arthroplasty, the bone fragment technique has the ability to heal with bone-to-bone healing, with retention of the native tendon-to-bone interface. This type of healing would be expected to be superior to the scar tissue that typically forms with a tendon-to-bone repair. The use of latissimus tendon transfers has become less common because of the relatively high rate of poor results associated with the procedure. In the authors' study, they still had 10% poor results with the bone fragment technique, which was a drastic improvement from 27% poor results with a standard tenotomy technique. The current indications for latissimus tendon transfer for massive rotator cuff tears are limited to young patients with irreparable supraspinatus and infraspinatus tears with intact teres minor and subscapularis tendons.

T. Duquin, MD

Development of Fatty Atrophy After Neurologic and Rotator Cuff Injuries in an Animal Model of Rotator Cuff Pathology

Rowshan K, Hadley S, Pham K, et al (Univ of California at Irvine)
J Bone Joint Surg Am 92:2270-2278, 2010

Background.—Detachment of a tendon from its osseous insertion, as can be the case with severe rotator cuff injuries, leads to atrophy of and increased fat in the corresponding muscle. We sought to validate a rotator cuff injury model in the rabbit and to test the hypothesis that tenotomy of a rotator cuff tendon would consistently create muscle atrophy and fatty degeneration analogous to the changes that occur after injury to a nerve innervating the same muscle.

Methods.—New Zealand white rabbits were divided into three groups: (1) partial rotator cuff tear without retraction of the muscle, (2) complete rotator cuff tear with retraction of the muscle, and (3) nerve transection of the subscapular nerve. Animals were killed at two or six weeks after injury, and the muscles were analyzed for weight, cross-sectional area, myosin fiber-type composition, and fat content. In addition, the subscapular nerve was harvested at two weeks and evaluated for neuronal injury.

Results.—At six weeks after injury, the rabbit muscles in the complete tenotomy and nerve transection groups had significant decreases in wet mass and increases in fat content relative to the control groups. Fat accumulation had a similar spatial pattern at six weeks in both the nerve transection and complete tenotomy groups. Such changes were not seen in the partial tenotomy group. No change was found in muscle myosin fiber-type composition. At two weeks after injury, subscapular nerves in the complete tenotomy group showed gross evidence of neuronal injury.

Conclusions.—This study establishes the rabbit subscapularis muscle as a valid model to study the muscular changes associated with rotator cuff tears. Our data suggest that the muscular changes associated with complete tenotomy are comparable with those seen with denervation of the muscle and suggest that chronic rotator cuff tears may induce a neurologic injury.

▶ This is an interesting, well-designed study showing that when a rotator cuff tendon is cut and released, the atrophy pattern is similar to nerve input transection. Massive retracted rotator cuff tears that are chronic develop atrophy, and this study supports the concept of nerve compromise as a possible cause or at least contributor of the atrophy. This is supported by what one finds clinically in the chronic rotator cuff tear setting. Many shoulder surgeons used to do meticulous interval releases to advance chronic tears to the footprint or at least the articular margin, and we saw a very high failure rate. If there is neural input compromise, possibly from compression at the suprascapular notch, then even the best interval releases and tension-free repairs will fail. I rarely do interval releases at this time unless there is less than 50% atrophy on sagittal T1 MRI and intraoperative quality appears satisfactory. Even with this situation, one should consider suprascapular nerve release, as this can be a pain generator. This study supports this concept and can be used as a model in future studies to further improve our understanding of if and when atrophy will occur after rotator cuff tears.

T. R. McAdams, MD

Reverse Shoulder Arthroplasty for the Treatment of Irreparable Rotator Cuff Tear without Glenohumeral Arthritis
Mulieri P, Dunning P, Klein S, et al (Florida Orthopaedic Inst, Tampa; Foundation for Orthopaedic Res and Education, Tampa, FL)
J Bone Joint Surg Am 92:2544-2556, 2010

Background.—The purpose of the present study was to evaluate the indications for, and outcomes of, reverse shoulder arthroplasty in patients with massive rotator cuff tears but without glenohumeral arthritis.

Methods.—From December 1998 to December 2006, sixty-nine patients (seventy-two shoulders) were managed with reverse shoulder arthroplasty for the treatment of irreparable rotator cuff dysfunction without glenohumeral arthritis. The indications for reverse shoulder arthroplasty were persistent shoulder pain and dysfunction despite a minimum of six months of nonoperative treatment, the presence of at least a two-tendon tear, and Hamada stage-1, 2, or 3 changes in a patient for whom a non-arthroplasty option did not exist. Fifty-eight patients (sixty shoulders) had a minimum of two years of follow-up. Thirty-four shoulders had had no previous surgery (Group A), and twenty-six shoulders had had at least one previous surgical procedure (Group B). Postoperatively, patients were prospectively followed both clinically and radiographically. Survival analysis was performed, with the end points being removal or revision of the implant, radiographic loosening, and declining American Shoulder and Elbow Surgeons score.

Results.—Common characteristics of patients managed with reverse shoulder arthroplasty in this study were pain and (1) <90° of arm elevation at the shoulder without anterosuperior escape (n = 40; 66.6%); (2) <90° of elevation with anterosuperior escape (n = 16; 26.7%); or (3) irreparable rotator cuff tear and pain with >90° of elevation (n = 4; 6.7%). The average duration of follow-up was fifty-two months (range, twenty-four to 101 months). All measured outcomes improved postoperatively. For all patients, the average American Shoulder and Elbow Surgeons score improved from 33.3 to 75.4 (p < 0.0001), the average Simple Shoulder Test score improved from 1.6 to 6.5 (p < 0.0001), the average visual analog score for pain improved from 6.3 to 1.9 (p < 0.0001), the average visual analog score for function improved from 3.2 to 7.1 (p < 0.0001), the average forward flexion improved from 53° to 134° (p < 0.0001), the average abduction improved from 49° to 125° (p < 0.0001), the average internal rotation improved from S1 to L2 (p < 0.0001), and the average external rotation improved from 27° to 51° (p = 0.001). There were a total of twelve complications in eleven patients (prevalence, 20%).

The survivorship at a mean of fifty-two months (range, twenty-four to 101 months) was 90.7% for all patients, 91.8% for Group A, and 87% for Group B.

Conclusions.—When non-arthroplasty options either have failed or have a low likelihood of success, reverse shoulder arthroplasty provides reliable pain relief and return of shoulder function in patients with massive rotator cuff tears without arthritis at the time of short to intermediate-term follow-up.

▶ The authors present 60 shoulders that were treated with a reverse total shoulder arthroplasty (RTSA) for an irreparable rotator cuff tear without arthritis. They had 2 groups, one that had no previous attempt at rotator cuff repair, and one that had at least one attempt at cuff repair. Outcome measures all improved over preoperative measures, including internal and external rotation. There was no difference between groups. Final active forward flexion returned to 134°, external rotation to 51°, and internal rotation to L2. The implant survivorship was 91% at 4 years follow-up.

It is difficult to advocate removing a nonarthritic joint to treat a soft tissue problem, rotator cuff disease. The authors have clearly shown that this is a viable option in patients with irreparable symptomatic rotator cuff tears (2 tendon chronic tear with atrophy in the older patient). It would be impossible to duplicate these results with any kind of cuff repair or tendon transfer in this patient population. The authors have nicely shown that an RTSA is an excellent option for this group of patients no matter what parameter is measured: motion, pain, satisfaction, or function. In our series, massive irreparable cuff tears in patients with chronic pain and no arthritis is the second most common indication for RTSA, which is second only to cuff tear arthropathy.

T. W. Wright, MD

Symptomatic Progression of Asymptomatic Rotator Cuff Tears: A Prospective Study of Clinical and Sonographic Variables
Mall NA, Kim HM, Keener JD, et al (Washington Univ School of Med, St Louis, MO; et al)
J Bone Joint Surg Am 92:2623-2633, 2010

Background.—The purposes of this study were to identify changes in tear dimensions, shoulder function, and glenohumeral kinematics when an asymptomatic rotator cuff tear becomes painful and to identify characteristics of individuals who develop pain compared with those who remain asymptomatic.

Methods.—A cohort of 195 subjects with an asymptomatic rotator cuff tear was prospectively monitored for pain development and examined annually for changes in various parameters such as tear size, fatty degeneration of the rotator cuff muscle, glenohumeral kinematics, and shoulder function. Forty-four subjects were found to have developed new pain, and the parameters before and after pain development were compared. The forty-four subjects were then compared with a group of fifty-five subjects who remained asymptomatic over a two-year period.

Results.—With pain development, the size of a full-thickness rotator cuff tear increased significantly, with 18% of the full-thickness tears showing an increase of >5 mm, and 40% of the partial-thickness tears had progressed to a full-thickness tear. In comparison with the assessments made before the onset of pain, the American Shoulder and Elbow Surgeons scores for shoulder function were significantly decreased and all measures of shoulder range of motion were decreased except for external rotation at 90° of abduction. There was an increase in compensatory scapulothoracic motion in relation to the glenohumeral motion during early shoulder abduction with pain development. No significant changes were found in external rotation strength or muscular fatty degeneration. Compared with the subjects who remained asymptomatic, the subjects who developed pain were found to have significantly larger tears at the time of initial enrollment.

Conclusions.—Pain development in shoulders with an asymptomatic rotator cuff tear is associated with an increase in tear size. Larger tears are more likely to develop pain in the short term than are smaller tears. Further research is warranted to investigate the role of prophylactic treatment of asymptomatic shoulders to avoid the development of pain and loss of shoulder function.

▶ This is a National Institutes of Health—sponsored research project with its main purpose to elucidate the natural history of asymptomatic rotator cuff tears. To be included in the study, the patient had to have one shoulder with a symptomatic rotator cuff tear and the contralateral one with an asymptomatic rotator cuff tear as demonstrated by sonography. One hundred ninety-five patients met these criteria. The end point was 2 years or the presence of new onset significant pain for greater than 6 weeks. Based on this short-term natural history study, the authors show that 44 of 195 of these patients ultimately developed symptomatic rotator cuff pain in the previous asymptomatic rotator cuff tear shoulder. They then compared a subset of the persistently asymptomatic shoulders with the ones that developed pain. They found that asymptomatic shoulders with a larger cuff tear to begin with were at higher risk of extending that tear and becoming symptomatic.

This is an outstanding study that attempts to ask the question of which cuff tear will ultimately become symptomatic. The ultimate implications are which shoulders should be operated on, maybe even when they are asymptomatic with a rotator cuff tear, and which ones can be left alone. The duration of this study is too short to answer this question, but it is a very important question that needs to be answered. There may be selection bias in this study, as only patients with one shoulder with a known painful rotator cuff tear are enrolled. It is probable that this group is prone to rotator cuff disease (maybe more than the population in general) and in particular to painful rotator cuff disease. A better population group would be a random group of age-matched patients with no shoulder complaints. It was also not clear in the body of the article if the patient was blinded to the findings of the sonographic results on the asymptomatic shoulder. It is possible that if the patients know they have a rotator cuff tear on the asymptomatic shoulder, they may be more prone to the perception of pain in that shoulder. Despite these limitations, the authors are adding in a significant fashion to our knowledge of the natural history of rotator cuff disease.

T. W. Wright, MD

27 Shoulder: Trauma

Method of Subcoracoid Graft Passage in Acromioclavicular Joint Reconstruction

George MS, Jorgensen JR (KSF Orthopaedic Ctr, Houston, TX)
Orthopedics 33:812, 2010

Background.—Surgical reconstruction is recommended for the treatment of severe acromioclavicular separation type IV and V injuries as well as symptomatic type III injuries that have not resolved with nonoperative approaches. Several surgical techniques can be used, including primary ligament repair, modified Weaver-Dunn reconstruction, and free soft tissue transfer passed either through or around the coracoid process. Reconstruction using free soft tissue grafts passed around the coracoid process is more biomechanically stable than modified Weaver-Dunn reconstruction. Passing the suture and/or graft material under the coracoid process is the most technically demanding aspect of this approach because of limited exposure, proximity to neurovascular structures, width of the conjoined tendon, and thickness of fascia adjacent to the coracoid process. The 45° Suture Lasso offers the surgeon a readily available, appropriately curved, and sharp tool to pass sutures and/or soft tissue grafts safely, simply, and efficiently.

Methods.—Six patients (mean age 41 years) with chronic type V acromioclavicular separation had reconstruction with semitendinosus allograft using the Suture Lasso to pass the graft under the coracoid process. Follow-up was a minimum of 6 months, with postoperative radiographs obtained 2 weeks after surgery.

Technique.—With the patient positioned in the beach-chair position, the affected arm is draped free. A 5-cm incision follows Langer's line over the acromioclavicular joint. The deltotrapezial fascia is elevated off the anterior and posterior aspects of the distal clavicle and acromion process. Having palpated the coracoacromial ligament under the anterior acromion, it is sharply elevated from the acromial insertion, and the coracoacromial ligament is freed to the coracoid process level. An oscillating saw is used to excise the distal 1 cm of the clavicle. The intramedullary canal of the distal clavicle is prepared using a high-speed bur. Coracoacromial ligament transfer and transosseous free ligament passage are assured. The coracoid process is palpated, then the Suture Lasso is passed from medial to lateral just adjacent to and below the coracoid, posterior to the conjoined tendon insertion. The Suture Lasso is passed along the bony surface of the coracoid, avoiding neurovascular entanglement. The wire is passed through the Suture Lasso and reacquired on the coracoid process' lateral aspect. The wire is used to move the semitendinosus graft under the coracoid process and out two drill holes in the distal clavicle. The graft is knotted over the top of the distal clavicle, then nonabsorbable sutures are placed in the knot portion of the graft for security. Braided absorbable suture is used to repair the deltotrapezial fascia. The wound is closed, then the shoulder is placed in a 15° external rotation abduction sling to minimize tension on the repair.

Results.—Excellent pain relief was reported by all patients at least 6 months postoperatively. No clinical deformities recurred, nor were there any complications or neurovascular injuries.

Conclusions.—Passing the graft under the coracoid when performing acromioclavicular reconstruction is the most challenging part of the process. Use of the Suture Lasso to make the subcoracoid passage avoids extensive dissection and neurovascular involvement. Operating room time is reduced, along with patient morbidity.

▶ This article describes the surgical technique for reconstruction of severely displaced acromioclavicular joint separations, using a tendinous graft passed under the surface of the coracoid and around the distal end of the clavicle, and the transfer of the distal aspect of the coracoacromial ligament to the distal end of the clavicle.

The article focused, as a surgical tip, on the value of using a 45° Suture Lasso (Arthrex, Naples, Florida) to pass grafts (technique described in the article) or sutures (modified Weaver-Dunn technique) under the surface of the coracoid because of its appropriate curvature and sharp end.

The technique consisted on the passage of the Suture Lasso from medial to lateral, immediately adjacent and below the coracoid and posterior to the insertion of the conjoined tendon. They tested this technique on 6 patients with chronic type V acromioclavicular separations without complications. No control group was used.

Theoretical advantages of the use of the mentioned instrument include the following:

1. Elimination of the necessity of any dissection under the coracoid avoiding damage to the neurovascular structures, as the sharp end of the Suture Lasso can directly pierce the soft tissues around the coracoid. This is particularly true if only sutures are to be passed, but some additional dissection might be needed to pass a graft wider than the hole made by the instrument.

2. Faster technique for the reasons exposed above, but the authors did not provide the time used in this step of the surgery or compare it with other nonexpensive options, such as using right-curved hemostats.

Disadvantages may include the following:

1. The possibility of piercing neurovascular structures with the Suture Lasso if it was not passed just around the bone and if a too medial or inferior insertion of the instrument was used.

2. The added price of the instrument.

A. M. Foruria, MD, PhD

Risk of axillary nerve injury during percutaneous proximal humerus locking plate insertion using an external aiming guide

Saran N, Bergeron SG, Benoit B, et al (McGill Univ Health Centre, Montreal, Quebec, Canada; Univ of Montreal, Quebec, Canada)
Injury 41:1037-1040, 2010

Objectives.—The purpose of this study was to determine which screws could be safely inserted percutaneously into a proximal humerus locking plate using a new external aiming guide without injuring the axillary nerve. We also sought to evaluate that all the screws could be accurately inserted in a locked position with the external guide.

Methods.—Eight cadaveric specimens were implanted with a proximal humerus locking plate using a minimally invasive direct-lateral deltoid splitting approach using an attached external aiming guide for screw insertion. The anatomic proximity of the axillary nerve to the guidewires and screws was measured following soft tissue dissection and inspection of the nerve.

Results.—The two superior holes (C1 and C2) were proximal to the axillary nerve with an average distance of 15.1 mm. Screw F was on average 6.6 mm distal to the axillary nerve but within 2 mm of the nerve in two specimens. In all specimens, the locking screws were appropriately seated in a locked position using the external aiming guide.

Conclusions.—This study suggests that percutaneous fixation of a proximal humerus locking plate with an external aiming guide can be safely used for proximal humerus fractures. The limited number of screws that can be inserted into the proximal fragment using the current external guide arm may compromise fixation of more unstable fractures. Therefore, the indications for percutaneous locking plate fixation of the proximal humerus using an external aiming guide should be limited to stable fracture patterns that can be anatomically reduced.

▶ Recently developed minimally invasive techniques for proximal humeral fracture fixation have attempted to improve the biology of fracture healing. A minimally invasive lateral deltoid splitting approach has been described using a proximal humeral locking plate that has shown good results for 2-part and 3-part valgus-impacted proximal humerus fractures. However, the accurate insertion of the locking screws without a percutaneous guide may be technically difficult, as the traditional screw insertion guide block cannot be used percutaneously without risk of stretching the axillary nerve. External guides have been designed to overcome this potential problem when inserting a proximal humerus locking plate through a minimally invasive approach. The authors conclude from their study that the external guide, which is commercially available, can be safely used for fracture fixation without injury of the axillary nerve. The closest drill hole to the nerve was located about 1 cm from the nerve. One of the limitations of the study was that the specimens were intact humerii, not fractured humerii. In the fracture situation, the relative distances between the anatomical structures and the nerve may be altered. For example, during reduction through the surgical neck, there may be impaction across the fracture site because of the osteopenic nature of the bone at the surgical neck. Thus, the distances to the axillary nerve may well be closer than one might expect. Another limitation of the study is that the cadaveric humerii size, length, and height from which the specimens were harvested may have implications in reference to the proximity of the axillary nerve. This was not documented in the study. However, it is helpful for the surgeon to realize that this technique is well described and the tools are available, if he/she wishes to attempt this technique. The surgeon should still be very cognizant of the potential for axillary nerve injury despite the findings described in this article.

E. Cheung, MD

Sub-muscular plating of the humerus: An emerging technique
Ziran BH, Kinney RC, Smith WR, et al (Atlanta Med Ctr, GA; Geisinger Health Ctr, Danville, PA; et al)
Injury 41:1047-1052, 2010

Objective.—The purpose of the present study was to evaluate percutaneous sub-muscular internal fixation using a locked screw methodology for treatment of diaphyseal humeral fractures.

Methods.—Inclusion criteria were multiple extremity fractures, open fractures, neurovascular injuries, additional ipsilateral upper extremity fractures, the inability to obtain a satisfactory closed reduction and isolated fractures with circumstances that prevented effective bracing. Exclusion criteria were immaturity, neoplasm, infection and intra-articular extensions in the same bone. Outcome measures included clinical and radiographic healing, complications, elbow and shoulder symptoms, range of motion (ROM) and Constant—Murley (CM) scores.

Results.—Thirty-one patients with 32 fractures were evaluated with a mean follow-up of 16 months (3—38 months). There was radiographic healing in 31 out of the 32 fractures; the non-union was revised to open plating at 6 months and healed uneventfully. Hardware complications included two construct disengagements; one patient was revised and healed, and the other achieved union with bracing. Neurovascular complications included one preoperative nerve palsy that recovered by 3 months, two partial to complete postoperative nerve palsies that recovered by 6 months, and one intact-to-complete nerve palsy due to a bone fragment that required decompression with full recovery by 3 weeks. All patients had functional ROM with a mean CM score of 88. There were no elbow complaints and minor shoulder dysfunction occurred in two patients with ipsilateral shoulder injuries. The rate of neurovascular complications was comparable to open plating techniques and all patients had full recovery.

Conclusion.—We feel sub-muscular anterior plating of the humerus using locking screw technology is a viable and useful method for diaphyseal humeral fractures.

▶ The authors describe their technique and outcomes using anterior submuscular plating for the treatment of midshaft humeral fractures. The technique uses a 2-pin external fixator, which was used to help maintain a closed reduction during the procedure, much like a femoral distractor is used for the lower extremity. Two Schanz pins were then placed into the humerus, anteriolateral in the proximal segment and posteriolateral in the distal segment. A bolster was used to prevent sagging at the fracture site, while the distractor maintained length and alignment. Once reduction was verified, the plate was centered over the fracture with fluoroscopic assistance. The ends of the plate were marked, and 2 small incisions were centered over the second-to-last hole on each side of the plate. Distally, the radial nerve and lateral antebrachial cutaneous nerve were identified and protected. The lateral antebrachial cutaneous nerve exits the biceps brachii and was protected during the initial exposure. The interval between the brachioradialis and brachialis was then developed and the radial nerve was identified. Once identified, a separate transmuscular interval was created by splitting the lateral third of the brachialis to center the bone in the portal. Proximally, the interval between the pectoralis major and the long head of the biceps brachii was identified and developed. The deltoid and pectoralis major were retracted lateral, while the biceps brachii and coracobrachialis were retracted medial to expose the anterior proximal diaphysis of the humerus. The plate was inserted and centered in each operative portal with fluoroscopic guidance. Once reduction and plate placement were achieved, fixation could be performed.

One potential concern with any submuscular technique for these fractures is that of the radial nerve. In each case, the authors dissected out the nerve and they felt that it was not at risk. The authors believe that the temporary nerve palsies may have been caused by reductive manipulation. It should also be noted that this method is much more challenging to use with distal third fractures because there is a flare of the humerus that may lateralize the retractor and bring it closer to the course of the radial nerve. Limitations were the retrospective nature and lack of control in the study. This prevents direct comparison to other methods of fixation, such as open plating and intramedullary (IM) nailing. The authors acknowledge that a future prospective randomized study comparing this submuscular plating technique with open plating or IM nailing as controls would enable better assessment of effectiveness of the technique.

E. Cheung, MD

The Clavicle Hook Plate for Neer Type II Lateral Clavicle Fractures

Renger RJ, Roukema GR, Reurings JC, et al (Hosp de la Santa Creu i Sant Pau, Barcelona, Spain; Med Ctr Haaglanden, Den Haag, The Netherlands; St Elisabeth Hosp, Tilburg, The Netherlands; et al)
J Orthop Trauma 23:570-574, 2009

Objective.—To evaluate functional and radiologic outcome in patients with a Neer type II lateral clavicle fracture treated with the clavicle hook plate.

Design.—Multicenter retrospective study.

Setting.—Five level I and II trauma centers.

Patients.—Forty-four patients, average age 38.4 years (18—66 years), with a Neer type II lateral clavicle fracture treated with the clavicle hook plate between January 1, 2003, and December 31, 2006.

Intervention.—Open reduction and internal fixation with the clavicle hook plate. Removal of all 44 implants after consolidation at a mean of 8.4 months (2—33 months) postoperatively.

Main Outcome Measurements.—At an average follow-up of 27.4 months (13—48 months), functional outcome was assessed with the Constant-Murley scoring system. Radiographs were taken to evaluate consolidation and to determine the distance between the coracoid process and the clavicle.

Results.—The average Constant score was 92.4 (74—100). The average distance between the coracoid process and the clavicle was 9.8 mm (7.3—14.8 mm) compared with 9.4 mm (6.9—14.3 mm) on the contralateral nonoperative side. We observed 1 dislocation of an implant (2.2%), 2 cases of pseudarthrosis (4.5%), 2 superficial wound infections (4.5%), 2 patients with hypertrophic scar tissue (4.5%), and 3 times an acromial osteolysis (6.8%). Thirty patients (68%) reported discomfort due to the implant. These implant-related complaints and the acromial osteolysis disappeared after removal of the hook plate. With all the patients, direct functional aftercare was possible.

Conclusions.—The clavicle hook plate is a suitable implant for Neer type II clavicle fractures. The advantage of this osteosynthesis is the possibility of immediate functional aftercare. We observed a high percentage of discomfort due to the implant; therefore, we advise to remove the implant as soon as consolidation has taken place.

▶ This retrospective multicenter study evaluated the clavicle hook plate for treatment of Neer type II lateral clavicle fractures in 42 patients. All plates were removed at an average of 8.4 months (2-33 months) postoperatively after X-ray documentation of fracture healing. Surgery was performed by experienced trauma surgeons in 5 separate institutions. Outcomes were evaluated by the Constant score, which averaged a very acceptable 92 (74-100) with the worst results occurring in older patients (> 60 years). Radiographic results revealed a coracoclavicular distance of 9.8 mm (7.3-14.8 mm) versus 9.4 mm (6.9-14.3 mm) on the nonoperative side. Complications were minimal and

disappeared following plate removal. Importantly, postoperative immobilization was kept to a minimum and allowed for early return to daily activities. No mention was made concerning the time before returning to sports or overhead activities. Impingement symptoms were the most problematic issue while the plate remained in, all of which resolved following plate removal. This is an important study because it is the first multicenter study showing good to excellent results for the clavicle hook plate used to treat these lateral clavicle fractures. Most importantly, it documents the need for plate removal in all patients after fracture healing. Also, it is important to discuss with the patient preoperatively the very high probability that they may experience impingement symptoms while the plate is in place and that they should expect to have the plate removed at some point, requiring a second operation. This is a great option for treating these hard-to-fix fractures in the right patient.

J. C. Macy, MD

Biomechanical evaluation of a new fixation technique for internal fixation of three-part proximal humerus fractures in a novel cadaveric model
Brianza S, Plecko M, Gueorguiev B, et al (AO Res Inst, Davos Platz, Switzerland; Unfallkrankenhaus Graz der AUVA, Austria)
Clin Biomech 25:886-892, 2010

Background.—The optimal surgical treatment for displaced proximal humeral fractures is still controversial. A new implant for the treatment of three-part fractures has been recently designed. It supplements the existing Expert Humeral Nail with a locking plate. We developed a novel humeral cadaveric model and the existing implant and the prototype were biomechanically compared to determine their ability in maintaining interfragmentary stability.

Methods.—The bone mineral density of eight pairs of cadaveric humeri was assessed and a three-part proximal humeral fracture was simulated with a Greater Tuberosity osteotomy and a surgical neck wedge ostectomy. The specimens were randomly assigned to either treatment. A bone anchor simulated part of a rotator cuff tendon pulling on the Greater Tuberosity. Specimens were initially tested in axial compression and afterward with a compound cyclic load to failure. An optical 3D motion tracking system continuously monitored the relative interfragmentary movements.

Findings.—The specimen stabilized with the prototype demonstrated higher stiffness ($P = 0.036$) and better interfragmentary stability (P values<0.028) than the contralateral treated with the existing implant. There was no correlation between the bone mineral density and any of the investigated variables.

Interpretation.—The convenience of this new IM-nail and locking plate assembly must be confirmed in vivo but the current study provides a biomechanical rationale for its use in the treatment of three-part proximal humeral fractures. The improved stability could be advantageous in particular when medial buttress is missing, even in osteoporotic bone.

▶ The authors present a biomechanical study comparing 2 proximal humeral nails for fixation of 3-part proximal humeral fractures. Eight cadaveric humeri, normalized for bone density, were used in the model. A 3-part fracture model was utilized, including a surgical neck and greater tuberosity osteotomy. The greater tuberosity fragment was fixed with a custom anchor, reinforced with polymethylmethacrylate to assist in mechanical testing.

Each humerus was fixed with either a standard humeral nail (Expert Proximal Humeral Nail) or a new nail with locking plate (Expert Proximal Humeral Nail with Locking Plate for Humeral Nail). Biomechanical testing was performed for axial stiffness and cyclic loading in compression and angular/rotational displacement through the greater tuberosity.

The proximal humeral locking plate and humeral nail had significantly greater axial stiffness, with greater load and cycles to failure compared with the proximal humeral nail. At 10 000 cycles, there was less displacement and rotation through the greater tuberosity in the proximal humeral locking plate and humeral nail.

This biomechanical study confirms that the addition of a proximal humeral locking plate to a proximal humeral nail significantly increases the biomechanical strength of the construct. The clinical utility remains unknown, as most surgeons prefer to avoid damage to the rotator cuff during insertion of the nail and elect to perform proximal locked plating.

J. Jacobson, MD

A Prospective Clinical Study of Proximal Humerus Fractures Treated With a Locking Proximal Humerus Plate

Yang H, Li Z, Zhou F, et al (Med School of Nantong Univ, Jiangyin City, Jiangsu Province, China)
J Orthop Trauma 25:11-17, 2011

Objectives.—The purpose of this prospective study was to evaluate the safety, efficacy, and functional outcome of the locked proximal humerus plate (LPHP) to treat proximal humerus fractures.

Design.—Prospective clinical trial.

Setting.—University orthopedic center.

Patients.—Over a 25-month period, 64 consecutive patients were treated with a LPHP for an unstable or displaced proximal humerus fracture.

Intervention.—Demographic data, trauma mechanisms, surgical approaches, and postoperative complications were collected from medical records. Fracture classification according to the Neer classification, radiographic head—shaft angle, and screw tip—articular surface distance in true anteroposterior and axillary lateral radiographs of the shoulder were measured postoperatively.

Main Outcome Measurements.—The functional Outcome was evaluated with a Constant—Murley (CM) evaluation. The CM score is a validated shoulder-specific scoring system in which patients report subjective findings. The physician reported the objective measurements of the shoulder.

Results.—Follow-ups were completed for all of the patients. The overall complication rate was 35.9%, with screw penetration into the glenohumeral joint as the most frequent problem (7.6%). Deep wound infections were observed in 3.1% (n = 2) of the cases and avascular necrosis in 3.1% (n = 2). All complications occurred in 4-part fractures. Subacromial impingement, frozen shoulder, rotator cuff rupture, and wound dehiscence were observed in 3.1% (n = 2), 3.1% (n = 2), 1.6% (n = 1), and 1.6% (n = 1) of the cases, respectively. Multivariate linear regression analysis revealed that the fracture pattern and the presence or absence of medial support were significant predictors of functional Outcome ($P = 0.026$ and $P = 0.003$, respectively). Patient age ($P = 0.581$), sex ($P = 0.325$), and initial tuberosity displacement (varus/extension or valgus/impaction; $P = 0.059$) were not significantly associated with the CM score.

Conclusions.—The LPHP seems to be a promising implant for the fixation of proximal humerus fractures. However, there are certain limitations that should be mentioned. The number of cases in our study was small, and no safe conclusions can be extracted regarding the rate of avascular necrosis. Additional studies with larger cohorts and longer follow-ups are necessary to better define the appropriate indications for and expected Outcomes of this technology.

▶ This article is a prospective case series with level IV evidence of patients who underwent open reduction and internal fixation (ORIF) of displaced 2-, 3-, and 4-part proximal humerus fractures with a locking proximal humerus plate. The period of collection was from 2005 to 2007. Strengths of this study include a relatively large patient cohort (64), prospective data collection, and the use of a validated shoulder outcome score (Constant-Murley [CM] score). Patients in this series underwent ORIF through a deltopectoral approach with suture fixation of the tuberosities and application of a locked proximal humerus plate. Allografting of the humeral head defect (cancellous chips or calcium phosphate cement) was also routinely used. Follow-up was a minimum of 1 year with the primary outcome being the CM score. All patients had union of their fracture at final follow-up. According to CM scores, 3 were excellent, 28 were good, 29 were moderate, and 4 had poor outcomes. Significant predictors of outcome (CM score) after multivariate linear regression analysis were fracture pattern (2- and 3-part fractures did better than 4-part fractures) and the presence or absence of medial calcar support for the humeral head. Patient age, sex, and initial tuberosity displacement were not found to be predictive of outcome. Complications occurred in 35.9% of patients with screw penetration after humeral head collapse (7.6%) being most common, followed by malunion

(4.6%), and deep infection (3.1%). The rate of avascular necrosis was low at 3.1% and seen exclusively in 4-part fractures. Five patients required reoperation for complications in this series. All complications occurred in 4-part fractures. The authors felt that achieving adequate medial support was key to preventing collapse and screw cutout and improving clinical outcomes, specifically strength and range of motion.

This study adds little new information to the body of literature on the use of locking plates for the treatment of proximal humerus fractures. Clinical and radiographic outcomes and complication rates were similar to other series. One of the most difficult aspects of treating 3- and 4-part fractures is the management of the displaced tuberosities. Unfortunately, the authors do not describe their technique for repair and fixation of the tuberosities, and they fail to adequately report the healing status of the tuberosities in their series. Also, the study could have been improved with a detailed description of their medial support classification system and technical tips to improve medial support in unstable fractures.

J. M. Wiater, MD

The Biomechanics of Locked Plating for Repairing Proximal Humerus Fractures With or Without Medial Cortical Support
Lescheid J, Zdero R, Shah S, et al (Univ of Toronto, Ontario, Canada; St Michael's Hosp, Toronto, Ontario, Canada; et al)
J Trauma 69:1235-1242, 2010

Background.—Comminuted proximal humerus fracture fixation is controversial. Locked plate complications have been addressed by anatomic reduction or medial cortical support. The relative mechanical contributions of varus malalignment and lack of medial cortical support are presently assessed.

Methods.—Forty synthetic humeri divided into three subgroups were osteotomized and fixed at 0 degrees, 10 degrees, and 20 degrees of varus malreduction with a locking proximal humerus plate (AxSOS, Global model; Stryker, Mahwah, NJ) to simulate mechanical medial support with cortical contact retained. Axial, torsional, and shear stiffness were measured. Half of the specimens in each of the three subgroups underwent a second osteotomy to create a segmental defect simulating loss of medial support with cortex removed. Axial, torsional, and shear stiffness tests were repeated, followed by shear load to failure in 20 degrees of abduction.

Results.—For isolated malreduction with cortical contact, the construct at 0 degrees showed statistically equivalent or higher axial, torsional, and shear stiffness than other subgroups examined. Subsequent removal of cortical support in half the specimens showed a drastic effect on axial, torsional, and shear stiffness at all varus angulations. Constructs with cortical contact at 0 degrees and 10 degrees yielded mean shear failure forces of 12965.4 N and 9341.1 N, respectively, being statistically higher

($p < 0.05$) compared with most other subgroups tested. Specimens failed primarily by plate bending as the humeral head was pushed down medially and distally.

Conclusions.—Anatomic reduction with the medial cortical contact was the stiffest construct after a simulated two-part fracture. This study affirms the concept of medial cortical support by fixing proximal humeral fractures in varus, if absolutely necessary. This may be preferable to fixing the fracture in anatomic alignment when there is a medial fracture gap.

▶ This article uses a synthetic proximal humerus model to show that medial cortical support may be important to the overall construct stability when one particular type of locked proximal humerus plate technique is used to stabilize 2-part proximal humerus fractures with medial comminution and varus angulation. Osteotomies were performed at various angles simulating varus malreductions, with and without medial cortical support. Construct failure was documented, and plate failure was described. The article suggests that fixing a proximal humerus fracture in varus may be preferable to anatomic alignment to prevent construct failure. In this model, no attempt was made to adjust for proximal humerus muscle attachment forces, which may influence the forces seen by the fracture in vivo. Also, the segmental defect used to produce the medial comminution in this study does not coincide with commonly found medial comminution of typical proximal humerus fractures, and plate bending is not the typical mode of failure for these constructs, that is, screw cutout is usually seen clinically. Overall, however, this concept of medial metaphyseal support makes sense, and complications relating to lack of this support (hardware failure and loss of reduction) are not seen infrequently. Several recent studies have shown that medial support is critical to successful treatment of these particular proximal humerus fractures.

J. C. Macy, MD

Biomechanical Comparison of Contemporary Clavicle Fixation Devices
Renfree T, Conrad B, Wright T (Univ of Florida, Gainesville)
J Hand Surg 35A:639-644, 2010

Purpose.—Because recent studies have shown that malunited or nonunited clavicle fractures treated nonsurgically have poor outcomes, early fixation of certain clavicle shaft fractures using contemporary implants has become more common. Little is known about the physiologic loading of these implants. This study was designed to observe the biomechanical behavior and strength of implants used for fixation of the clavicle shaft.

Methods.—We used synthetic clavicle bones that were produced in 2 pieces to replicate the conditions of a transverse fracture. Ten specimens per group were tested using 3 clavicle fixation constructs: precontoured clavicle plates with unicortical locking, precontoured clavicle plates with bicortical nonlocking screws, and intramedullary Rockwood clavicle pins. Two loading conditions were used: cantilever bending and 3-point bending.

Results.—For cantilever bending, both plate groups failed by fracture at the most medial screw hole. The pin group was unable to resist the small torque associated with off-axis loading. The pin group failed at a lower maximum load, which occurred with a greater maximum displacement. The pin group was also less stiff than the plate group. In the 3-point bending test, the pin group was significantly more flexible and achieved higher failure loads than the plate groups. There were no significant differences between the unicortical and bicortical screws for any of the measured variables with either loading condition.

Conclusions.—Both locking and nonlocking constructs appear to provide similar rigid fixation under the tested mechanical conditions. The intramedullary pin can provide high resistance to failure loads in situations when rigidity and rotational stiffness are not required. Intramedullary pin fixation appears to be inadequate where rotational stiffness is required.

▶ The authors present a well-designed biomechanical comparison of 3 types of clavicle fixation in a synthetic clavicle fracture model. Specifically, the authors compared locked unicortical plate fixation, unlocked bicortical plate fixation, and intramedullary Rockwood clavicle pin fixation of midshaft clavicle fractures in cantilever bending and 3-point bending loading conditions. Not surprisingly, the authors found increased resistance to loading and stiffness of both plate groups when compared with the pin fixation. Resistance to off-axis loading was significantly worse in the pin group when compared to both plate groups. However, the pin fixation was more flexible and therefore led to higher failure loads in the 3-point bending setting than the plate groups. This suggests that clavicles fixed with intramedullary pins will allow for more displacement prior to failure in the clinical setting, which may be beneficial for resistance to failure following postoperative motion or trauma. However, this level of displacement may impact overall union rates, which was not evaluated in this study, and clinical relevance of the study is limited as a result.

In my practice, I prefer the application of a precontoured clavicle plate with hybrid (locking and unlocking) fixation placed superiorly on the clavicle, and this has led to outstanding results in my hands. The ability to use unicortical locking screws in a plate, especially medially, is attractive so that injury to the major neurovascular structures due to inadvertent plunging with the drill or placement of screws that are too long is avoided. However, as the authors of this study point out, the main point of failure from cantilever bending of these plates is with loss of fixation medially, so I continue to use hybrid fixation and bicortical fixation (either locked or nonlocked) medially when possible.

J. Yao, MD

Trends and Variation in Incidence, Surgical Treatment, and Repeat Surgery of Proximal Humeral Fractures in the Elderly

Bell J-E, Leung BC, Spratt KF, et al (Dartmouth-Hitchcock Med Ctr, Lebanon, NH)

J Bone Joint Surg Am 93:121-131, 2011

Background.—The treatment of proximal humeral fractures in the elderly remains controversial. Options include nonoperative treatment, open reduction with internal fixation (ORIF), and hemiarthroplasty. Locking plate technology has expanded the indications for ORIF for certain fracture types in osteoporotic bone. This study was performed to characterize the incidence, treatment, and revision surgery of proximal humeral fractures according to geographic region both before (1999 to 2000) and after (2004 to 2005) the introduction of locking plates.

Methods.—We used a 20% sample of Medicare Part-B data and the Medicare denominator file for the years 1998 to 2006. Proximal humeral fractures were identified by Common Procedural Terminology codes for treatment, categorized as nonoperative, ORIF, or hemiarthroplasty. Geographic variation in treatment type was determined with use of 306 hospital referral regions. Odds ratios for revision surgery were calculated by the need for repeat surgery within one year of the index procedure. Rates were adjusted for age, sex, race, and comorbidities.

Results.—There were 14,774 proximal humeral fractures in the 20% sample from 1999 to 2000 (an estimated total of 73,870 fractures) and 16,138 fractures in the sample from 2004 to 2005 (an estimated total of 80,690 fractures). The overall age, sex, and race-adjusted incidence of proximal humeral fractures was unchanged from 1999 to 2005 (2.47 vs. 2.48 per 1000 Medicare beneficiaries; p = 0.992). However, the absolute rate of surgically managed proximal humeral fractures rose 3.2 percentage points from 12.5% to 15.7%, a relative increase of 25.6% (p < 0.0001). The relative increase in the percentage of fractures treated with ORIF was 28.5% (p < 0.0001), while the percentage of fractures treated with hemiarthroplasty increased 19.6% (p < 0.0001). There were large regional variations in the proportion treated surgically (range, 0% to 68.18%). The rates of repeat surgery were significantly higher in 2004 to 2005 compared with 1999 to 2000 (odds ratio = 1.47, p = 0.043).

Conclusions.—Although the incidence of proximal humeral fractures in the elderly did not change from 1999 to 2005, the rate of surgical treatment increased significantly. The marked regional variation in the rates of surgical treatment highlights the need for better consensus regarding optimal treatment of proximal humeral fractures. Additional research is needed to help to determine which fractures are best treated operatively in order to maximize outcome and minimize the need for revision surgery.

Level of Evidence.—Therapeutic Level II. See Instructions to Authors for a complete description of levels of evidence.

▶ The authors demonstrated that the incidence of open reduction with internal fixation for proximal humerus fractures has risen significantly (29%) since proximal humeral locking plates have been introduced. Unfortunately, they were unable to show that the rise was due solely to fixation with locking plates, rather than with other fixation techniques, such as percutaneous pin fixation, which has also gained in popularity. They also showed a wide geographic variation in surgical treatment of these fractures but were unable to demonstrate whether there was a similar geographical difference in the number of fellowship-trained surgeons, the density of orthopedic surgeons, or the number of years that surgeons in those areas had been in practice. Certainly in my practice (limited to upper extremity), my threshold for operating on proximal humerus fractures has been lowered since the introduction of proximal humeral locking plates. The percentage of patients who I may have been more inclined to treat nonoperatively prior to the introduction of these plates (severe osteopenia, comminution of medial calcar, etc) because of poor fixation methods may be reflective of the difference in numbers shown in this study.

K. J. Renfree, MD

Proximal humeral fractures: current concepts in classification, treatment and outcomes
Murray IR, Amin AK, White TO, et al (Edinburgh Shoulder Clinic, UK)
J Bone Joint Surg [Br] 93-B:1-11, 2011

Most proximal humeral fractures are stable injuries of the ageing population, and can be successfully treated non-operatively. The management of the smaller number of more complex displaced fractures is more controversial and new fixation techniques have greatly increased the range of fractures that may benefit from surgery.

This article explores current concepts in the classification and clinical aspects of these injuries, reviewing the indications, innovations and outcomes for the most common methods of treatment.

▶ The article by Murray and coauthors presents a review of the most recent available information on the treatment of proximal humerus fractures. This group of surgeons has shown great interest in this topic, and during the past years, they have explored and presented their experience in different aspects of this injury.

When considering the best option for a patient with a proximal humerus fracture, the authors, in addition to the type of fracture, emphasize the importance of taking into account factors related to a patient's comorbidities and expectations, but also those related to the surgeon experience. In this regard, they suggest that the difficulties in dealing with complex humerus fractures might suggest that this problem should be treated in tertiary referral centers.

It seems appropriate to divide these fractures into those which should clearly be treated conservatively, those in which surgery is essential, and those situated in the gray zone of lack of evidence. Unfortunately, many of our patients fall in the latter category. It is honest to recognize that surgery is only mandatory in less than 1% of the fractures (open, floating shoulder, vascular injury, etc).

Assuming that the great majority of patients may be better off with conservative treatment, especially the elderly, if one decides that surgery is required, open reduction and internal fixation should be the procedure of choice in the vast majority of cases. This is true in the young and active patient. Hemiarthroplasty should be reserved for head splitting fractures and comminuted fractures in the elderly. Tuberosity nonunion is the feared complication that is being solved by some surgeons with the use of reverse arthroplasty. This concept should clearly stand the test of time before it can be openly recommended.

The conclusion of this review seems wise: "The challenge for the future is to select those patients who are going to be at increased risk of developing complications or a poor functional result after non-operative treatment"; only these should undergo operative management.

S. A. Antuña, MD, PhD

Clavicular Fractures Following Coracoclavicular Ligament Reconstruction with Tendon Graft: A Report of Three Cases
Turman KA, Miller CD, Miller MD (Univ of Virginia Health System, Charlottesville)
J Bone Joint Surg Am 92:1526-1532, 2010

Background.—Over 60 techniques have been developed to surgically manage severe acromioclavicular joint separations. An anatomic reconstruction of both the conoid and the trapezoid coracoclavicular ligament is especially appealing because these ligaments act synergistically to limit displacement of the acromioclavicular joint, improving the stability of the joint and enhancing clinical outcome. Few reports note the complications associated with newer techniques such as this. Seven patients had reconstruction of the coracoclavicular ligaments with an anatomic tendon graft technique, and three suffered complications related to the clavicular fixation.

Case Reports.—*Case 1*: Man, 26, had a Rockwood type-V acromioclavicular separation after a bicycle accident. Tibialis anterior allograft reconstruction was done, including clavicular tunnels 7 mm in diameter to accommodate the graft. Two weeks later there was anatomic reduction of the acromioclavicular joint, but the patient did not return until 4 months postoperatively, when he had reinjured the shoulder while white-water rafting a month earlier. There was a healing clavicular fracture through the lateral bone tunnel with minimal displacement and visible callus formation. The acromioclavicular joint reduction was maintained. Conservative treatment was undertaken.

Case 2: Man, 48, had chronic type-V acromioclavicular separation 2 years after a motorcycle accident. A tibialis anterior allograft reconstruction was done with 6-mm clavicular tunnels. He was instructed to perform passive range-of-motion exercises for 6 weeks, then begin strengthening exercises at 3 months. At 4 months he reinjured the shoulder while bow hunting. The atraumatic injury caused sudden pain in the shoulder after the patient tried to pull the bowstring. Minimally displaced clavicular fracture through the medial bone tunnel was managed conservatively.

Case 3: Woman 37, had a type-V acromioclavicular separation after an all-terrain-vehicle accident. A semitendinosus autograft reconstruction was done through 5.5-mm clavicular tunnels 3 months after injury. Clinical and radiographic evidence of failure with recurrent acromioclavicular joint deformity was found 6 weeks after surgery. Revision reconstruction of the coracoclavicular ligaments with a tibialis anterior allograft was performed. A "blowout" of the posterior wall of the medial clavicular tunnel had caused loss of fixation and loss of reduction of the acromioclavicular joint. Pins were placed in the joint and a suture anchor was placed in the coracoid to supplement the reconstruction through new holes. Supported range of motion was advised for 3 months.

Analysis.—Repair techniques were designed to keep the acromioclavicular joint reduced long enough to permit primary healing of the coracoclavicular ligaments. Failure to address the acromioclavicular ligaments and capsule may have increased the forces across the coracoclavicular ligament reconstruction, raising the risk for failure. Contributing to the complications and failure of fixation were technical factors such as excessively large tunnels done to accommodate large grafts, modification of the technique to add the coracoid suture anchor, factors related to placing the interference screws, poor patient compliance, and poor patient-surgeon communication.

Conclusions.—Risk of fracture may be reduced by proper preoperative counseling coupled with surgical modifications. The latter include the intraoperative use of smaller-diameter bone tunnels, the maintenance of an adequate bone bridge between the tunnels, the use of a single bone tunnel, and the avoidance of posterior cortical breach or blowout by precise placement of tunnels. Postoperative management should include clearly conveyed goals and sufficient communication between the surgeon, the patient, and the physical therapist.

▶ Primum non nocere, or first, do no harm, is the phrase that always comes to mind when discussing reconstruction of acromioclavicular (AC) separations.

The authors present 3 patients with clavicle fracture complications from the anatomic reconstruction, which was recently popularized. Unfortunately, techniques that work on cadaveric specimens may have other problems in vivo. The stresses placed across the AC/coracoclavicular joints after reconstruction are significant, and one should expect that whatever fixation method is chosen, it will be stressed and postoperative radiographs will often be humbling. This is why I have evolved to a technique for AC reconstruction, which is a primum non nocere approach. A static anchor (metallic 4 pronged) in the coracoid loaded with 2 large sutures passed through 2-mm drill holes in the anatomic positions of the clavicle, combined with a semitendinosus allograft around both the coracoid and clavicle. In this way, the small drill holes are less of a fracture risk (vs 5.5- to 6-mm holes in this case series), no bioabsorbable implants are used (to lessen cystic lesion risk), the sutures do not cross around the coracoid or clavicle (so if a fracture does occur, reduction and clavicle alignment remain stable), and if the anchor pulls out then this is a simpler fix than fixing a coracoid fracture. I have not had one of these anchors pull out, but I have treated outside cases with coracoid fractures when suture was placed all the way around the base. It does not mean that my technique is the only way to do it; failures can still occur, but I am comfortable that I will have adequate bone stock if I were to have to revise it. As we look for improved biomechanical stability for this injury, we must keep in mind the challenges of revision of a particular technique if it were to be needed.

T. R. McAdams, MD

Surgical treatment of chronic acromioclavicular dislocation: Comparison between two surgical procedures for anatomic reconstruction
Fraschini G, Ciampi P, Scotti C, et al (San Raffaele Scientific Inst, Via Olgettina, Milan, Italy; Univ of Milan, Italy)
Injury 41:1103-1106, 2010

Introduction.—Surgical treatment of chronic complete acromioclavicular (AC) joint dislocation is still debated and no gold standard surgical procedure has been identified.

Materials and Methods.—A retrospective series of 90 patients treated for AC dislocations is reported here. Patients were divided into three groups: group 1 receiving AC reconstruction with a Dacron vascular prosthesis; group 2 receiving AC reconstruction with LARS® artificial ligament; group 3 receiving conservative treatment. Follow-up was performed after 1, 6 and 15 months with plain radiographs, UCLA, SPADI and modified UCLA acromioclavicular rating scales.

Results.—Patients treated surgically presented significant better functional outcome compared to patients treated conservatively with overall positive results in 93.3% of patients for group 2 and 53.3% of patients for group 1. However, reconstruction with Dacron vascular prosthesis presented an unacceptable high complications rate (43.3%).

Conclusion.—Our results show that anatomic AC reconstruction with LARS® artificial ligament resulted in both satisfactory functional outcome and low complication rate. Therefore, we recommend this procedure for the treatment of chronic complete AC dislocations.

▶ The authors in a retrospective manner report on the surgical outcomes for 2 types of late acromioclavicular (AC) reconstructions and compare them with nonoperative management of types III and IV dislocations. This was a nonrandomized study. One group was treated with a Dacron graft looped around the coracoid and clavicle, and the other was treated with a ligament prosthesis called a Ligament Augmentation and Reconstruction System (LARS) placed around the coracoid and through 2 holes in the clavicle fixed with interference screws. Both surgical groups had better functional outcome than the control nonoperative group; however, the Dacron graft had a 43% complication rate, mostly failure of the construct. The LARS group had only 1 ligament rupture. The authors feel that interference screw fixation through 2 screw holes is superior to loop fixation, as it spreads the forces out about the distal clavicle.

In reviewing this article, I was disadvantaged, not being familiar with the LARS artificial ligament. It is not clear to me if it is designed to assist and support the AC joint indefinitely or if it is ultimately replaced by fibrous tissue. This is a short-term study, and indeed, if the LARS will experience the major share of the AC load indefinitely, one would have to postulate that it will ultimately fail. It is possible, however, that if the AC joint is reduced long enough, fibrous tissue will eventually load share and protect the LARS even in these chronic reconstructions.

T. W. Wright, MD

28 Arm and Humerus

Surgical treatment of pathologic fractures of humerus
Piccioli A, Maccauro G, Rossi B, et al (CTO Hosp, Rome, Italy; Catholic Univ, Rome, Italy; et al)
Injury 41:1112-1116, 2010

This study evaluates different operative treatment options for patients with metastatic fractures of the humerus focusing on surgical procedures, complications, function, and survival rate.

From January 2003 to January 2008, 87 pathological fractures of the humerus in 85 cancer patients were surgically treated in our institutions. Histotypes were breast ($n = 21$), lung ($n = 14$), prostate ($n = 5$), bladder ($n = 4$), kidney ($n = 13$), thyroid ($n = 7$), larynx ($n = 1$), lymphoma ($n = 5$), myeloma ($n = 8$), colon-rectum ($n = 1$), melanoma ($n = 1$), testicle ($n = 1$), hepatocellular carcinoma ($n = 1$) and unknown tumours ($n = 3$). Lesions of the proximal epiphysis were treated with resection and endoprosthetic replacement ($n = 30$). The remaining 57 fractures were stabilized with antegrade unreamed intra-medullary locked nailing without (9 cases) or with resection and use of cement (48 cases). The function of the upper limb was assessed using the Musculo-Skeletal Tumor Society (MSTS) rating scale and survival rate was retrospectively analysed.

The mean survival time of patients after surgery was 8.3 months. Complications of endoprosthetic replacement recorded included disease relapse ($n = 3$), soft tissue infection ($n = 2$) and palsy of musculocutaneous nerve ($n = 1$) whereas, for intra-medullary locked nailing there were three cases of soft tissue infection and one case of radial nerve palsy. The mean MSTS score at follow-up was 73% for endoprosthesis and 79.2% for locked intra-medullary nailing.

Endoprosthetic replacement of the proximal humerus provides a good function of the upper limb, a low risk of local relapse with a low complication rate at follow-up. Unreamed nailing provides immediate stability and pain relief, minimum morbidity and early return of function.

▶ This well-done retrospective cohort study evaluated pathologic humerus fractures in a large group of patients treated with endoprosthetic replacement (one-third of cohort, proximal epi/metaphyseal lesions) or intramedullary (IM) nailing (two-thirds of cohort, diaphyseal lesions). There were multiple primary sites for the metastatic disease. Highly vascularized tumors were embolized prior to surgery. Indications for surgery (impending fracture, size and location, pain) were not discussed. However, surgery was performed based on previously described criteria. The evaluation of complications, functional outcome using the Musculoskeletal Tumor Society rating scale, and survival rates was performed. Survival rates averaged 8.3 months. Complications were limited. Recurrence rates were low. Functional scores were respectable at 73% for endoprosthesis and 79% for IM nailing. Restoring proximal humeral muscle attachments, such as the rotator cuff, deltoid, and pectoralis, were found to be important in improving function after endoprosthetic reconstruction. Pain was completely or significantly reduced in all but 2 patients, and overall quality of life was dramatically improved. This study confirms that appropriate surgical treatment of pathologic humerus fractures using selection criteria based on lesion location can improve the overall quality of life for patients with metastatic disease to the proximal or diaphyseal humerus.

J. C. Macy, MD

Functional bracing of humeral shaft fractures. A review of clinical studies
Papasoulis E, Drosos GI, Ververidis AN, et al (Democritus Univ of Thrace, Alexandroupolis, Greece)
Injury 41:e1-e7, 2010

Functional bracing has been widely accepted as the gold standard for treating humeral shaft fractures conservatively. We conducted a literature review to verify the efficacy of this treatment method. Sixteen case series and two comparative studies fulfilled the criteria set. Analysis of these clinical studies showed that humeral shaft fractures when treated with functional bracing heal in an average of 10.7 weeks. Union rate is high (94.5%). Statistical analysis showed that proximal third fractures and AO type A fractures have a higher non-union rate although this is not statistical significant. Residual deformity and joint stiffness are considered the main drawbacks of conservative treatment. Angulation — usually varus — rarely exceeded 10°, while full shoulder and elbow motion was achieved in 80% and 85% of the patients, respectively. Nevertheless, in the few studies that subjective parameters such as functional scores, pain and quality of life were assessed results were not so promising.

▶ This article looks at functional bracing for humeral shaft fractures. Specifically, the authors performed a literature review of 16 case series and 2 comparative studies. Based on this collection, they noted that the average humeral fracture treated with functional bracing healed in 10.7 weeks. Specifically, they noted that there was a higher nonunion rate in more proximal fractures and that 80% to 85% of patients retained full shoulder and elbow range of motion. Most of the studies did not include subjective parameters, such as functional scores or pain scores. Of the nonunions, they noted that spiral fractures had a significantly higher nonunion rate. Most authors noted that up to 20° of varus angulation could be accepted functionally and cosmetically. Of note was that despite early immobilization of the shoulder and elbow, some range of motion loss could be expected in as much as 15% to 20% of patients.

Given the heterogeneity of these studies and their results, it is difficult to have any final conclusions. None of these studies had a routine Constant score or Disabilities of the Arm, Shoulder, and Hand score performed. It appears overall, though, that at this time functional bracing offers a reasonable rate of union and acceptable functional results at a lower cost and complication rate than surgery. However, this remains a gray zone of when and what fractures specifically can or should be treated with bracing. Overall, this collective summary really did not shed any new light for what are essentially already established standards of care. It did prove, though, that a good randomized study would be of benefit in relation to this topic.

S. F. M. Duncan, MD, MPH, MBA

The external fixation in the treatment of humeral diaphyseal fractures: Outcomes of 84 cases
Catagni MA, Lovisetti L, Guerreschi F, et al ("A. Manzoni Hosp", Lecco, Italy; et al)
Injury 41:1107-1111, 2010

We retrospectively review 84 cases of diaphyseal humeral fractures (24 type A, 38 type B, 22 type C of the AO/OTA classification) treated with external fixation (Hoffmann II frame) between 1995 and 2007. Six of these fractures were complicated with radial nerve palsy. Four cases were open fractures. All reductions were achieved closely or through minimal open approaches. All fractures achieved consolidation with an average of 95 days (range 58—140). The six radial nerve palsies had complete spontaneous recovery. According to the Constant score excellent shoulder function was recorded in 54.6% of the cases, good results in 25%, fair in 13.6% and poor in 6.8%. The elbow function according to the Mayo elbow performance index was excellent in 81.8% of cases, good in 13.6%, fair in 2.3%, and poor in 2.3%. We observed superficial pin tract infections in 12% of the patients. There was no cases of deep infection.

External fixation of humeral diaphyseal fractures as recorded in this case series, represents a management option, which allows straightforward fracture reduction and adequate stability, with a short operative time, excellent consolidation rate and good functional results with no major complications secondary to this type of surgery.

▶ The article looks at 84 cases of patients treated with external fixation for humeral diaphyseal fractures. The article is interesting because I believe that in most countries the gold standard is really open reduction and internal fixation based on AO principles. Other possible techniques include intramedullary nailing. In most practices, external fixation is probably used much less commonly. In this study, they looked at their results and they had surprisingly good results. They had no nerve injuries. The preoperative nerve palsies that were present all resolved. Elbow function in general appeared to be better than shoulder function. They only had some cases of superficial pin infections that were easily treated with oral antibiotics. Their operative time was averaged only 30 minutes, which is actually quite impressive, considering these usually take much longer with open reduction and internal fixation. They did have a case where they had to reapply the frame. The X-rays they show do show good approximation of the fracture fragments but definitely are not completely anatomic. However, whether this makes significant clinical evidence is unlikely. They do talk about that the current accepted upper limits of angular deformities are 20° of procurvatum, 30° of varus, up to 4 cm of shortening, and at 1 cm of translation. The authors note that external fixation has the advantages of nonoperative treatment by retaining the fracture hematoma, the vascularity of the periosteum and endosteum, as well as the advantage of internal fixation, which allows for improved alignment of the fracture and sufficient stability for rehabilitation.

Overall, this is a reasonable technique to consider. However, nerve injuries are still possible, especially with proximal pins causing injury to the axillary nerve and the distal pins causing injury to the radial nerve. This technique should be kept in mind, but at this time, I do not believe it is going to cause a paradigm shift in the treatment of these injuries.

S. F. M. Duncan, MD, MPH, MBA

29 Arthritis

Prospective Outcomes of Stage III Thumb Carpometacarpal Arthritis Treated With Arthroscopic Hemitrapeziectomy and Thermal Capsular Modification Without Interposition
Edwards SG, Ramsey PN (Georgetown Univ Hosp, Washington, DC)
J Hand Surg 35A:566-571, 2010

Purpose.—To prospectively evaluate the subjective and objective results of Eaton stage III thumb carpometacarpal arthritis treated with arthroscopic hemitrapeziectomy and thermal capsular modification without interposition.

Methods.—Twenty-three patients with Eaton stage III thumb carpometacarpal arthritis had arthroscopic hemitrapeziectomy without interposition and were evaluated with regard to grip and pinch strength, digital and wrist motion, Disabilities of the Arm, Shoulder, and Hand (DASH) questionnaire, analog pain scores, and radiographic findings before surgery, 3 months after surgery, and at a minimum of 4 years after surgery.

Results.—At 3 months after surgery, average DASH score improved from 61 to 10, and pain scores decreased from 8.3 to 1.5. Grip and key pinch strength improved 6.8 kg and 1.9 kg, respectively, and wrist and digital motion were unchanged. Proximal migration of the first metacarpal averaged 3 mm, and translation decreased from 30% to 10%. Nineteen of 23 patients were pleased with their overall outcomes. After 3 months, DASH scores, grip and pinch strengths, motion, patient satisfaction, and radiographic subsidence and translation remained unchanged for a minimum of 4 years.

Conclusions.—Arthroscopic hemitrapeziectomy and thermal capsular modification offers patients with Eaton stage III arthritis a minimally invasive alternative that can provide increased function and decreased pain by 3 months after surgery. These results appear to last for a minimum of 4 years and are comparable to those reported for open techniques involving complete trapeziectomy. Substance interposition does not appear to be necessary.

▶ Edwards and Ramsey present a prospective outcomes study of the largest cohort of patients with Eaton stage III thumb carpometacarpal (CMC) joint arthritis treated with arthroscopic hemitrapeziectomy and thermal capsular modification without interposition. As seen in multiple other reports of treatment modalities for this very common disorder, the authors of this study show very compelling results with their technique. However, the caveat to interpreting the results of this study is that the authors attempt to compare the outcomes of their patients with those of historical studies, which may be misleading because the cohorts may be different. Nevertheless, the results are impressive and confirm what I have hypothesized for years: that arthroscopic treatment of thumb CMC arthritis is a useful option with short recovery periods and that interposition of any substance between the remaining hemitrapezium and the thumb metacarpal is not necessary. As Kuhns and others have proposed,[1] the body is capable of creating its own natural interposition in the form of an organized hematoma. The key to the success of this technique, either done open or arthroscopically, is to adequately suspend the thumb metacarpal while the hematoma is maturing. This may be done with a Kirschner wire (K-wire) (as described in this study), or to avoid complications or irritation from the K-wire, suspension may be achieved through other means (Cox et al[2]), which is my current preference.

J. Yao, MD

References

1. Kuhns CA, Emerson ET, Meals RA. Hematoma and distraction arthroplasty for thumb basal joint osteoarthritis: a prospective, single-surgeon study including outcomes measures. *J Hand Surg Am.* 2003;28:381-389.
2. Cox CA, Zlotolow DA, Yao J. Suture button suspensionplasty after arthroscopic hemitrapeziectomy for treatment of thumb carpometacarpal arthritis. *Arthroscopy.* 2010;26:1395-1403.

Wrist Tendon Forces During Various Dynamic Wrist Motions
Werner FW, Short WH, Palmer AK, et al (SUNY Upstate Med Univ, Syracuse, NY)
J Hand Surg 35A:628-632, 2010

Purpose.—A common treatment of arthritis of the thumb carpometa-carpal joint requires all or a portion of the flexor carpi radialis tendon (FCR) to be used as an interpositional graft. The purpose of this study was to examine the *in vitro* tendon forces in 6 wrist flexors and extensors to determine whether their force contribution changes during various dynamic wrist motions along with a specific application to the FCR.

Methods.—We tested 62 fresh-frozen cadaver wrists in a wrist joint motion simulator. During wrist flexion-extension, radioulnar deviation, dart throwing, and circumduction motions, the peak and average tendon forces were determined for the extensor carpi ulnaris, extensor carpi radialis brevis and longus, abductor pollicis longus, flexor carpi radialis, and flexor carpi ulnaris.

Results.—During a dart-throwing motion, the mean and peak FCR forces were statistically less than during the other 3 motions. Conversely, the mean and peak flexor carpi ulnaris forces were statistically greater during the dart-throwing motion than during the other 3 motions.

Conclusions.—Patients who have undergone a surgical procedure in which all or a portion of the FCR has been harvested may experience a decrease in wrist strength with wrist motion, as the FCR tendon normally applies force during wrist motion. The motion least likely to be affected by such surgery is the dart-throwing motion when the force on the remaining FCR is minimized.

▶ This article makes a quantitative contribution to what has typically been a qualitative assumption in hand surgery but with limited data to support it. Hand surgeons frequently harvest the flexor carpi radialis (FCR) tendon, most commonly for thumb basilar joint surgery. The size of the tendon and volume of the muscle suggest a sizable contribution of the FCR to wrist motion. However, authors have almost universally reported not only excellent clinical results but also subtle deficits, if any, after tendon harvest. This apparent contradiction has been investigated relatively recently by Naidu et al[1] demonstrating a decrease in wrist flexion fatigue resistance and a decrease in wrist flexion/extension torque ratio.

The authors of this article quantitatively investigated the in vitro contribution of the FCR in various motions about the wrist. The findings were that during the dart-throwing plane of motion, forces on the FCR tendon were significantly less than those in other planes (flexion/extension, circumduction, and radioulnar deviation). Given our increasing knowledge of the role of the dart-throwing motion in hand and wrist function and rehabilitation, this article is a contribution to our understanding of why harvesting a tendon of this anatomically apparent importance leads to relatively subtle changes for so many of our patients. Furthermore, it suggests that in patients engaged in occupations that require forceful or prolonged motions in the planes of significant FCR contribution, surgeons look for alternative tendons to harvest. It is my practice that in this (albeit unusual) situation, I avoid harvesting the FCR and use an alternative (eg, abductor pollicis longus).

P. Blazar, MD

Reference

1. Naidu SH, Poole J, Horne A. Entire flexor carpi radialis tendon harvest for thumb carpometacarpal arthroplasty alters wrist kinetics. *J Hand Surg Am.* 2006;31: 1171-1175.

30 Arthroscopy

Anatomic Course of the Superficial Branch of the Radial Nerve in the Wrist and Its Location in Relation to Wrist Arthroscopy Portals: A Cadaveric Study
Kiliç A, Kale A, Usta A, et al (Taksim Education and Res Hosp, Istanbul, Turkey; Istanbul Univ, Turkey)
Arthroscopy 25:1261-1264, 2009

Purpose.—The aim of this study was to assess the course of the superficial branch of the radial nerve (SBRN) at the level of the wrist and its branches in relation to wrist arthroscopy portals.

Methods.—Dissections were performed on 11 hands from 6 cadavers in the section starting from the point where the SBRN begins to emerge and ending at the terminal branches of the dorsal hand. The distribution of the SBRN, the distance from the superficial branch to the dorsal portals used in wrist arthroscopy, and the distance from the superficial branch to the anatomic determinants (styloid process of the radius, Lister tubercle) were studied.

Results.—At the level of the wrist, the nerve bifurcated into 2 branches in 8 of 11 wrists (73%) and into 3 branches in 3 of 11 wrists (27%). The mean distance from the SBRN where it was first detected proximal to the Lister tubercle was 73 mm. The mean distance between the styloids was 52 mm; the distance between the Lister tubercle and styloid process of the radius was 23 mm. At the wrist level, the distance from the branch closest to the radial side to the Lister tubercle was 28 mm (L-D1), 21 mm (L-D2/3), and 7 mm (RS-D1). The distance of the closest nerve branch to the 3-4 portal was 9 mm. The distances of the other portals were 5 mm (1-2RMC–D1), 8 mm (1-2RMC–D2/3), 8 mm (1-2P–D1), and 9 mm (1-2P–D2/3).

Conclusions.—The limited size of the area where portals can be positioned and the anatomic variations between individuals are major obstacles in developing a guideline for reducing the risk of SBRN injury in wrist arthroscopy.

Clinical Relevance.—Great care must be taken when using the 1-2 portal. We suggest making a skin-only incision for this portal and then using blunt dissection to help prevent injury to the SBRN.

▶ The authors report on their cadaveric study of the location of the superficial branch of the radial nerve with respect to common wrist arthroscopic portals. Their main conclusion was that the 1-2 portal is very close to the superficial branch of the radial nerve, and they suggest a skin-only incision followed by blunt dissection to prevent injury to the nerve. The distance of the nerve relative to the 1-2 portal was found to be less than 1 mm. This study was based on preserved cadaveric hands, which included 11 wrists of 6 cadavers. Their findings also suggest a common occurrence of the superficial nerve branching into 2 branches in 8 of the 11 wrists compared with 3 branches in 3 of the 11 wrists.

There are some limitations with the study. One is that they describe the size of the hands used in the study as small. Certainly, this could affect the distances measured relative to the general population. These cadavers were preserved specimens, not fresh frozen soft tissue, which may alter the mobility of the tissues and the distances that were measured. I think that ideally this type of study might be done under 10 to 12 lb of traction in the position that we normally perform wrist arthroscopy. Traction may shift the position of the nerves either closer or farther away from the portals. The authors do also remind us that the distances that they measured were from the needle marking the portal location to the nerve as opposed to the size of the true portal (several millimeters in diameter). This basically would include some variation, probably upward of 2 to 3 mm of difference in the distance based on the diameter of the arthroscopic trocar or portal compared with the size of the needle.

Nonetheless, the authors remind us of the importance of understanding the location of the superficial branch of the radial nerve and its usual variability. We must keep in mind the location of the nerve and the variability of the nerve (bifurcation or trifurcation). When preparing arthroscopic portals at the wrist, it is important to incise the skin only and to protect the soft tissue down to the retinacular or capsular level to minimize injury to any superficial nerve branches.

D. G. Dennison, MD

Arthroscopic Resection of Dorsal Wrist Ganglia: 114 Cases With Minimum Follow-Up of 2 Years
Gallego S, Mathoulin C (Universidad de Antioquia, Medellín, Colombia; Institut de la Main—Clinique Jouvenet, Paris, France)
Arthroscopy 26:1675-1682, 2010

Purpose.—The objective of this study was to review the results of arthroscopic resection of dorsal wrist ganglion (DWG), as well as to describe the senior author's technique and technical details to minimize potential complications.

Methods.—Between September 1999 and May 2004, 114 patients underwent arthroscopic resection of DWG with a minimum follow-up of 24 months. We describe the surgical technique and discuss our results and complications.

Results.—A total of 114 patients (87 female patients and 27 male patients) with a mean age of 33.1 years were treated with our operative technique. The symptoms at presentation were unsightly appearance in 63 (55.2%), pain in 33 (28.9%), and both unsightly appearance and pain in 18 (15.8%). The patients presented between 1 and 96 months before surgery (mean, 17.81 months). Of the patients, 66 (57.9%) had been treated previously with nonsurgical modalities (aspiration) and 1 had undergone open surgery. The origin of the DWG was more commonly related to the midcarpal joint (85 patients [74.6%]). Our surgery brought about a significant improvement in flexion and extension after surgery ($P < .005$). Similarly, our surgery brought about a significant improvement in grip strength ($P < .005$). In patients with preoperative pain, treatment also showed a significant impact. At 2 years' follow-up, there were 14 recurrences (12.3%), diagnosed at a mean of 16.86 months after surgery (range, 2 to 25 months). Complications were identified in 6 patients (5.26%), and the mean time off work was 11 days, with a majority of patients returning in less than 1 week.

Conclusions.—Arthroscopic DWG resection showed an improvement in functional measurements in addition to relief of pain in a significant proportion of patients. Complications related to the operative technique did not cause any significant long-term functional deficit. The recurrence rate was 12.3%, and patient satisfaction was high. Arthroscopic technique allows patients to use their hand immediately. The results of this study support the use of arthroscopy as primary treatment for DWG resection.

Level of Evidence.—Level IV, therapeutic case series.

▶ Gallego and Mathoulin have presented on 114 cases of arthroscopic dorsal wrist ganglion excision with a minimum of 2-year follow-up, likely the largest such series in the literature to date. Not surprisingly, they have found recurrence rates (12.3%) comparable to the low end of those seen with open dorsal wrist ganglion excision (up to 40%) and with those previously published for arthroscopic ganglion excisions (from 1% to 20%). They also report a high level of patient satisfaction with few surgical complications.

This is exactly what I find in my patient population. I prefer not to perform ganglion excisions open unless the cyst is extremely large, and I am concerned that I will not be able to fully excise the sac arthroscopically. Otherwise, in most cases, I (and my patients and my residents and fellows) prefer to resect these arthroscopically, with comparable recurrence and satisfaction rates as those published in this study. What I found interesting was that any recurrences were also treated with arthroscopic re-excision in this series, whereas in my practice, I find patients with recurrence with arthroscopic excision wish to try a different approach and elect to undergo the open procedure for re-excision.

What the authors don't discuss in this article is the occasional difficulty in visualizing the stalk of the ganglion as it arises (usually) from the dorsal aspect of the scapholunate ligament. It has been reported in the literature to be visible anywhere from 20% to 100% of the time. In my practice, I believe the number is on the lower end of that range. What I have done recently to help with visualization of the stalk is a percutaneous intralesional injection of a dye (indigo carmine) to help visualize the cyst and stalk. The stalk is clearly visible after the dye has been injected, and I can confidently excise everything that is stained with it, including (most importantly) the stalk. To date, I have not had any recurrences I know of using this adjunct to the arthroscopic ganglionectomy.

J. Yao, MD

Comparison of Arthroscopic and Open Treatment of Septic Arthritis of the Wrist: Surgical Technique
Sammer DM, Shin AY (Mayo Clinic, Rochester, MN)
J Bone Joint Sur Am 92:107-113, 2010

Background.—Open irrigation and débridement is the standard of treatment for septic arthritis of the wrist. Although isolated cases of arthroscopic irrigation and débridement have been reported, a comparison of arthroscopic and open techniques has not been performed, to our knowledge. The purpose of this study was to compare the two methods of management.

Methods.—A retrospective comparison of patients with septic arthritis of the wrist initially treated, over an eleven-year period, with open or arthroscopic irrigation and débridement was undertaken at a single institution. The clinical presentation, laboratory and microbiological findings, hospital course, complications, and outcomes were compared between the two groups.

Results.—Between 1997 and 2007, thirty-six patients with septic arthritis involving a total of forty wrists were identified. Nineteen wrists (seventeen patients) were initially treated with open irrigation and débridement, and twenty-one wrists (nineteen patients) were initially treated arthroscopically. Eleven wrists in the open-treatment cohort required repeat irrigation and débridement, and eight wrists in the arthroscopy cohort required a repeat procedure. If a repeat irrigation and débridement was required, it was performed in an open fashion in all but two cases. When the comparison included all of the patients in the series, no difference between the two cohorts was found with regard to the number of irrigation and débridement procedures required or the length of the hospital stay. However, when the comparison was limited to the patients with isolated septic arthritis of the wrist, it was found that only one of seven wrists in the open-treatment cohort but all eight wrists in the arthroscopy cohort had been successfully managed with a single irrigation and débridement procedure (p = 0.001). No patient in whom isolated septic arthritis of the wrist had been treated with arthroscopic irrigation and débridement required a second operation. The patients in whom isolated septic arthritis of the wrist was treated with the open method stayed in the hospital for an average of sixteen days compared with a six-day stay for those in whom isolated septic arthritis of the wrist was treated with the arthroscopic method (p = 0.04). The ninety-day perioperative mortality rate in the series was substantial (18% [three patients] in the open-treatment cohort and 21% [four patients] in the arthroscopy cohort).

Conclusions.—Arthroscopic irrigation and débridement is an effective treatment for patients with isolated septic arthritis of the wrist; these patients had fewer operations and a shorter hospital stay than did patients who had received open treatment. However, these benefits were not seen in patients with multiple sites of infection.

▶ This study is significant in that it compares 2 different techniques for the treatment of septic arthritis of the wrist. Strengths of the article include the relatively large number of patients in the study, especially given the uncommon occurrence of this condition, and that all were from a single institution. One particular weakness of the article, in this reviewer's opinion, is that although the authors state "broad-spectrum intravenous antibiotics tailored to the culture results were administered postoperatively" and "an infectious disease consultation was obtained to assist with determining the appropriate antibiotic(s) and duration of treatment," nowhere do they mention the type and duration of antibiotics that were used. Antibiotics are arguably just as important as the method of irrigation and debridement chosen for the treatment of a septic wrist. Although the arthroscopic technique may result in fewer operations and shorter hospital stay, it is important for the reader to also know which antibiotics were used and for how long. The article would have been strengthened by this information and would then be even more useful to the reader. Regardless, I do believe that this study is important in describing the effectiveness of arthroscopic irrigation and debridement of the isolated septic joint. The decrease in days of hospital stay and number of operations not only benefit the patient but also are cost-effective. This technique is also my treatment of choice for the occasional septic wrist that I see in my practice.

S. S. Shin, MD, MMS

31 Neural Integration, Pain and Anesthesia

Changes in Tissue Substance P Levels in Patients With Carpal Tunnel Syndrome
Öztürk N, Erin N, Tüzüner S (Akdeniz Univ, Antalya, Turkey)
Neurosurgery 67:1655-1661, 2010

Background.—Although carpal tunnel syndrome (CTS) is the most common entrapment neuropathy in adults, its etiology is not completely known. Chronic inflammation, fibrosis of the transverse carpal ligament (TCL), and altered sensory response contribute to the symptoms.

Objective.—Because substance P (SP) is known to be involved in neuropathic pain, chronic inflammation, and fibrosis, the present study evaluated changes in SP levels in patients with CTS.

Methods.—TCL, median nerve adventitia, and synovial connective tissue of the middle flexor digitorum superficialis tendon samples from patients (n = 42) with CTS and healthy control subjects (n = 13) who were operated on for hand wounds were obtained at surgery. A group of these patients with CTS (n = 9) had received meloxicam treatment for 10 days before surgery. A 2-step acetic acid extraction was used to determine changes in SP levels in free nerve endings (neuronal) and in nonneuronal cells.

Results.—Changes in SP levels were observed in both neuronal and nonneuronal tissues. SP levels increased in extracts of the TCL and synovial connective tissue of the middle flexor digitorum superficialis tendon but not in the median nerve adventitia of patients with CTS. Meloxicam pretreatment increased SP levels in nonneuronal components of the TCL.

Conclusion.—These findings suggest that SP contributes to the pain and inflammation associated with CTS. Further studies are required to evaluate the therapeutic potentials of SP receptor (NK1R) antagonists in CTS.

▶ This study tests the hypothesis that substance P may play a role in the pathogenesis and symptoms of carpal tunnel syndrome. Substance P is a neuropeptide that is involved in pain and inflammatory pathways. This study compared substance P levels in the wrist tissues of people who underwent carpal tunnel release, patients treated with meloxicam and then underwent carpal tunnel release, and a control group that was operated on for traumatic wrist injuries.

This study found higher levels of substance P in the carpal tunnel patients when compared with the controls.

These are interesting preliminary data because they suggest that substance P may play a role in the pain of carpal tunnel syndrome and that through its proin-flammatory effects may even contribute to the pathogenesis. If future studies bear this out, it opens the door to possible medical treatments of carpal tunnel syndrome through the use of substance P antagonists. However, this study must be taken with caution because of some methodologic concerns. Most importantly, the control group was very different from the carpal tunnel groups (younger and far higher percentage of men), which weakens the comparison between groups. Second, given the small numbers, it is not possible to under-stand at what role substance P elevation occurs in the process: is it a promoter of carpal tunnel syndrome or simply a byproduct of chronic nerve compression? This evocative study points to new potential ways of understanding and possibly treating carpal tunnel syndrome.

C. Curtin, MD

32 Peripheral Nerve Injury and Repair

Glatiramer Acetate Immune System Augmentation for Peripheral Nerve Regeneration in Rat Crushed Sciatic Nerve Model
Luria S, Waitayawinyu T, Conniff J, et al (Univ of Washington School of Medicine, Seattle)
J Bone Joint Surg Am 92:396-403, 2010

Background.—Protective antiself response to nervous system injury has been reported to be mediated by a T-cell subpopulation that can recognize self-antigens. Immune cells have been shown to play a role in the regulation of motor neuron survival after a peripheral nerve injury. The objective of the present study was to evaluate the effects of immune system augmentation with use of the antigen glatiramer acetate, which is known to affect T-cell immunity, on peripheral nerve regeneration.

Methods.—Wild-type and nude-type (T-cell-deficient) rats underwent crush injury of the sciatic nerve. Three and six weeks after the injury, the sciatic nerve was examined, both functionally (on the basis of footprint analysis and the tibialis anterior muscle response and weight) and histologically (on the basis of axon count).

Results.—Significantly greater muscle responses were measured after three weeks in the group of wild-type rats that were treated with glatiramer acetate (control limb:injured limb ratio, 0.05 for the glatiramer acetate group [n = 9], compared with 0.51 for the saline solution group [n = 8]; $p < 0.05$). Higher axon counts were also found in this group (control limb:injured limb ratio, −0.07 for the glatiramer acetate group [n = 10], compared with 0.29 for the saline solution group [n = 8]; $p < 0.05$). The nude-type rats showed no response to the intervention after three weeks but showed a delayed response after six weeks. A second dose of glatiramer acetate, delivered forty-eight hours after the injury, did not result in an improved response as compared with the control groups.

Conclusions.—We found that a single treatment with glatiramer acetate resulted in accelerated functional and histological recovery after sciatic nerve crush injury. The role of T-cell immunity in the mechanism of glatiramer acetate was suggested by the partial and late response found in the T-cell-deficient rats.

▶ The authors investigate using the antigen glatiramer acetate that suppresses T-cell reaction to peripheral nerve injury in an effort to improve nerve regeneration. The authors cited a previous study in which T-cells recognize the site of nerve injury and retard nerve regeneration by an antiself response. The use of this antigen was postulated by the authors to improve nerve regeneration by blocking the T-cell immune response. The authors used the rat model for this experiment and found that after crush injury of the sciatic nerves, the treated group had increased weight of the tibialis anterior muscle and increased axon count. The authors concluded that single treatment using glatiramer acetate resulted in functional and histological recovery after a sciatic nerve crush injury in the rat model.

The elusiveness of improving nerve regeneration continues to baffle scientists. Many compounds have been used, and most of them can show an improvement in nerve regeneration in the murine model. The most difficult part of this exercise is that regeneration of nerves in rats is quite rapid, and it will be difficult to translate this model to a primate model and ultimately to human trials. Therefore, this compound is certainly a promising avenue for local immune modulation to improve nerve recovery. However, the enthusiasm should be tempered by using this compound for a nerve transection model in which recovery is more clinically relevant. Nerve crush injuries will usually recover to reasonable function, but nerve transections often leave patients with devastating residual effects. Therefore, the next extension of this study is to use the nerve transection model. Whether this compound will improve nerve regeneration remains to be seen. However, this study is certainly a first step in an innovative approach to evaluating nerve regeneration by modulating the immune response.

K. Chung, MD

Nerve Grafts and Conduits
Colen KL, Choi M, Chiu DTW (New York Univ School of Medicine; Columbia Univ, NY)
Plast Reconstr Surg 124:386e-394e, 2009

Peripheral nerve defects are common. The surgeon faced with these problems must provide the best functional recovery for the patient with the tools provided. The ideal nerve reconstruction would create a tensionless repair with direct coaptation. However, this is not always possible and other techniques must be employed. The alternatives to direct coaptation include nerve autografts, nerve conduits, and tissue-engineered constructs. This article reviews commonly used autogenous nerve grafts and conduits. Autogenous nerve grafts have been utilized in various techniques which include the trunk graft, cable graft, interfascicular graft, and vascularized graft. The nerve conduits reviewed fall into the category of autogenous biological conduits, nonautogenous biological conduits, and nonbiological conduits. New technologies are being developed to enhance peripheral nerve regeneration with the concept that conduits can be enriched and manipulated in the laboratory to promote regeneration of the peripheral nerve. Further clinical studies hold the promise of successful alternatives for treating peripheral nerve injuries.

▶ The article dealing with nerve grafts and conduits presents an overview about the surgical alternatives that we have to bridge a nerve defect. The senior author, Dr Chiu, has popularized the clinical use of veins as nerve graft substitutes with his publications.

Nerve conduit research has shifted from single materials, such as vein, muscle, silicone tube, polyglactin, or polyglycolic acid, to the combination of different materials or to enrichment of diverse tubes with either growth factors or cells that enhance nerve regeneration. Many of these newer concepts are very promising. But clinical long-term results will have to show that these combinations are at least functionally equal or superior to the gold standard of nerve reconstruction, the autologous nerve graft. Another major step that has to be taken is to show that these methods can also favorably be applied in defects longer than 3 cm and—even more interestingly—in the reconstruction of motor nerves, as most of the existing studies report only on results with sensory nerve restoration.

The authors state that sacrificing the posterior interosseous nerve (PIN) as a graft would not cause any deficit. A recent publication, however, shows that the PIN plays an important role in the proprioception of the wrist and that resection of this nerve may lead to proprioceptive imbalance in the wrist.[1] This new functional aspect of the PIN should be considered when choosing a nerve graft.

Like many researchers before them, the authors of this study mistakenly cite Gluck's publication from 1880 as the first report of nerve reconstruction with a conduit.[2] While it was indeed Gluck who first reported about bridging nerve defects with Danish leather, bone drains, catgut, and muscle in animals, he actually did so in a separate publication in 1881.[3]

M. S. S. Choi, MD

References

1. Hagert E, Persson JKE. Desensitizing the posterior interosseous nerve alters wrist proprioceptive reflexes. *J Hand Surg Am.* 2010;35:1059-1066.
2. Gluck T. Ueber Neuroplastik auf dem Wege der Transplantation. *Arch Klin Chir.* 1880;25:606-616.
3. Gluck T. Ueber Transplantation, Regeneration und entzündliche Neubildung. *Arch Klin Chir.* 1881;26:896-915.

Relationships Among Pain Disability, Pain Intensity, Illness Intrusiveness, and Upper Extremity Disability in Patients With Traumatic Peripheral Nerve Injury

Novak CB, Anastakis DJ, Beaton DE, et al (Univ of Toronto, Ontario, Canada; York Univ, Toronto, Ontario, Canada; Washington Univ School of Medicine, St Louis, MO)

J Hand Surg 35A:1633-1639, 2010

Purpose.—In patients with a peripheral nerve injury, a simple conceptualization assumes that pain disability is determined by pain intensity. This study evaluated the relationships among pain intensity, illness intrusiveness, and pain disability.

Methods.—After we obtained ethics board approval, we enrolled English-speaking adult patients who had experienced an upper extremity peripheral nerve injury 0.5 to 15 years previously. Patients completed the Disabilities of the Arm, Shoulder, and Hand (DASH), Illness Intrusiveness Scale, Pain Disability Index, and McGill Pain questionnaires. We used multivariate linear regression to evaluate the variables that predicted pain disability.

Results.—There were 124 patients (41 women, 83 men; mean ± SD, 41 ± 16 y of age). The median time since injury was 14 months (range, 6–145 months), and there were 43 brachial plexus nerve injuries. Mean ± SD scores were: pain disability, 29 ± 18; illness intrusiveness, 40 ± 18; DASH, 45 ± 22; and pain intensity, 4.6 ± 3.0. The pain disability, DASH, and illness intrusiveness scores were significantly higher in patients with brachial plexus injuries than in those with distal nerve injuries (p<.05). There was strong correlation between pain disability and DASH (r = 0.764, p<.001) and illness intrusiveness (r = 0.738, p<.001) and a weaker correlation with pain intensity (r = 0.549, p<.001). The final regression model predicting pain disability scores explained 70% of the variance with these predictors: DASH (β = 0.452, p<.001), illness intrusiveness (β = 0.372, p<.001), and pain intensity (β = 0.143, p=.018).

Conclusions.—Pain disability was substantial after nerve injury, and pain intensity explained the least variance among the model variables.

TABLE 3.—Correlation Coefficients Between PDI Scores and Other Questionnaires

	PDI	IIRS	VAS Pain	DASH
PDI				
IIRS	0.738*			
VAS pain	0.549*	0.500*		
DASH	0.764*	0.653*	0.487*	
Age	0.008	0.023	−0.056	0.054
Time since injury	0.037	0.056	0.203†	−0.130

PDI, Pain Disability Index; IIRS, Illness Intrusiveness Rating Scale.
*Level of significance, p<.001.
†Level of significance, p=.020.

Pain intensity should be considered only one component of pain, and the impact of pain in the context of disability should be considered in patients with chronic nerve injury.
Type of Study/Level of Evidence.—Prognostic IV (Table 3).

▶ The authors designed this study to identify the factors that interfere with life domains in patients with chronic upper extremity peripheral nerve injury. Factors associated with pain disability, pain intensity, illness intrusiveness, and upper extremity disability were measured using the Pain Disability Index (PDI), visual analog scale (VAS) pain score, Illness Intrusiveness Rating Scale (IIRS), and Disabilities of the Arm, Shoulder, and Hand (DASH) score, respectively. The authors found strong correlations between pain disability and DASH scores and illness intrusiveness, and a weak correlation between pain disability and pain intensity (Table 3). The final regression model predicting the PDI score explained 70% of the variance of the predictors of DASH, IIRS, and VAS scores.

The impact of pain should be considered within the context of disability. However, it may be too early to conclude that pain disability is substantial after nerve injury, because when the PDI is used in patients with both motor paralysis and pain, it measures both the extent of disability associated with pain and motor dysfunction. Many patients with chronic nerve injuries show a discrepancy between pain and motor dysfunction. We often see patients with C5-C6 brachial plexus nerve root injury who complain of severe motor disability of the affected upper extremities in activities of daily living because of dysfunction of the shoulder and elbow, but these patients do not experience significant pain. Few people with brachial plexus avulsion injury complain of pain throughout the day. Most patients with such injury feel severe pain at night and experience mainly disability in activities of daily living during the day because of the paralyzed upper extremity. In patients with such motor-sensory discrepancy who have high PDI scores and low VAS scores, motor dysfunction is substantial after nerve injury. The strong correlation between the PDI, DASH, and IIRS scores can be explained by frequent overlapping of the same kinds of questions among the 3 questionnaires.

R. Kakinoki, MD, PhD

Modern surgical management of peripheral nerve gap
Pabari A, Yang SY, Seifalian AM, et al (Royal Free Hampstead NHS Trust Hosp, London, UK; Univ College London, UK)
J Plast Reconstr Aesthet Surg 63:1941-1948, 2010

The management of peripheral nerve injury requires a thorough understanding of the complex physiology of nerve regeneration. The ability to perform surgery under magnification has improved our understanding of the anatomy of the peripheral nerves. However, the level of functional improvement that can be expected following peripheral nerve injury has plateaued. Advancements in the field of tissue engineering have led to an

TABLE 3.—Summary of FDA-Approved Nerve Conduits and Clinical Outcomes in Humans

Composition	Nerve Conduits	Authors	Nerve Repair	Clinical Data		Outcome
				Length	Follow up (Months)	
Type I Collagen	NeuraGen® Integra NeuroSciences	Lohmeyer et al., 2009[41]	Digital nerves (12)	Up to 18 mm	12	4/12 excellent, 5/12 good, 1/12 poor, 2/12 none
	Degradation: 48 months	Bushnell et al., 2008[42]	Digital nerves (12)	Up to 20 mm	12–22	4/9 excellent, 4/9 good, 1/9 fair
		Farole et al., 2008[43]	Lingual and inferior alveolar nerves (9)	15 mm	12–30	4/9 good, 4/9 some, 1/9 none
		Ashley et al., 2006[44]	Brachial plexus birth injury (7)	Up to 20 mm	24	4/5 good, 1/5 poor
		Taras et al., 2005[45]; 2008[46]	Median, ulna, radial, posterior interosseous, common digital, superficial radial nerves (75)			Ongoing clinical study.
	NeuroMatrix NeuroFlex® Collagen Matrix, Inc. Degradation: 7 months					
Polyglycolic Acid	Neurotube®	Rosson et al., 2009[47]	Spinal accessory,[52] median,[53] ulna nerves (6)	Up to 40 mm	4–66	6/6 return of motor function.
	Synovis Degradation: 6 months	Dellon et al., 2006[48]	Digital nerves in toe to thumb transfer (1)	25–30 mm	30	Return of sensory function.
		Navissano et al., 2005[49]	Facial nerve (7)	Up to 30 mm	7–12	1/7 very good, 4/7 good, 2/7 fair

Poly-DL-lactide-caprolactone	Neurolac® Polyganics Degradation: 16 months	Battiston et al., 2005[50]	Digital nerve (17)	Up to 40 mm	6–74	13/17 very good, 3/17 good, 1/17 poor
		Kim et al., 2001[51]	Neuroma of medial plantar nerve (1)	20 mm	10	Pain resolved.
		Bertleff et al., 2005[54]	Digital nerve (21)	Up to 20 mm	12	Sensory recovery seen.

Editor's Note: Please refer to original journal article for full references.

exciting complement of commercially available products that can be used to bridge peripheral nerve gaps. However, the quest for enhanced options is ongoing. This article provides a review of the current treatment options available following peripheral nerve injury, a summary of the published studies using commercially available nerve conduits and nerve allografts in humans and the emerging hopes for the next generation of nerve conduits with the advancement of nanotechnology (Table 3).

▶ The authors have provided a comprehensive review of peripheral nerve injury, regeneration, and the management of these injuries when associated with loss of nerve substance or a nerve gap that cannot be overcome by end-to-end suturing. The greater part of their discussion focuses on the use of nerve conduits as substitutes for the standard nerve autograft. They provide a balanced review of the published experience, both in animal models and clinical studies, with currently approved and commercially available conduits, including collagen, polyglycolic acid, and poly-DL-lactide-caprolactone conduits. They mention a more recent addition to the surgical armamentarium, a decellularized nerve allograft, although they do not include this device in their summary Table 3. More recent laboratory[1] and clinical studies of this device suggest that it outperforms previous conduits. The need still exists for a successful substitute for autografts for patients with long nerve gaps. This seems most likely to be achieved by melding biologics, such as stem cells that ultimately become Schwann cells, with newly developing biocompatible materials.

V. R. Hentz, MD

Reference

1. Johnson PJ, Newton P, Hunter DA, Mackinnon SE. Nerve endoneurial microstructure facilitates uniform distribution of regenerative fibers: a post hoc comparison of midgraft nerve fiber densities. *J Reconstr Microsurg*. 2011;27:83-90.

33 Diagnostic Imaging

Abnormal Microarchitecture and Reduced Stiffness at the Radius and Tibia in Postmenopausal Women With Fractures

Stein EM, Liu XS, Nickolas TL, et al (Columbia Univ College of Physicians and Surgeons, NY; et al)
J Bone Miner Res 25:2296-2305, 2010

Measurement of areal bone mineral density (aBMD) by dual-energy x-ray absorptiometry (DXA) has been shown to predict fracture risk. High-resolution peripheral quantitative computed tomography (HR-pQCT) yields additional information about volumetric BMD (vBMD), microarchitecture, and strength that may increase understanding of fracture susceptibility. Women with ($n = 68$) and without ($n = 101$) a history of postmenopausal fragility fracture had aBMD measured by DXA and trabecular and cortical vBMD and trabecular microarchitecture of the radius and tibia measured by HR-pQCT. Finite-element analysis (FEA) of HR-pQCT scans was performed to estimate bone stiffness. DXA *T*-scores were similar in women with and without fracture at the spine, hip, and one-third radius but lower in patients with fracture at the ultra-distal radius ($p < .01$). At the radius fracture, patients had lower total density, cortical thickness, trabecular density, number, thickness, higher trabecular separation and network heterogeneity ($p < .0001$ to .04). At the tibia, total, cortical, and trabecular density and cortical and trabecular thickness were lower in fracture patients ($p < .0001$ to .03). The differences between groups were greater at the radius than at the tibia for inner trabecular density, number, trabecular separation, and network heterogeneity ($p < .01$ to .05). Stiffness was reduced in fracture patients, more markedly at the radius (41% to 44%) than at the tibia (15% to 20%). Women with fractures had reduced vBMD, microarchitectural deterioration, and decreased strength. These differences were more prominent at the radius than at the tibia. HR-pQCT and FEA measurements of peripheral sites are associated with fracture prevalence and may increase understanding of the role of microarchitectural deterioration in fracture susceptibility.

▶ This study examined bony microarchitecture in 169 postmenopausal women. Patients with a history of fragility fracture had lower density, cortical and trabecular thickness, and number, and higher trabecular separation than those without a history of fracture. There was no difference in bone mineral density (BMD) as measured by dual-energy x-ray absorptiometry (DXA) between groups.

251

Although measurement of BMD by DXA is currently the gold standard for the diagnosis of osteoporosis, BMD does not always accurately reflect fracture risk. As such, recent efforts have focused on more sophisticated imaging technology to more accurately assess the determinants of bone strength and fracture risk. The authors used high-resolution peripheral quantitative CT (HR-pQCT) to examine bone microarchitecture and stiffness and were able to detect differences between fracture and nonfracture patients, which were not evident by DXA scan. This article builds on prior work examining HR-pQCT as a useful imaging modality in assessing skeletal fragility and fracture risk. As of yet, no guidelines exist for its use in clinical practice or its ability to accurately predict fracture risk. This study, however, supports treating patients with fragility fractures for underlying abnormalities in bone metabolism despite a normal DXA scan.

T. D. Rozental, MD

Comparative Evaluation of Postreduction Intra-Articular Distal Radial Fractures by Radiographs and Multidetector Computed Tomography
Arora S, Grover SB, Batra S, et al (Maulana Azad Med College & Lok Nayak Hosp, New Delhi, India)
J Bone Joint Surg Am 92:2523-2532, 2010

Background.—Computed tomography can be an adjunct to radiographs when evaluating intra-articular fractures of the distal part of the radius. Acute-phase multidetector computed tomography has better temporal, spatial, and contrast resolution than a conventional scanner has. The aim of this study was to determine prospectively whether the addition of a multidetector computed tomography scan (with various reconstructions) results in changes in the evaluation of intraarticular distal radial fractures and thus changes in the plans for further management.

Methods.—Radiographs and multidetector computed tomography scans were compared prospectively in the evaluation of 117 patients (120 wrists) with acute intra-articular distal radial fractures. The parameters that were measured included the ability to detect intra-articular step and gap displacements, central articular depression, coronal plane fracture, the number of articular fragments, comminution, and associated injuries in the wrist region (carpal bone fractures, distal radioulnar joint disruption, and ulnar styloid fracture).

Results.—The average measurements for intra-articular step and gap were 0.4 mm and 0.9 mm, respectively, on postreduction radiographs and 1.3 mm and 2.4 mm, respectively, on sagittal multidetector computed tomography images (p < 0.0001 for each). Central articular depression was found in twenty-one wrists (18% of the total) on radiographs, but on multidetector computed tomography it was found to be present in seventy-four wrists (62% of the total) (p < 0.0001). Twenty-six radiographically occult injuries in the wrist region, including six scaphoid fractures, were detected with the help of multidetector computed tomography. Overall, the recommended treatment plan changed in 23% of the cases when the evaluation included multidetector computed tomography images in addition to conventional radiographs. Interobserver and intraobserver agreements were significantly increased when radiographs and multidetector computed tomography images both were available for evaluation ($\kappa = 0.73$ and 0.91, respectively) as compared with interobserver and intraobserver agreement with radiographs alone ($\kappa = 0.43$ and 0.69, respectively).

Conclusions.—Multidetector computed tomography provides more accurate information regarding the anatomy of intra-articular distal radial fractures than radiography provides. The addition of multidetector computed tomography to plain films frequently changes the therapeutic recommendations for such cases.

▶ The authors present a comparison of plain radiographs and multidetector CT in evaluating reductions for displaced distal radius fractures. CT scans were more accurate in determining residual displacement. This study reinforces prior work identifying 2-dimensional CT as a more accurate method of judging fracture fragment step-off and gapping than conventional radiographs. The study is most useful in that it includes a clinical component by determining how often the treatment method was changed following review of the CT images. We are not able, however, to determine whether patient outcomes (clinical or radiographic) were different for patients in whom treatment changed as a result of the CT. In addition, the authors do not discuss the cost associated with obtaining the more sophisticated imaging. I typically reserve CT scans for comminuted fracture patterns in which the treatment algorithm remains in question. In my hands, the number of patients who would benefit from a multidetector scan remains relatively small.

T. D. Rozental, MD

34 Flaps, Vascular and Microvascular Topics

Transplanted Fingerprints: A Preliminary Case Report 40 Months Posttransplant

Szajerka T, Jurek B, Jablecki J (St Hedwig's Hosp, Trzebnica, Poland; Metropolitan Police Headquarters, Wroclaw, Poland)
Transplant Proc 42:3753-3755, 2010

For the past century, fingerprints have been considered permanent and specific for each individual. However, with the advances in transplantology, fingerprints have lost their permanence. Because no study has yet been described, we examined possible changes in the fingerprint pattern of a transplanted hand.

In 2006, we performed a hand transplantation on a 32-year-old man. The donor was revealed to have had a criminal record; his fingerprints were stored in the Polish automated fingerprint identification system. A forensic technician fingerprinted the transplanted hand nine times between June 2006 and September 2009. The appearance of minutiae and white lines and the change in the distance between papillary ridges were assessed in the thumbprints of the transplanted hand. The appearance of white lines was only temporary; at no point did they impair fingerprint identification. No significant changes occurred in the distance between the friction ridges. The observed small differences were ascribed to the two techniques used to collect the prints (spoon vs rolling). The number of minutiae ranged from 1 to 3, reaching a maximum in the third posttransplant month.

A 40-month observation showed no significant changes in the fingerprints of the transplanted hand. Nevertheless, a long-term study is needed because of the risk of chronic rejection. The noninvasiveness of dactylography argues for inspecting its application to diagnose acute rejection. Finally, lawmakers should be made aware of the personal-protection issues related to the growing number of hand-transplant recipients.

▶ This interesting case report studies the effects of hand transplantation at 40 months on the fingerprints of the transplanted hand. This is an interesting article for a quick review. The use of dactylography could have future application in studying acute rejection in the transplantation patient. The fingerprints did not appear to change in a significant fashion over time. The personal

255

protection issues also are interesting to consider, as more hand transplants will be performed in the years to come.

C. Carroll IV, MD

35 Tumors

Solitary Intra-Articular Osteochondroma of the Finger
Baek GH, Rhee SH, Chung MS, et al (Seoul Natl Univ College of Medicine, South Korea)
J Bone Joint Surg Am 92:1137-1143, 2010

Background.—A solitary osteochondroma of the finger occasionally occurs intra-articularly and may cause clinical symptoms, including limited motion and deformity. The present report describes the clinical features and the results of operative treatment for a series of patients who had a solitary intra-articular osteochondroma of the finger.

Methods.—Ten patients with a solitary intra-articular osteochondroma of a phalanx of a finger were managed surgically. Eight patients were male, and two were female. The average age at the time of surgery was fourteen years. Treatment consisted of mass excision for three patients and mass excision with corrective osteotomy for six. One additional patient had a boutonniere deformity and underwent extensor tendon reconstruction combined with mass excision. The average duration of follow-up was forty-four months.

Results.—The proximal phalanx was affected in six patients, and the middle phalanx was affected in four. All tumors involved the distal epiphysis. All patients had postoperative improvement in terms of deformity and/or limitation of motion. Six patients had a preoperative mean coronal plane deformity of 29°, which improved to 4° after surgery. The preoperative mean arc of flexion-extension improved from 54° to 78° in four patients who had a motion deficit at the proximal interphalangeal joint and from 60° to 80° in one patient who had a motion deficit at the distal interphalangeal joint. Two patients had a residual flexion contracture, one with preexisting osteoarthritis and one with a longstanding progressive boutonniere deformity. There were no other complications or recurrences.

Conclusions.—Isolated intra-articular osteochondroma of the finger can cause deformity and/or motion limitation. Early mass excision and corrective osteotomy when indicated are recommended to restore full range of motion and to prevent osteoarthritis and secondary deformity.

▶ This report is a retrospective case series of 10 patients with intra-articular solitary osteochondromas. There was appropriate follow-up of minimum 21 months and average of 44 months. Despite the limited evidence ranking of this type of article, there are a number of important lessons:

- The majority was found in children but also in young adults.
- This entity can be confused with clinodactyly or camptodactyly and hence is an indication for plain radiographs in cases where those diagnoses are in the differential diagnosis.
- Osteotomy was required in most cases to correct malalignment in addition to removal of the osteochondroma.
- The limitation of motion in these patients is greater than that typically seen in extra-articular osteochondromas.

This is a useful article, and the point that more aggressive surgical intervention in contrast to an extra-articular osteochondroma is compelling.

P. Blazar, MD

36 Miscellaneous

Effects of Workers' Compensation on the Diagnosis and Surgical Treatment of Patients with Hand and Wrist Disorders
Day CS, Alexander M, Lal S, et al (Beth Israel Deaconess Med Ctr and Harvard Med School, Boston, MA)
J Bone Joint Surg Am 92:2294-2299, 2010

Background.—Workers' Compensation differs from standard insurance, and it is unclear how or if Workers' Compensation insurance influences the diagnosis and treatment of hand and wrist disorders. The aim of this study was to compare the diagnosis and course of treatment of hand disorders between patients with Workers' Compensation insurance and patients with standard insurance.

Methods.—The complete medical records of patients who visited an academic orthopaedic hand clinic between January 2005 and January 2007 were reviewed, and information on patient history, utilization of diagnostic tests, diagnosis, surgery, and wait-time to surgery was collected. Patients with Workers' Compensation insurance and those with other, third-party coverage were analyzed and compared. Patients without insurance were excluded from this study.

Results.—1413 patients (representing 2121 diagnoses) were included in the study. One hundred and sixteen patients (8%) had Workers' Compensation insurance and 1297 patients (92%) had standard insurance. Patients with Workers' Compensation insurance were younger than patients with standard insurance (mean age, forty-three years compared with fifty years, respectively; p < 0.05) and were also more likely to be male (50% compared with 40%, respectively; p = 0.04). Generally, Workers' Compensation patients more often had neurological conditions (p < 0.01), but there was no significant difference in the most common diagnoses between the two groups. Patients with Workers' Compensation underwent surgery slightly more often than did patients with standard insurance (44% compared with 35%, respectively; p = 0.07) and had a higher average number of visits before undergoing surgery (2.3 visits compared with 1.2 visits, respectively; p < 0.05). Twenty-three (45%) of the fifty-one patients with Workers' Compensation insurance who received a diagnosis indicating the need for surgery underwent surgery after the first visit, compared with 316 (69%) of 458 patients with standard insurance (p < 0.05). Patients with Workers' Compensation insurance were more likely than patients with standard insurance to undergo electrodiagnostic testing (26% compared with 15%, respectively; p < 0.01) or magnetic resonance imaging (16% compared with 9%, respectively; p = 0.02).

Conclusions.—Compared with patients receiving standard insurance, patients receiving Workers' Compensation insurance have a greater number of clinic visits before undergoing surgery and receive more diagnostic testing. More research is needed to explore these differences and their potential clinical and economic consequences.

▶ The authors retrospectively evaluated the medical records of 1413 patients at an academic center orthopedic hand clinic over the course of 2 years to evaluate the clinical differences between patients with Workers' Compensation insurance and those with standard insurance in terms of the use of electrodiagnostic testing or MRI. In this cohort, 8% had Workers' Compensation and the rest had standard insurance. The authors found that patients with Workers' Compensation have a greater number of clinic visits before undergoing surgery and receive more diagnostic tests.

It is intriguing to imply that patients with Workers' Compensation may be systematically different from those with standard insurance. It has always been hypothesized that patients with Workers' Compensation may have other issues when placed in a relatively adversarial relationship between the patient and the employment environment. Because Workers' Compensation system is not a no-fault system, these patients may seek to magnify their symptoms and perhaps delay recovery to return to the workplace, which may not be a pleasant atmosphere for the workers. This observational study, although potentially confounded by many variables because of the retrospective chart review process, is consistent with what is suggested in the literature, but the exact factors that affect the treatment of patients with Workers' Compensation are still unknown.

K. Chung, MD

Sternoclavicular Joint Infection: A Comparison of Two Surgical Approaches
Puri V, Meyers BF, Kreisel D, et al (Washington Univ, St Louis, MO)
Ann Thorac Surg 91:257-262, 2011

Background.—This study compares conventional open debridement with the recently proposed flap closure technique for sternoclavicular joint infection.

Methods.—This is a retrospective review of patients undergoing surgery for sternoclavicular joint infection during the last 7 years.

Results.—Twenty patients underwent 35 operations for sternoclavicular joint infection from 2002 to 2009. The debridement and open wound procedure (10 of 20 patients, 50%) involved debridement of the clavicle, manubrium, and first rib and open wound care. The joint resection and flap closure procedure (10 of 20 patients, 50%) involved partial resection of the clavicle, manubrium, and first rib, with immediate (9 of 10) or early

(1 of 10) wound closure with pectoralis major advancement flap. The two groups were comparable in comorbidities, duration of symptoms, radiologic findings, and microbiologic results. Despite an approach of planned reoperation for wound care, the open group had fewer mean procedures performed per patient (1.6 ± 0.7 versus 1.9 ± 1.6), owing to fewer unplanned procedures (0 versus 0.8 procedures/patient) than the flap group. The incidence of wound complications (hematoma, seroma) was lower in open patients (0 of 10 versus 5 of 10). The median length of hospitalization was shorter in the open group (5.5 versus 10.5 days), but all open patients (10 of 10; 100%) required prolonged wound care compared with 2 of 10 (20%) in the flap group. The only hospital mortality occurred in the flap group. Eventual wound healing was satisfactory in all survivors.

Conclusions.—For sternoclavicular joint infection, a single-stage resection and muscle advancement flap leads to a higher incidence of complications. Debridement with open wound care provides satisfactory outcomes with minimal perioperative complications but requires prolonged wound care.

▶ The article by Puri et al presents the results of 2 different approaches for treating sternoclavicular joint infections.

Twenty patients with acute septic arthritis were included in the study. Patients with postoperative infections were excluded. Diabetes, immunosuppressive treatments, or intravenous drug abuse were common.

Once the diagnosis was confirmed by laboratory parameters and CT/MR imaging, the patients were treated surgically. In 10 patients, the joint was resected, debrided, and the wound was left open and managed with negative pressure wound therapy for secondary closure. In 10 patients, the debridement was followed by primary closure with the aid of a pectoralis major advancement flap.

The results showed that even though the open wound treatment group had a higher number of patients requiring prolonged wound care (longer than 2 weeks), this group showed a significantly lower degree of complications.

This article may be quite useful for upper extremity surgeons because it gives clear guidance on how to deal with this quite uncommon but potentially dangerous infection. This is a very superficial joint that benefits from simpler procedures. Although the limited number of patients in this series does not allow us to definitively accept their conclusions, their results enlighten us to the use of the simple open approach with negative pressure wound therapy.

S. A. Antuña, MD, PhD

Article Index

Chapter 5: Hand: Congenital Differences

Chapter 6: Hand: Microsurgery and Flaps

Chapter 7: Hand: Peripheral Nerve

Chapter 8: Hand: Tendon

Chapter 17: Elbow

Chapter 18: Elbow: Arthroplasty

Chapter 19: Elbow: Trauma

Chapter 20: Brachial Plexus

Chapter 21: Elbow: Cubital Tunnel Syndrome and Ulnar Nerve

Chapter 22: Shoulder: Anatomy and Instability

Chapter 23: Shoulder: Arthroplasty

Chapter 24: Shoulder: Arthroscopy

Chapter 28: Arm and Humerus

Chapter 29: Arthritis

Chapter 30: Arthroscopy

Chapter 31: Neural Integration, Pain and Anesthesia

Chapter 32: Peripheral Nerve Injury and Repair

Chapter 33: Diagnostic Imaging

Chapter 34: Flaps, Vascular and Microvascular Topics

Chapter 35: Tumors

Chapter 36: Miscellaneous

Author Index

Printed and bound by CPI Group (UK) Ltd, Croydon, CR0 4YY

08/05/2025

01864677-0004